The Christian Woman's Guide

to Personal Health Care

The Christian Woman's

Guide to Personal

Health Care

DEBRA EVANS

CROSSWAY BOOKS • WHEATON, ILLINOIS
A DIVISION OF GOOD NEWS PUBLISHERS

The Christian Woman's Guide to Personal Health Care

Copyright © 1998 by Debra Evans

Published by Crossway Books
a division of Good News Publishers
1300 Crescent Street
Wheaton, Illinois 60187

Cover illustration: FPG International

First printing 1999

Printed in the United States of America

A substantial portion of the material in this book was previously published in *The Woman's Complete Guide to Personal HealthCare,* copyright © 1991 by Debra Evans. This new edition has been revised and thoroughly updated.

This book was current to the best of the author's knowledge at the time of its publication, but before following any advice contained within it you should, of course, verify information with an appropriate health-care provider or agency. All medical decisions should be made with the guidance and advice of the reader's own health-care provider. The information presented in this book is based on an in-depth review of recent medical literature. It is intended only as an informative resource guide and is not intended to replace the advice of anyone's own health-care agency or provider, with whom one should always confer before starting any medical treatment, herbal therapy, diet, or exercise program.

Scripture references marked NEB are taken from *The New English Bible* © The Delegates of the Oxford University Press and The Syndics of the Cambridge University Press, 1961, 1970.

Scripture references marked NLT are taken from the *Holy Bible,* New Living Translation, copyright © 1996. Used by permission of Tyndale House Publishers, Inc., Wheaton, Ill., 60189. All rights reserved.

Scripture verses marked PHILLIPS are from *The New Testament in Modern English*, translated by J. B. Phillips © 1972 by J. B. Phillips. Published by Macmillan.

Unless otherwise designated, Scripture is taken from the *Holy Bible: New International Version.* Copyright © 1973, 1978, 1984 by International Bible Society. Used by permission of Zondervan Publishing House. All rights reserved.

The "NIV" and "New International Version" trademarks are registered in the United States Patent and Trademark Office by International Bible Society. Use of either trademark requires the permission of International Bible Society.

Library of Congress Cataloging-in-Publication Data
Evans, Debra.
    The Christian woman's guide to personal health care / Debra Evans.
       p.   cm.
    Rev. and updated version of: The woman's complete guide to personal healthcare.
    Includes bibliographical references and index.
    ISBN 1-58134-020-6 (pbk. : alk. paper)
    1. Women—Health and hygiene. 2. Christian life. I. Title. II.
Series: Evans, Debra. Woman's complete guide to personal healthcare.
  RA778.E915 1998
  613'.04244—dc21   98-30000
                                                      CIP

15	14	13	12	11	10	09	08	07	06	05	04	03	02	01	00	99
15	14	13	12	11	10	9	8	7	6	5	4	3	2	1		

$\mathscr{D}$ EDICATION

For
HELEN WESSEL
1924-1998

women's health pioneer, advocate, author, and educator,
loving friend and servant of our Lord Jesus Christ—
with lasting gratitude for her work and witness.

$\mathscr{C}$ONTENTS

$\mathcal{L}$ IST OF FIGURES

$\mathcal{A}$CKNOWLEDGMENTS

I give thanks to God for the many friends, colleagues, authors, and mentors who have shown me, by their teaching and example, why we need to understand (and, when necessary, challenge) cultural assumptions about women's health care. Among these cherished companions, I especially want to recognize the contributions made by Karen Pryor; Rea and Loren Siffring, M.D.; Percy Marsa, M.D.; Marian Thompson; Mary and Gregory White, M.D.; Cheryl Bauman; Sheila and John Kippley, Ph.D.; Evelyn Billings, M.D.; Ingrid Trobisch; Anne Marie Mitchell, Ph.D., C.N.M., M.S.N.; Sidney Callahan, Ph.D.; Selma Fraiberg, Ph.D.; Doris Haire; Brigitte Jordan, Ph.D.; Dana Raphael, Ph.D.; David Gustafson, M.D.; Lee and David Stewart, Ph.D.; Helen Wessel; Kathy Nesper; Martha and William Sears, M.D.; Herbert Ratner, M.D.; Jan Barger, R.N., I.B.C.L.C.; Tryn Clark, B.S.N., M.S.W.; Phyl Kenney, R.N.; Samuel Fuenning, M.D.; Ann Figard, I.C.C.E.; Barbara Bernard, I.B.C.L.C.; Thomas Hilgers, M.D.; and Kathleen Raviele, M.D.

PREFACE

With information about women's health care widely available through doctors' offices, magazines, Internet Web sites, libraries, and local booksellers, why do we need yet another resource guide? I asked myself this question when my publisher approached me last year and inquired about my interest in revising an earlier text. Was it worth the effort? Weren't there already more than enough books on the topic?

While I looked through the stacks of the largest bookstores in Austin, scanned the shelves of our community library, and browsed the Web, I realized that even though nearly nine years had passed since the first edition of this book was published, there still was no other women's health guide that covered the same material. So I began to pray. It didn't take long to get an answer. The book you are now holding—*The Christian Woman's Guide to Personal Health Care*—is the result.

This guide, as you will soon discover, isn't so much an encyclopedic reference work as it is a hefty dose of encouragement. What it says is that learning about the way your body works can help you obtain the kind of health care that will benefit you most. It supports your right and responsibility to make informed choices concerning the drugs, devices, technologies, and surgeries your health-care provider recommends. It offers a positive, life-affirming, Christ-centered view of women's reproductive health. And it comprehensively provides practical ways for you to manage your personal health on a month-by-month basis.

Being a woman is an amazing experience. Coping with our biological complexity can be exhilarating, exasperating, even exhausting. The recurring reproductive issues we face aren't always easy to understand or cope with. It's my hope that you'll feel wiser and more confident concerning your personal health after you become well acquainted with the material in this book.

As Christians, we find it difficult to sort out the good from the bad in this

God-created yet fallen world we live in. The call to be consistently Christ-centered in our approach to caring for our bodies often conflicts with the spirit of our age.

Nevertheless, our charge to "rule and subdue the earth" has not changed. We are the image-bearers of our Creator, granted dominion over His creation, accountable to the Giver of Life for how we carry out this amazing responsibility.

The Christian Woman's Guide to Personal Health Care is dedicated to enabling you to perform this task. It is a uniquely Christian, practical guide to navigating the stormy waters of reproductive health care, from menarche until menopause.

Each chapter covers a wide variety of general reproductive health concerns. It explains what kinds of questions to ask and things to consider in order to obtain excellent medical treatment. Also, possible alternative remedies and home treatments are presented, emphasizing that there is rarely just one way of dealing with a specific symptom or concern. All of this information is presented from a point of view that recognizes the extraordinary value of human life as a reflection of God's image from the moment life begins.

Yes, there are some information-packed women's health books on the market. But a number of them also contain information that conflicts with classic Christianity. I make no apologies for this book. It doesn't tell you how to engage in a way of life or promote alternative "health treatments" that don't conform to what the Bible teaches us about reproductive health.

As Christ's followers, we need information on women's health care, too—but not from a point of view that bends our beliefs about women's physical, emotional, and spiritual makeup. What does this mean from a practical standpoint? I believe it means:

- Reevaluating our deepest attitudes and beliefs about ourselves as women.
- Guarding our reproductive health by understanding what the Bible says about women's sexuality and then living out our convictions.
- Accepting and honoring our biological complexity and individual distinctiveness as we responsibly assume stewardship of our bodies.
- Discovering how we can consistently honor human life in our approach to personal health care and medical treatment.
- Learning ways to minimize the health risks as we cope with the common physical challenges related to being a woman.

Before you begin reading *The Christian Woman's Guide to Personal Health Care*, please take a moment to look at the table of contents to gain a general idea of what lies ahead. Additional resources and readings on these topics are listed at the end of the book.

Notice that Part I of this book gives information unique to women's menstrual experience—menstrual physiology, female sexual anatomy, PMS, painful periods, and variations of menstrual bleeding patterns. Specific health concerns are presented along with a general overview of each subject.

Part II of the book discusses family-planning issues, including ovulation, fertility-awareness methods, child-spacing concerns, and infertility treatments. If you are single, you may still want to read about ovulation and start charting your menstrual cycles to gain a better understanding of your body— a truly fascinating and illuminating endeavor.

Part III is about becoming your own health-care advocate. If I sound critical in this book at times, it's simply because there is a genuine crisis in reproductive medicine today. The fact is, every woman needs to become actively involved in making health-care decisions because of the rapid seismic changes that have taken place in women's health care over the past thirty to forty years.

Part IV provides detailed information on coping with endometriosis, doctors' exams, diagnostic surgeries, hysterectomy, and sexually transmitted diseases. Every effort has been made to ensure that benefits and risks related to various treatment options have been listed as accurately as possible to help you make informed choices. An overview of the prevention and diagnosis of women's cancers is also included as a general introduction to a topic that each one of us profits from learning about. Finally, the notes, glossary, and resource sections make it easier for you to find what you are looking for exactly when you need it.

That's it—from understanding and coping with the ups and downs of the menstrual cycle and menopause, to facing the challenge of living with our fertility, to dealing with doctors, to getting the right kind of care when we need it—*The Christian Woman's Guide to Personal Health Care* covers all of these topics and more.

Through determining what alternatives are available, deciding what course of action to take, and directing our health management in cooperation with our health-care team, we become active participants in a dynamic process—the care and healing of our bodies.

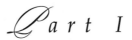

Part I

THE

MENSTRUAL CYCLE

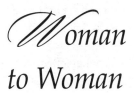

Have you found that coping with your body's cycles can be an interesting challenge? Or have you ever wished you were a little *less* biologically complex?

Without looking at a calendar, most of us know when we are about to start our periods, whether we like it or not. Breast tenderness, water retention, abdominal discomfort, fatigue, and a wide variety of stress-related symptoms are experienced by nearly 75 percent of menstruating women. For others, menstrual discomforts are more severe.

It makes sense to learn about the rhythms and reactions of our bodies to fluctuating hormones. Doing what we can to alleviate cyclical discomforts is an ongoing responsibility for each one of us. Knowing God's strength in the midst of our most aggravating moments doesn't mean denying our symptoms or pretending we aren't designed to experience our sexuality in a multidimensional way. Instead, it means learning to live wisely with our bodies—a lifelong process for every woman.

At face value, being a woman is, at least in a biological sense, more complicated than being a man. Only a woman can fully understand what it's like to live with the predictable unpredictability of a cyclical nature. Ask any woman, and she will describe days when she is more sensitive to stress, tense times that tend to accompany ovulation, menstruation, and menopause. Reactions vary from mild irritability to near-suicidal despair and are *real*. (Do I hear an "Amen"?)

Coping constructively with the ups and downs of the menstrual cycle—or the absence of it—requires stamina and smart thinking. Vitamin supplements, hormonal preparations, herbal remedies, and special dietary regimens may be used with success to reduce the severity of associated symptoms. Stress management techniques, when effectively employed, can significantly relieve hormonally related tension. Prayer, use of Scripture, positive self-statements, and other cognitive strategies have been especially helpful approaches for countless women. In later chapters of this book, you will have the opportunity to consider these coping measures and more.

Yet hormonal levels *will* fluctuate through each phase of a woman's life, regardless of what we do, say, or think about our bodies. These unseen chemical messengers trigger multiple activities in hundreds of thousands of cells, month after month, intricately orchestrating a harmony between a woman's mind and body that at times seems to slip irritatingly out of tune.

What should we say then? Is living with a cyclical nature a blessing or a curse? Where do we turn when we need advice on how to cope? From whom do we learn the wisdom that will help us to understand the way our bodies were designed to work?

Twenty-five years of work and research in the field of reproductive health have convinced me that you don't need an M.D. or a Ph.D. to be knowledgeable and discerning about women's health issues. It has never been easier to become informed about our bodies than it is right now. Browse through a local newsstand, bookstore, or the World Wide Web, and you'll quickly discover an abundance of accessible information.

Even so, when my daughters were growing up, I often felt frustrated that there weren't more materials written from a clear Christian perspective to help me teach my children about their sexual design. I grew tired of "picking out the bones and chewing the rest." I wanted a book that would encourage me to pass on important truths about women's health to Joanna and Katherine. But I never found a book written by a women's health advocate for Christian women that contained the information they will need to make the best health-care choices possible.

That's why I wrote *The Christian Woman's Guide to Personal Health Care*. My daughters always deserve the best from me, including an honest "realness" and comforting openness about God's good design for women's sexuality.

First and foremost, I want my daughters to know that:

— God created our bodies to bear His image (Genesis 1:27; Psalm 8:3-8);

— we have been created females by God's design for His glory (Genesis 1:26; Ephesians 2:10);

— we belong to God, not to ourselves (Psalm 100:3; 1 Corinthians 6:19-20);

— our lives are a priceless gift, bestowed upon us by a loving Creator who has watched over us from the moment we were conceived in our mothers' wombs (Psalm 139:13-16; Jeremiah 1:5);

— we affirm God's good gift of our sexuality as we worship our Creator, abiding by His precepts and commands (Psalm 27:1-5; Psalm 34:5; Romans 10:9-11; 1 John 3:18-24); and,

— as each of us experiences the joys and challenges of living life as a woman, we do so with the understanding that our lives have meaning, value, and purpose both here and in eternity. How we invest our time and talent matters to our Maker (Ephesians 5 and 6; 1 Peter 1:3-9; 1 John 3:1-2).

Oswald Chambers, a teacher and evangelist widely known for his devotion to Christ, believed that the call to dominion is also reflected in ancient Christian teachings concerning self-control and stewardship of one's body. "I have to account to God for the way in which I rule my body under His domination," he writes in *My Utmost for His Highest*. "The point to decide is this— 'Do I agree with my Lord and Master that my body shall be His temple?' If so, then for me the whole law for the body is summed up in this revelation, that my body is the temple of the Holy Ghost."[1]

For those belonging to the first generation in world history to be taught that our personal reproductive rights take precedence over any "outside control," this kind of thinking may come as a shock. The idea that "I am not my own—I have been bought with a price" is uncomfortable for many women today, and not without reason. Our ability to control reproduction—through drugs, devices, and surgery—has changed many of our basic assumptions about our reproductive health over the past twenty-five years.

As a result, the challenge facing Christian women today as we learn to approach health care in an attitude of stewardship is to care for ourselves in a way that is pleasing and responsible to God—to whom our bodies belong. Acceptance can lead to appreciation, as well as understanding, of the many details and infinite wisdom that went into creating our natural design.

BEGINNING WITH THE BASICS

This next section is full of amazing details that aren't boring at all if you have a healthy curiosity about how your reproductive system works. Read it as though you were taking a refresher course. I realize you may be weary of seeing starkly scientific anatomical charts and diagrams, but it's vital that we share a common language with our physicians—and I have no way of telling how much or little you may know about your body at this point. Please feel free to skip over some areas.

For those readers who may feel embarrassed by some of this information, I understand your discomfort. It wasn't easy for me to say *cervical mucus* for the first time either. This book occasionally requires me to be almost embarrassingly blunt. My husband sometimes cringes in mock disgust when I use anatomically correct language, but I also know he's used to it by now. He has read—and benefited—from this book, too. I encourage you to pass it on to your husband if you are married; he may be interested.

If you have a daughter who soon will learn about her cyclical nature for the first time, think about how you will share the information with her when the right time arrives. For example, did you ever consider that the menstrual cycle normally revolves around ovulation rather than menstruation?

Yet how many girls, when they have their first periods, are told by their mothers, "Honey, isn't this wonderful? This means that you may become a *mother* someday. Now each month an egg is being released from one of your ovaries. Your period means that the egg has passed through your body. But when the time is right, when you are married and ready to start a family, the amazing moment will come when a baby may grow from one of your eggs— and then a brand-new life will begin."

It's really all a matter of our perspective, isn't it?

THE ROLE OF SEX HORMONES

About half of all American girls are believed to begin menstruating between the ages of twelve and a half and fourteen and a half. The onset of menstruation, called *menarche*, follows about two years of breast development and other changes associated with *puberty* and normally takes place anytime between the ages of ten and sixteen and a half. About a century ago, the average age of menarche in middle class American girls was fifteen and a half. But today, due to improved diet and health care, the average age has fallen to twelve and a half. By the time most young women start their periods, they are typically within an inch or two of their adult height.

What triggers menarche isn't known, but nutrition, health, and genetic factors are believed to play a role. This monthly process continues until pregnancy, lactation, or menopause interrupt the hormonal events required to make changes in the uterine lining, or *endometrium.*

Primary sex hormones are largely responsible for this process (Figure 1). Secreted by the ovaries, *estrogen* and *progesterone* govern a wide range of reproductive functions, as well as our *secondary sexual characteristics.* These characteristics include:

— amount and location of body hair growth;
— breast development;
— widening of the hips;
— thickening of the vaginal lining, with an increase in cervical mucus production;
— location of body fat deposits—breasts, buttocks, thighs;
— sex drive;
— changes in external genitalia;
— timing and amount of bone growth; and
— development of smooth, soft skin.

Effects of Estrogen and Progesterone
Figure 1

HORMONE	SOURCES	EFFECTS
Estrogen	Ovary (egg follicle); placenta during pregnancy	Growth of the female sexual organs and promotion of secondary sexual characteristics of the female, such as breasts, hair distribution, voice, bone structure. Growth of the endometrium; inhibits production of FSH; increases production of LH.
Progesterone	Ovary (corpus luteum, the ruptured egg follicle); placenta during pregnancy	Primary function is to maintain endometrium of uterus for fertilized egg. Causes swelling of breasts but not milk production. Causes salt and water retention in body. Inhibits production of LH.

"While hormones are invisible, their effects are observable, and understanding them explains many of the important ways our bodies function," explains developmental endocrinologist Dr. Geoffrey Redmond. "Hormones are especially important in the processes in our bodies that change from day to day."[2]

In males, *testosterone* is the principal sex hormone. It is produced by the testes. The testes are the masculine equivalent to the ovaries. Both are sets of glands that secrete the hormones responsible for the sexual functions and characteristics behind our biological differences.

At an early stage of prenatal development, a group of cells organizes into two identical structures called *gonads*. The male gonads, or testes, begin to secrete testosterone by the seventh or eighth week after conception. In the developing female, the gonads start to change into ovaries by the tenth or eleventh week, developing high in the abdomen near the kidneys. The testes eventually descend into a pouch of skin outside the body called the *scrotum*. The ovaries, however, move slightly downward and outward, ending up near the rim of the pelvis inside the abdominal cavity.

THE OVARIES AND OVULATION

Each mature ovary, resembling an almond in shape and appearance, is about one inch wide, one and a half inches long, and one-quarter of an inch thick. The ovaries are smooth and pink in younger women; in older women they are pitted and gray. This change is due to ovulation. Repeated discharges of *ova*, or eggs, through the surface of the ovaries cause these glands to become wrinkled up and puckered looking as successive scars form.

At a baby girl's birth, each ovary holds precious cargo—about one-quarter of a million small saclike structures called *primary follicles*. Many of these follicles contain immature ova. When the girl reaches puberty, all but approximately ten thousand of these primary follicles degenerate. By the time a woman is fifty, most have disappeared.

Around the age of eight, girls start to secrete a "hormonal messenger" from the pituitary gland that prepares their bodies for other reproductive functions (Figure 2). Once called into action, the pituitary gland steps up its production of hormones when a girl is between the ages of eleven and fourteen, causing the onset of puberty.

During the stage of puberty, the ovaries begin releasing estrogen into the bloodstream. Increased estrogen levels then cause the *fallopian tubes*, *uterus*, and *vagina* to mature, increasing the size and functional ability of these important structures (Figures 3 and 4).

Female Hormone Production
Figure 2

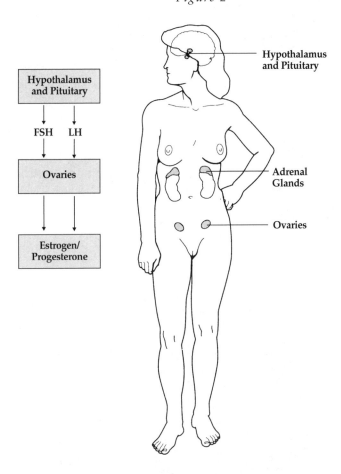

Primary follicles lying in the ovaries develop and mature in response to two very specific hormones released by the pituitary gland: *follicle-stimulating hormone* (FSH) and *luteinizing hormone* (LH) (Figure 5). FSH brings about the growth of immature ova and enlargement of primary follicles each month. The follicle enlarges as fluids accumulate inside, similar to a skin blister. Fifteen to twenty of these immature primary follicles normally grow each month. Of these, just one bulges outward, getting ready to burst like a balloon lying on the side of an ovary. This mature follicle is called the *graafian follicle*. Remaining follicles simply degenerate and disappear.

Female Reproductive System: Front View
Figure 3

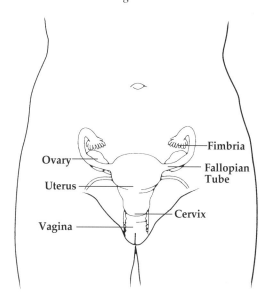

Female Reproductive System: Side View
Figure 4

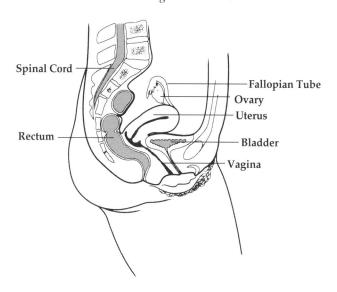

Effects of LH and FSH
Figure 5

HORMONE	EFFECTS
Follicle-stimulating hormone (FSH)	Directs the development and activity of the graafian follicles. Causes the follicles to secrete estrogen.
Luteinizing hormone (LH)	Works with FSH to stimulate continued estrogen production. Triggers ovulation, thereby initiating formation of the corpus luteum and causing it to begin secreting both estrogen and progesterone.

In the surface of the graafian follicle is a small nipplelike protrusion called a *stigma.* As the stigma develops, the pituitary gland increases its output of LH. When the LH level rises, the stigma disintegrates and causes the graafian follicle to burst (Figure 6). Some women actually feel this happen.

Graafian Follicle Bursts
Figure 6

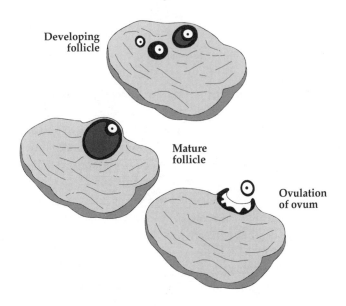

Developing follicle

Mature follicle

Ovulation of ovum

Called *mittelschmerz* after a German term that means "pain in the middle," a sharp sensation may be experienced in the middle of the abdomen toward either the right or left side, depending on which ovary has released an ovum through its graafian follicle. Cells remaining in the follicle are then stimulated by LH to change into a temporary gland called the *corpus luteum* (literally translated as yellow body in Latin) (Figure 7). The corpus luteum secretes two hormones that prepare the oviducts and uterus to receive the ovum.

Ovarian Changes During Menstrual Cycle
Figure 7

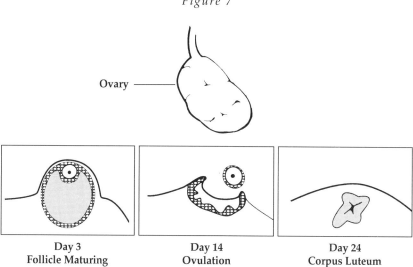

Day 3	Day 14	Day 24
Follicle Maturing	Ovulation	Corpus Luteum

The *ovum*, after it bursts forth from the follicle, is fragile yet resilient. It requires protection and nourishment during its journey down the fallopian tube, or *oviduct*, and can only be fertilized between twelve and twenty-four hours after ovulation. (I know what you may be thinking: How does anyone manage to get pregnant at all? And yet this extraordinary blueprint for human reproduction designed by God is precisely the way you and I entered into existence—a combination of God's hand working in our lives and the natural laws He has created). A discharge released with the ovum contains "nurse cells" that perform this vital function. Called *cumulus cells* because the cells look like a billowy cloud, they surround and sustain the egg on its way to the uterus.

The fallopian tubes are trumpet-shaped vessels, three to five inches long, extending from the upper corners of the uterus toward the ovaries (Figure 8). Although it is not completely understood how the ovum enters the fallopian tubes, it is thought that muscles within the walls of the tubes begin to contract rhythmically around the time of ovulation, thereby creating internal suction.

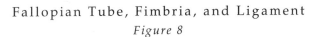

Fallopian Tube, Fimbria, and Ligament
Figure 8

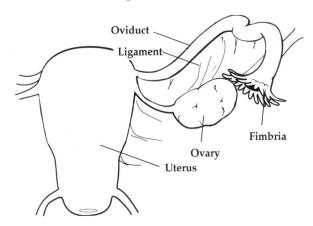

Ligaments attached to the uterus support the fallopian tubes, drawing the fingerlike ends of the tube (*fimbria*) toward the ovary. The fingers then literally "pick up" the egg for deposit. It's an intricate, elegant process, don't you think? There are even recorded cases of the oviduct of one side reaching over to the left (and vice versa) in order to retrieve an egg on the other side. Amazing!

Once inside the fallopian tube, the ovum is guided by thousands of tiny hairlike projections called *cilia* (from the Latin for eyelid, presumably in reference to the eyelashes). Beating in unison the cilia create a one-way route, also aided by muscular contractions. "Come on down!" the cilia seem to shout, guided by an irresistible urge to get the egg down to its nest, or womb.

Occasionally, a follicle ripens but does not contain an egg. Termed *empty follicle syndrome*, this condition has recently been discovered and can be a key in understanding certain types of infertility and how to treat it. *Sonograms* (ultrasound scanning) and *hormonal assays* (blood sample checks for hormone levels) are used to diagnose this condition, which can often by remedied through hormone therapy.

When the fallopian tubes are scarred by sexually transmitted infection (*pelvic inflammatory disease*, or PID) or severed by surgery, the egg cannot pass through. The result is reproductive impairment or *sterility*.

THE UTERUS

The *uterus,* or womb, is a hollow muscular pear-shaped pouch that lies in the pelvic cavity between the bladder and the rectum. It is about three inches long and two inches wide at the top. The uterus becomes more narrow toward the *cervix* (Latin for neck), where it's normally about a half to one inch across (Figure 9).

Divisions of the Uterus
Figure 9

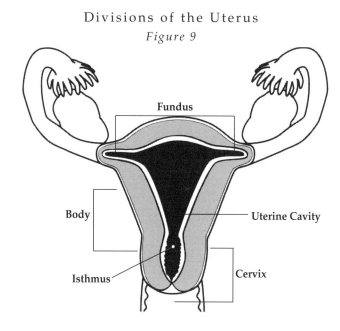

The uterus is divided into three distinct parts:

The fundus. The upper part of the uterus lies between the fallopian tubes. Extremely muscular, it is responsible for the strong contractions during labor that press the baby down through the pelvis during childbirth.

The body. Situated beneath the fundus, this portion makes up the largest section of the uterus. Along with the fundus, it is capable of great expansion and enlarges enormously during pregnancy. The body of the uterus narrows near its base at a place called the *isthmus* (Latin for narrow passage). The isthmus thins out and lengthens during pregnancy, aiding uterine growth. The attachment of the embryo inside the uterus following fertilization normally takes place here.

The cervix. The lowest part of the uterus, the cervix is attached to the front wall of the vagina and is about an inch long. The cervix has fewer muscle cells than the uterus and more collagen fibers. *Collagen,* the word taken from the

Greek word for glue, is a fibrous protein found in cartilage, bone, and connective tissue within the body. Within the cervical canal, a mucous membrane contains glands that secrete a fluid (cervical mucus) that changes in appearance and chemical composition each cycle as ovulation approaches. (For a more detailed description, please refer to chapters 6 and 7.)

The uterus is normally maintained in its position within the abdominal cavity by the muscles of the *pelvic floor* (Figure 10). The cervix is the only "fixed portion" of the uterus—that is, the only part of the uterus that stays put while the womb changes positions during exercise, lovemaking, and pregnancy. The rest of the womb is capable of a wide range of movement. It is free to expand, contract, tip forward or backward, and be pushed upward by a full bladder or downward by a distended rectum. During sexual response, the uterus changes position several times and contracts during the phases of sexual arousal that accompany orgasm.

Uterine Muscle Support
Figure 10

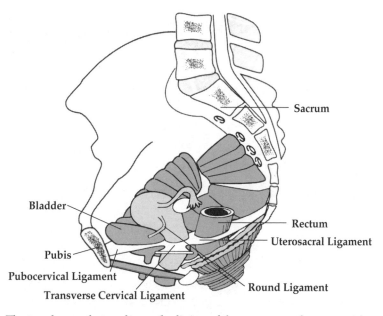

The two layers that make up the lining of the uterus are the *myometrium*, or "muscle layer," and the *endometrium*, or "inside layer." The myometrium consists of many interwoven fibers of muscle tissue and accounts for seven-eighths of the uterine wall's thickness. The outermost layer is called the *perimetrium* (Figure 11).

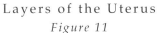

Layers of the Uterus
Figure 11

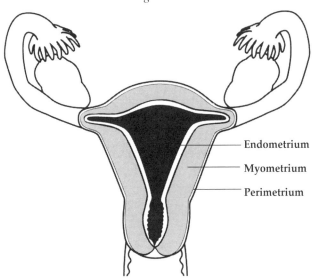

Endometrium

Myometrium

Perimetrium

There are three layers of muscle in the myometrium: an *inner layer* of circular fibers; a *middle layer*, laid out in a figure-eight pattern around blood vessels in order to stop the flow of blood after a baby is born; and an *outer layer* that extends lengthwise across the uterus like wide rubber bands (Figure 12). The outer layer is four times more plentiful in the area of the fundus to aid in the expulsion of a baby during labor.

The Endometrium and Menstruation

The endometrium lines the body of the uterus and is richly supplied with blood vessels. About five-eighths of an inch thick, the endometrium is made up of soft, spongy tissue that multiplies for about two weeks before ovulation in preparation for the possible implantation of an embryo (Figure 13). An easy way to remember the difference between the layers of the uterus is this: myometrium=muscle supply; endometrium=blood supply.

During menstruation, the uppermost layer of the endometrium is shed like the peeling off of a layer of wallpaper. The four phases leading up to this event are as follows (Figure 14):

Regenerative Phase (not shown in Figure). As soon as menstruation stops, remaining glands and cells start to multiply and rebuild the

Muscles of the Uterus
Figure 12

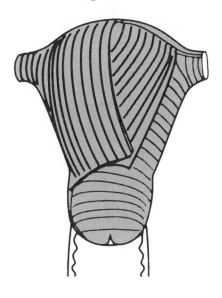

Monthly Changes in Uterine Lining
Figure 13

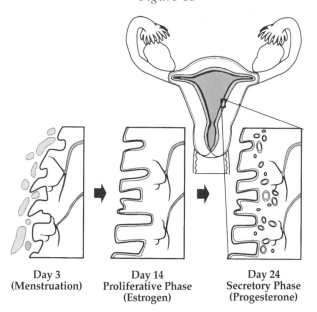

| Day 3 (Menstruation) | Day 14 Proliferative Phase (Estrogen) | Day 24 Secretory Phase (Progesterone) |

endometrium. Any leftover blood flow is reabsorbed, as in the healing of a wound. This phase lasts for two days.

Proliferative Phase. This phase begins two days after the end of menstruation and lasts until ovulation, sometime around the fourteenth day of the cycle. To proliferate (note the word *prolife* here) means "to grow rapidly in the pro-

Menstrual Cycle Events
Figure 14

Days	01	02	03	04	05	06	07	08	09	10	11	12	13	14	15	16	17	18	19	20	21	22	23	24	25	26	27	28
Phase	MENSTRUAL					PROLIFERATIVE PHASE									SECRETORY PHASE													

Physical / Emotional Events

MENSTRUAL	PROLIFERATIVE PHASE	OVULATION	SECRETORY PHASE
Frustration	Nausea		Spotting
Irritability	Pelvic Pain		Discharge
Anger	(sharp or dull)		Food Cravings
Anxiety	Abdominal Swelling		Bloating
Depression	Headaches		Anxiety
Fatigue	Depression		Depression
Relief	Spotting		Acne
Bleeding	Increased Sex Drive		Weight Gain
Diarrhea			Pelvic Pain
Abdominal Cramps			Constipation
Nausea			Headaches
Pelvic Pain			Fatigue
Back and Leg Pain			Frustration
Headaches			Swelling
Dizziness			Breast Changes
Acne			Change in Sex Drive
Nosebleeds			
Change in Sex Drive			
Increased Susceptibility to Infection			

Cervical / Mucus Events

MENSTRUAL	PROLIFERATIVE PHASE	SECRETORY PHASE
Thick	Thin	Thick
Cloudy	Clear	Cloudy
Dry	Wet	Dry
Tacky	Slippery	Tacky
Low Volume	High Volume	Low Volume
Low Elasticity	High Elasticity	Low Elasticity

duction of new cells." And that's exactly what happens as estrogen stimulates the lining of the endometrium to rebuild itself until it is about an eighth of an inch thick.

Secretory Phase. Starting after ovulation, the corpus luteum secretes progesterone, resulting in further growth in the cells of the endometrium, an increase in blood supply to this area, and the secretion of fluid from cells that have developed in the uterine lining. Also called the *Premenstrual Phase,* this is the time when women are most vulnerable to *premenstrual syndrome,* or PMS. When the lining of the uterus reaches a thickness of about one-quarter inch, it is a glistening red, having prepared itself to receive a fertilized ovum. High blood levels of progesterone and estrogen at this time in the cycle block the release of FSH and LH so that no new primary follicles start to mature.

Menstrual Phase. When fertilization does not take place, the fourth phase of the cycle is initiated. The corpus luteum begins to degenerate unless *human chorionic gonadotropin* (HCG)—the hormone secreted by a developing embryo—sends a message for progesterone levels to remain high. Without HCG, levels of estrogen and progesterone fall. The corpus luteum becomes a white scar, called the *corpus albicans* (white body), eventually ending up as a wrinkled indentation on the ovary.

About two days before the end of the normal menstrual cycle, the corpus luteum stops secreting hormones and the levels of estrogen and progesterone drop sharply, bottoming out on about the twenty-sixth day of a thirty-day cycle. When hormonal stimulation of the endometrium stops, the cells shrink to about two-thirds of their previous size. About one day prior to menstruation, blood vessels supplying the lining of the uterus are closed off. Without nutrients, cells lining the uterus die and separate from the endometrium. A little more than an ounce of body fluid and the same amount of blood leave the uterus in a flow that lasts between four and six days in most women (Figure 15).

To summarize, various events occur during the menstrual cycle, includ-

The Menstrual Flow

Figure 15

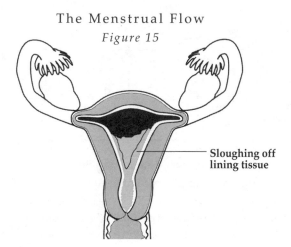

Sloughing off lining tissue

The Menstrual Cycle

Figure 16

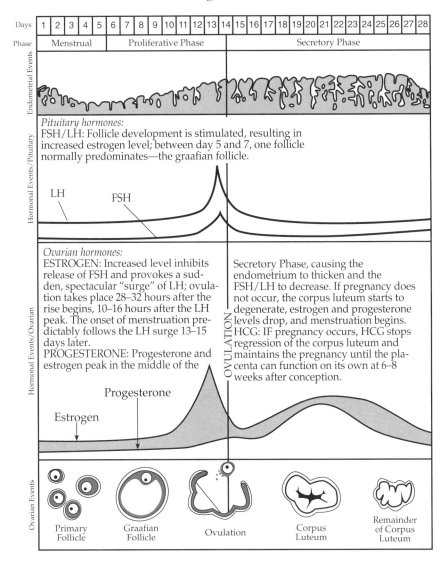

Days	1	2	3	4	5	6	7	8	9	10	11	12	13	14	15	16	17	18	19	20	21	22	23	24	25	26	27	28
Phase	Menstrual					Proliferative Phase									Secretory Phase													

Endometrial Events

Hormonal Events/Pituitary

Pituitary hormones:
FSH/LH: Follicle development is stimulated, resulting in increased estrogen level; between day 5 and 7, one follicle normally predominates—the graafian follicle.

LH   FSH

Hormonal Events/Ovarian

Ovarian hormones:
ESTROGEN: Increased level inhibits release of FSH and provokes a sudden, spectacular "surge" of LH; ovulation takes place 28–32 hours after the rise begins, 10–16 hours after the LH peak. The onset of menstruation predictably follows the LH surge 13–15 days later.
PROGESTERONE: Progesterone and estrogen peak in the middle of the

OVULATION

Secretory Phase, causing the endometrium to thicken and the FSH/LH to decrease. If pregnancy does not occur, the corpus luteum starts to degenerate, estrogen and progesterone levels drop, and menstruation begins.
HCG: IF pregnancy occurs, HCG stops regression of the corpus luteum and maintains the pregnancy until the placenta can function on its own at 6–8 weeks after conception.

Progesterone

Estrogen

Ovarian Events

Primary Follicle	Graafian Follicle	Ovulation	Corpus Luteum	Remainder of Corpus Luteum

ing changes in hormonal levels, ovarian activities, and endometrial appearance. Be sure you understand the complete cycle (Figure 16). In chapters to come, what you learn here will better enable you to accept—and understand—your own unique, God-given quirks and qualities.

Establishing
a Baseline

S ince most of us have short (*very* short) memories when it comes to being able to describe a history of our bodies' cycles, establishing a baseline can help us determine what's normal in our own situations. This is done best by recording the daily events related to one's menstrual cycle. If you are married, consider the advantages of sharing this information with your husband. Husbands, this is important!

These charts and records can later be interpreted by each of us, along with our health-care providers, to decide when and if medical intervention is necessary, as well as which home remedies may be effective. This is a great way to begin knowing and understanding our bodies better—an important step toward accepting ourselves as God has created us and assuming appropriate stewardship over His creation.

At least two methods can be used to arrive at this goal. The first is to take a menstrual profile (Figure 17) that asks specific questions about one's menstrual experience. The second is to keep a daily diary (Figure 18) in which the physical and emotional symptoms related to each monthly cycle are briefly charted.

Over time, certain patterns emerge that can be used to determine what's normal and what's not. Also these records are very helpful before and after pregnancy, lactation, and menopause—regular events in women's lives that commonly bring about the cessation of ovulation and menstruation.

Keeping a diary and recording a profile at the same time paints a more complete picture than if one is done without the other. Eventually, just the daily diary with notes on the back may be all that is needed. While it may seem odd at first to focus so much attention on this aspect of your life, this very focus—and the learning it produces—allows for greater comfort and freedom in living with the ups and downs of our menstrual cycles.

Menstrual charting may be entirely foreign to you. If it is, you will want to refer to other sections of this book for definitions and descriptions of some of the terms you will be using. For instance, what does it mean to have clear, stretchy vaginal secretions during the middle part of your cycle? What do the terms "wet" and "dry" mean? Read the chapter on fertility awareness (see chapter 6) before you begin charting if you aren't sure. For more information about menstruation, cramps, PMS, endometriosis, and other related topics, refer to the appropriate chapters.

Remember, we're *all* learning as we go. Each day, each month, and each year brings a deeper understanding and familiarity with our bodies, whether we are fourteen, forty-two, or seventy-four. That is one of the most interesting—and challenging—things about being a woman: *We're constantly changing*.

Consider the following suggestions help to diminish the frustration and discomfort of discordant days:

- Record, identify, and group your symptoms on a month-to-month basis.
- Become well informed about the menstrual cycle in general and how it effects your body in particular.
- Once you have established a baseline and discovered your own unique menstrual profile, meet with your health-care provider to create an individual program to fit your needs.
- Use a variety of relief measures.
- Use only the relief measures that work the best for you.
- Before abandoning a relief measure completely, modify it first or try it again at a later date.

Menstrual Profile

Figure 17

MY SAMPLE MENSTRUAL PROFILE

Age of first menstruation: _____

Dates of last menstrual period: _____

Length of menstruation: Note the number of days menstrual bleeding normally lasts. If cycle varies in length, what has been the range during the past two years? Does bleeding last longer than seven days? How often? When did this begin? Have you experienced bleeding between periods? When? Do you know why? Have you missed any periods?

_____

_____

_____

_____

Menstrual flow: On a scale of 1 (very scant) to 5 (very heavy), how would you rate your menstrual flow? Do you soak more than five pads per day? How many tampons per day do you use? Has your menstrual flow varied over the years? If so, what things might have affected it?

_____

_____

_____

_____

Menstrual pain: Do you have any cramping? If so, during which days of your period? How long does the cramping last? Have you experienced a change in menstrual discomfort over the years? List where you feel the cramps most. How strong are they? What do you do to manage your discomfort?

_____

_____

Ovulation: Do you experience midcycle pain or discomfort? At what point in your cycle? When did you first notice this? Identify where you feel the mittelschmerz ("middle pain"). How long does it last? How strong is it? What things seem to help relieve your symptoms?

_____

_____

_____

Premenstrual stress: Describe any premenstrual symptoms you currently experience prior to menstruation, such as tension, irritability, headaches, depression, anxiety, food cravings, breast fullness/tenderness, weight gain, water retention, or fatigue. When did you begin experiencing PMS? What seems to affect your symptoms most? How do you care for yourself during this time?

_____

_____

_____

Pregnancy and nursing: How many times have you been pregnant? Are you currently pregnant? How many children did you carry to term? How many children have you lost? In what ways have your pregnancies affected your menstrual periods afterwards? Describe the effect of breastfeeding on your cycles. Did you experience an absence of menstruation while nursing your child(ren)? For how long?

_____

_____

_____

Birth control: How have your menstrual cycles been affected by the use of birth control techniques? List the specific types of family planning methods you have used, including when and for how long you used them.

_____

_____

Sample Menstrual Diary
Figure 18

MY SAMPLE MENSTRUAL DIARY

DATES: NOVEMBER 26 — DECEMBER 21

Day 1:	Light flow, slight cramping. Began taking ibuprofen as needed.
Day 2:	Heavy flow with backache, diarrhea, cramping. Hot water bottle.
Day 3:	Heavy flow; noticed some clotting. Warm salt bath helped.
Day 4:	Flow subsiding, but still fairly heavy. Used usual comfort measures.
Day 5:	Light flow with weight loss; feeling great.
Day 6:	Some spotting; used mini-pads. Took morning and evening shower.
Day 7:	All is quiet! No discharge; dry.
Day 8:	Dry.
Day 9:	Nothing new to report.
Day 10:	Secretions beginning to change—milky colored.
Day 11:	Noticed increased, clearer secretions on tissue.
Day 12:	Lots of clear secretions. Also feeling some abdominal fullness.
Day 13:	Slippery, abundant; abdominal tenderness; mood swings.
Day 14:	Noticed abdominal pain/pressure about 10 P.M. Wet, clear, abundant.
Day 15:	Decreased, clear, less wet.
Day 16:	Decreased, cloudy, less wet.
Day 17:	Slight, creamy, wet.
Day 18:	Ditto.
Day 19:	Decreased, tacky, wet.
Day 20:	No change in secretions. Breasts tender; complexion changes.
Day 21:	Secretions changed—sticky, less clear, drier. Breasts sore.
Day 22:	Cloudy, drier, sticky. Feeling hungry a lot. Long walk and shower.
Day 23:	Scant, white, milky. Chocolate cravings; weight gain; bloating.
Day 24:	Same. Major mood swings. Had backrub, then took nap.
Day 25:	Dry. Breast tenderness and food cravings. Increased sexual desire.
Day 26:	Very slight spotting on tissue, increased clear secretions, wetness.

Some Helpful Hints

As you may have already discovered, it is vitally important to be sensitive to the ups and downs of female biological reality—your own as well as other women's. Here are some things to consider.

• Never say to a woman of any age, "Are you having your period?" This is a total mistake. Though you may be tempted at times when hormones are zooming, this is nevertheless the wrong thing to say, *especially* if you are the girl's mother. Since most females know the signs and symptoms, we rarely have to ask. Instead, try figuring it out some other way, maybe by keeping a mental calendar or becoming familiar with your daughter's (or your wife's) cycles through fertility awareness charts.

• Don't assume that all crying jags, intense irritability, and other strange behavior are related to the menstrual cycle. Are they? Of course not. Then why act as if they are? (Still, it's okay to be just a *little* suspicious. . . .)

• Accept the fact that the menstrual cycle is a normal daily physiological reality for most girls and women between the ages of fourteen and fifty. Note the word *accept* here. I didn't say "know" or "understand" or "realize." That's because acceptance is the first step toward understanding. You can't have one without the other, though many people try.

• Learn as much as you can about menstruation so that it seems more normal. As you cope with your cycle's daily demands, the physiological reality of your body's unique design will become more clear to you. The menstrual cycle is so much more than "the monthly shedding of the lining to the uterus," yet so few of us seem to fully realize it.

It's my belief that when we do realize this, we become more respectful of our bodies and are much less likely to abuse them through chronic dieting, overwork, harsh contraceptives, compulsive exercise, binge eating, and sex outside marriage, among other things. Making peace with our bodies—learning to be "at home" in the temporary tent God has given to us until we join Him in heaven, when we will receive brand-new bodies that will never perish—is no small thing for women living in our culture.

• Menstruation isn't a curse on womankind. Period. Anyone who believes this isn't reading the Bible correctly. And anyone who uses this to argue that women are somehow subhuman or dangerous is dreadfully wrong. The fact is this: Shedding of blood carries life-giving symbolism in Scripture. Think about it. *Without menstruation, there can be no children.*

As the world's first public health code, Levitical law protected God's people from infection and contamination because, without soap and water and other products essential to feminine hygiene, there would have been Big Trouble out there in the desert. Now that we have sanitary waste systems, clean water, and so on, healthy menstruation does not make a woman "unclean" in any way. (By the way, did you know that semen also was considered "unclean" according to Levitical law?) "Private" is a better way of describing menstruation today.

• Most menstrual difficulties are treatable. There is no reason any longer for women to "suffer" from PMS, pregnancy, and postmenopause when we have so many effective therapies to choose from. This is good news for both women *and* men. It's time everyone realized that menstruation is okay, that it's *normal* and not some nasty side effect of being a woman. With all of the excellent remedies, treatments, and products available to us, we can choose the best ways to improve our health and emotional well-being.

THE DEFINITION OF NORMAL

Since each of us has been created as a one-of-a-kind individual, naturally tremendous variety will exist between us. This seems to be especially true of menstruation. Consequently, if a woman compares herself too closely with her mother or a textbook or her best friend, she will start asking herself questions. Why do I have such heavy (or light or uncomfortable or long or . . .) periods when Carol's seem so easy? Why is Mom able to wear tampons and I'm not? Why do I have such terrible cramps and diarrhea the first day? Can anything be done to make me more *normal*?

We must look at the range of our symptoms instead. Any symptoms experienced from day to day in relation to our menstrual cycles can be broken down into four broad categories: First, some symptoms are normal, and treatment is not necessary. Second, others are normal, but treatment will help. Third, certain symptoms are abnormal, and treatment is needed. Fourth, for some individuals certain symptoms are abnormal, but treatment is currently unknown or not yet available. This way, we better "handle" or manage menstrual irregularities and discomfort while at the same time distinguishing between what's normal and abnormal in our own situations.

Not surprisingly, what we do to improve our reproductive health and whether we think we need medical treatment or not has a lot to do with how each of us defines normal. Individual women vary a great deal regarding their beliefs and attitudes in this regard. The more experienced and skilled a woman is in understanding her body's signals, the more likely she is to tolerate and accurately treat her own unique variations of normal.

The definition of normal, then, has a tremendous impact on a woman's reproductive health. If "normal menstruation" is defined, for example, as a twenty-eight day cycle including a five-day flow, a woman with a twenty-three day cycle with a six-day flow will have something to worry about. If her period is heavy, with some cramping and clotting, but she has not been adequately informed about how heavy or pain-free a "normal" period is "supposed" to be, she will be more likely to consider extreme or unusual measures to treat it.

What it all boils down to is this: *The more narrow our definition of normal, the more we suffer and the more reliant we are on expensive, extreme interventions to enable us to deal with menstruating* (Figure 19).

Range of Normalcy
Figure 19

NARROW RANGE

- Greater reliance on physician diagnosis and treatment
- Increased dependence on medical interventions
- More likelihood of side effects and other complications

WIDE RANGE

- Greater reliance on self-diagnosis and treatment
- Increased independence and freedom from unnecessary medical interventions
- Less likelihood of side effects and related complications

On the other hand, if our definition of normal is wide enough to include wide variations within a normal range of experience, we feel more comfortable accepting those variations and learning how to approach this aspect of our lives with the support of our friends, our family, and our health-care providers.

Into this scenario enters the modern health-care system, a complicated network of educators, nurses, doctors, and pharmaceutical companies. If our periods seem too heavy or too light, too short or too long, too late or too early, we look to professionals to provide the solutions. When we wonder if we have symptoms that need treatment, we phone a clinic. Who else can really tell us what's normal and what's not?

But are all health-care professionals equally qualified to help us? And, if not, how do we know which health-care providers to turn to?

What many of us have discovered is that our health-care providers can't always offer the cures we are seeking. Our physicians are not necessarily to blame for this. In fact, most doctors and nurses work diligently to apply their knowledge to our problems to the best of their ability. But when we expect them to know *everything* about our reproductive systems, we make our first mistake.

This assumption is entirely unrealistic for several obvious reasons: No one person knows everything that is currently known about reproductive health, and not everything is yet known about reproductive health. In addition, every woman is different, and so is what works for her.

Generally speaking, *the more experienced and knowledgeable a health-care provider is about reproductive health and the range of treatments available, the more flexible the provider will be in recommending a variety of treatment options—and encouraging you to become better educated about your health concerns.* Also health-care providers who are less financially motivated to schedule visits or write prescriptions (say, a physician's assistant employed by an HMO) will define "normal" in broader terms than private providers who derive income directly from their clients' phone calls, prescriptions, and visits (i.e., a physician who owns the clinic and the pharmacy you are visiting and is worried about the low volume of patients making office visits this month).

Now for the good news: You and I have a chance to make a difference. We can help ourselves and our health-care providers most by understanding ourselves best.

By working as full partners—instead of just as patients—within the health-care system, we obtain the greatest benefit from it. When we communicate clearly about our bodies by deciphering our doctors' "language" as they tell us what they are doing and what they need, we all benefit.

3

$\mathscr{P}$MS—

Its Signs, Symptoms, and Treatment

"There are two important realities to understand about PMS. They are: 1) Yes, it's real. 2) No, you're not crazy," says John R. Lee, M.D.[1] If you doubt that PMS is real, it's probably because you've never had it. It is real, and it's no joke.

PMS—sometimes called by the more accurate term, PMTS (*premenstrual tension syndrome*), or *congestive dysmenorrhea*—is defined as a group of symptoms that occur prior to the onset of menstruation and, for the most part, stop at the beginning of menstruation. Of course, those of us who experience PMS symptoms each month have been telling people this for years—we've just never gotten any credit for it.

Almost all women—up to 90 percent, in fact—experience one or more premenstrual symptoms at some point during their lives. And for those of us who may also be affected by PMS-like symptoms at a time other than just before our periods—after having a miscarriage, following hysterectomy or tubal ligation, during the postpartum period, or around the time of ovulation, for example—we know that the term PMS sometimes serves as a catchall diagnosis that doesn't entirely explain our condition.

In general, PMS takes place after ovulation during the time leading up to menstruation in what is called the *late luteal phase* of the menstrual cycle, at least three days prior to the beginning of one's period. Using this standard guideline enables us to more easily recognize the symptoms of PMS in ourselves and others. This does not mean that PMS-like symptoms will never happen at other times, because they can, for a variety of different reasons.

At least 75 percent of us experience minor or isolated premenstrual changes on a monthly basis. A number of studies on the specific incidence of a *regularly recurring cluster of premenstrual symptoms* have shown that somewhere between 20 and 50 percent of women report having a significant degree of PMS beyond the range of mild premenstrual symptoms, with an additional 3 to 5 percent experiencing a more serious condition called *premenstrual dysphoric disorder*, or PDD.[2]

In and of themselves, premenstrual symptoms do not comprise the condition known as PMS. As you can see from the following chart (Figure 20), a wide range exists between the mildest and most severe symptoms.

Premenstrual Symptoms and Conditions
(Range of Reported Severity)
Figure 20

Premenstrual dysphoric disorder

Premenstrual syndrome

Premenstrual symptoms

MILD   MODERATE   SEVERE

Severity of Symptoms

Of women reporting moderate to severe premenstrual symptoms, many are also likely to be approaching menopause; have experienced infertility, endometriosis, miscarriage, abortion, or stillbirth; have had their fallopian tubes "tied" (tubal ligation—see *post tubal ligation syndrome*) or their uterus and/or ovaries surgically removed; and/or have a history of depression, panic, anxiety, or eating disorders.[3] While these conditions are not believed to be the sole cause of PMS or PDD, they appear to affect the severity of symptoms.

By learning to identify the group of signs and symptoms associated with PMS and PDD, we no longer discount the impact these conditions have upon women's lives. We respond with greater wisdom to our bodies' needs for sleep, stress reduction, specific nutrients, and appropriate exercise. And we avoid ineffective treatments and misdiagnosis by helping our health-care providers eliminate other potential causes of our physical, behavioral, and emotional symptoms.

PMS AND PPD:
STILL CONTROVERSIAL AFTER ALL THESE YEARS

Although its specific causes are still unknown, PMS is a familiar term today. First identified as "premenstrual tension" by Dr. R. T. Frank in 1931, the term *premenstrual tension syndrome* was later popularized in the 1950s by Dr. Katherina Dalton of the Premenstrual Institute in the University College Hospital, London.[4]

According to Dr. Dalton, PMS is a cyclical condition that takes place no earlier than two weeks before menstruation and ends at the beginning of the next new cycle.[5] Her long-held theory has been that PMS is caused by a deficiency of the hormone progesterone. However, since "natural" progesterone treatment as advocated by Dr. Dalton and others has been tested in numerous double-blind, controlled clinical trials, and researchers were unable to find a difference between a placebo and the active drug, the assumption that the use of progesterone alone relieves PMS signs and symptoms has yet to be scientifically validated.[6] Even so, the use of natural progesterone in the treatment of premenstrual disorders continues to be a popular option among health-care providers who believe this is an effective treatment for some women.[7]

"To my mind, the hormone connection is most intriguing. It is obviously linked with the monthly hormone cycle; it never occurs prior to a year or so before menarche and never after menopause (unless you're on HRT [hormone replacement therapy])," author Dr. John R. Lee explains.[8] He adds:

> With ovulation, progesterone levels rise to assume dominance during the two weeks prior to menstruation. Progesterone blocks many of estrogen's potential side effects. A surplus of estrogen or a deficiency of progesterone during these two weeks allows an abnormal month-long exposure to estrogen dominance, setting the stage for the symptoms of estrogen side effects. . . . Low progesterone levels undoubtedly affect

hormone regulatory centers in the brain, resulting in increased production of hormones such as LH and FSH. These may also play a role in the complex symptomatology of PMS. However, for most women, simple correction of the progesterone deficiency will restore normal biofeedback and pituitary function.[9]

Sometimes the culprit isn't a hormonal imbalance at all. Other conditions can cause PMS-like symptoms as well. (See Figure 21.) Because medical research has yet to discover all the hormones and chemicals within the body related to sexuality and reproduction, our symptoms cannot be fully understood yet. In other words, no one knows what actually causes PMS.

Medical Problems That Can Mimic PMS
Figure 21

Fibrocystic breast changes
Endometriosis
Hormonal disorders
Viral and bacterial infections
Thyroid conditions
Chronic Fatigue Syndrome (CFS)
Fibromyalgia Syndrome (FMS)
Systemic yeast infection
Diabetes
Stress
Immune system irregularities
Pelvic infections
Dysmenorrhea (painful menstrual cramps)
Allergic reactions
Emotional disorders
Nutritional deficiencies

Possibilities still being investigated are:

- deficiency of progesterone during the premenstrual phase[10]
- imbalance of estrogen in relationship to progesterone[11]
- disruption in hormonal release and receptor sites (especially decreased levels of *sex hormone binding globulin,* or SHBG)[12]
- pituitary action[13]

- decreased levels of minerals (especially calcium, selenium, or magnesium) or vitamins (B6, A, or E), or essential fatty acids in the body[14]
- temporary alterations in ability to tolerate sugar and/or carbohydrates[15]
- decrease in levels of beta-endorphins (naturally occurring opiates produced in the brain)[16]
- prostaglandin excess[17]
- generalized yeast infection[18]
- abnormal essential fatty acid metabolism[19]

How all of these factors specifically affect those who experience PMS is currently unclear. But one thing *is* clear: PMS is not "all in your head." Only a part of it is. Recent research confirms that shifting levels of neurotransmitters, the brain chemicals that influence mood (serotonin, in particular) respond to hormonal changes, causing problems.[20]

It isn't necessary to know the exact causes of PMS before starting effective treatment. The good news is that placing a definitive label on this apparent hormonal disorder has allowed us, and our health-care providers, to understand something many women have in common—monthly chemical peaks and valleys related to the menstrual cycle.

These fluctuations create imbalances in the brain that, in turn, result in identifiable physical and emotional changes. Rather than viewing these changes as a disease, they can be seen as part of the rhythmical experience of menstruation. Because PMS is now treatable, this malady should not be used to justify treating women as incapable or incompetent members of society.

CHARTING PMS SIGNS AND SYMPTOMS

We do not need to simply tolerate PMS any longer. It is a widely recognized clinical condition even though not all doctors are familiar with its various guises. Since numerous home remedies, self-help strategies, and medical treatments are effective in treating most PMS symptoms, needless discomfort can now be eliminated.

Establishing a baseline and determining what's needed on an individual basis is essential to creating a personal plan. Few women have only one PMS symptom; most experience several. Generally speaking, PMS is marked by symptoms that:

- tend to increase in severity as the menstrual cycle advances;
- diminish or disappear when menstruation starts or soon after; and
- recur for at least three consecutive menstrual cycles.

PMS signs are usually unmistakable—irritability, bloating, backache, weight gain, headache, fatigue, depressive thoughts and feelings, forgetfulness, loss of coordination, food cravings, breast changes, and altered desire for sexual expression. These and other symptoms tend to reappear each month as menstruation approaches and estrogen predominates.

While more than two hundred symptoms associated with PMS have been identified, the most frequently reported are listed below (Figure 22). By dividing these signs into five general categories, health-care providers target PMS treatments at *clusters of symptoms* according to their *common characteristics and regularly recurring patterns* instead of at isolated, seemingly random complaints.

The five traditional PMS symptom classifications are pain, anxiety, craving, depression, and fluid retention. I have added a sixth group here for women whose monthly charts indicate they are more susceptible to infections and allergic reactions in the premenstrual phase of their cycles—classic signs of stress-induced suppression of the immune system.

PMS Signs and Symptoms
Figure 22

I. PMS PAIN GROUP

Increased pain sensitivity
Crampy discomfort
Headaches
Breast sensitivity, tenderness, and/or pain
Backache
Pelvic tenderness
Muscle or soft tissue soreness

II. PMS ANXIETY GROUP

Mood swings
Tension

Nervousness
Irritability
Panic attacks
Angry outbursts
Digestive system changes (nausea, constipation, diarrhea)

III. PMS CRAVING GROUP

Increased appetite
Food cravings—chocolate, sugar, carbohydrates (starchy foods), or salt
Fainting
Heart palpitations
Dizziness
Fatigue
Bingeing
Increased desire to use alcohol, mood-altering drugs

IV. PMS DEPRESSION GROUP

Insomnia
Forgetfulness, inability to concentrate
Frequent crying
Social withdrawal
Mental confusion
Accident proneness, decreased coordination, clumsiness
Loss of libido (sexual desire)
Lethargy accompanied by an increased need for sleep; difficulty waking
Irritability
Occasional thoughts of suicide

Note: If you have PMS Depression Group symptoms that do *not* markedly subside during the first two to three weeks of your menstrual cycles and/or are experiencing ongoing suicidal thoughts, *seek medical attention now.*

V. PMS FLUID RETENTION GROUP

Abdominal bloating and discomfort
Breast changes

Weight gain (two to five pounds or more)
Body image issues: low self-esteem, increased self-criticism
    related to one's physical appearance, avoidance of social contact
Swelling of joints, feet, ankles, legs, arms, hands, or eyelids

---

VI. PMS INFECTION / ALLERGY GROUP

Urinary tract infections
Skin changes such as cyclic acne, rashes, itching, or hives
Recurrent yeast infections; vaginitis
Diarrhea
Susceptibility to outbreaks of cold sores and herpes blisters
Frequent colds (starting late in the menstrual cycle), ear infections
Asthma, sore throats, sinus disorders
Stronger-than-normal allergic responses

Once you complete your menstrual profile and have kept a daily diary as presented in chapter 2, recurrent patterns in your own cycle will enable you to grade the length, severity, and timing of any PMS signs and symptoms. An important question to keep in mind when trying to determine the severity and duration of your PMS symptoms is this: *Do I primarily experience this recurring symptom during the premenstrual phase of my cycle?* If so, then your diagnosis and treatment options may differ from what they would be if you experience PMS-like symptoms at the beginning of your cycle or on a more continuous basis. In other words, it's important that your condition be diagnosed correctly. Don't assume that you have PMS just because that's what your symptom(s) seem to indicate: You may have another condition that needs to be diagnosed and treated differently.

Once you have a general idea of what your body is up to each month, make a specific chart (Figure 23) to fine-tune your analysis and enable your health-care provider to make an accurate assessment of your symptoms. Here's how:

Determine When and How Often PMS Signs Appear

Remember, you are the best evaluator of your own PMS signs. No other woman has felt exactly what you are feeling. If the symptoms recur regularly—that is, if they happen at about the same time in your cycle from month to month, then the symptoms are more likely to be related to your cycle. Otherwise there may be another cause for the signs you are interpreting.

Chart Signs of PMS

While some women do not require a chart to identify that they have PMS, it's beneficial to record PMS-related symptoms for at least two cycles to see how other events during the menstrual cycle—especially ovulation—affect your symptoms. Use the chart outlined on the following pages, rating each symptom separately.

Grade Your PMS Signs

In addition to recording the date you experience a specific symptom, it's also helpful to grade your symptom according to this scale:

0—*nonexistent* (no symptoms). "I don't have this symptom."

1—*mild* (symptom is present but does not interfere with normal daily activities). "This symptom is pretty mild and isn't a problem for me."

2—*moderate* (symptom is tolerable, though a little uncomfortable; it interferes somewhat with activities but is not disabling). "This symptom is moderate and manageable if I use basic coping techniques and health-maintenance strategies—exercise, a well-balanced diet, adequate rest, and relaxation."

3—*severe* (symptom is more than a little uncomfortable; it may interrupt activities, be somewhat disabling, and require medication and/or alternative treatments to reduce discomfort). "This symptom is severe enough that it causes me to seek over-the-counter treatments, self-help remedies, stress management, and alternative therapies to obtain relief."

4—*disabling* (symptom disrupts my life, causing me to miss work or school; medications and alternative treatments are necessary to decrease discomfort, but may be only partially effective). "This symptom is disrupting my life! Help!"

Total Your PMS Score

After filling in your score, add up the total for each day. The score is most likely to go up after ovulation during the premenstrual phase of your cycle if you have PMS.

The objective in completing these four steps is to *reduce the severity of PMS symptoms as naturally and effectively as possible.* By forming realistic expectations and goals for yourself, you can at the same time achieve greater peace of mind and bodily comfort from day to day. It's going to take some doing on your part, but I think you'll discover it's well worth the time and effort.

Charting PMS Signs
Figure 23

SYMPTOMS	DAY OF CYCLE																																		
---	01	02	03	04	05	06	07	08	09	10	11	12	13	14	15	16	17	18	19	20	21	22	23	24	25	26	27	28	29	30	31	32	33	34	35
Abdominal bloating																																			
Acne																																			
Aggressiveness																																			
Anger																																			
Antisocial feelings (desire to be alone)																																			
Anxiety																																			
Appetite shifts																																			
Backache																																			
Bladder irritability																																			
Bleeding gums																																			
Breast swelling																																			
Breast tenderness																																			
Body aches, pains																																			
Breathing difficulties																																			
Bruises																																			
Caffeine sensitivity																																			
Changes in sexual desire																																			
Chest pain																																			

SYMPTOMS   DAY OF CYCLE

Symptom	01	02	03	04	05	06	07	08	09	10	11	12	13	14	15	16	17	18	19	20	21	22	23	24	25	26	27	28	29	30	31	32	33	34	35
Cold sores																																			
Confusion																																			
Constipation																																			
Cramps																																			
Craving for chocolate																																			
Craving for alcohol																																			
Craving for salt																																			
Craving for starchy foods																																			
Craving for sugar, sweets																																			
Crying jags																																			
Decreased coordination																																			
Depression																																			
Diarrhea/ digestive upset																																			
Difficulty making decisions																																			
Distractibility																																			
Dizziness/faintness																																			
Eye infection, irritation																																			
Facial puffiness																																			
Fatigue																																			
Feeling fatter than usual																																			
Fibrocystic breast disease																																			

SYMPTOMS   DAY OF CYCLE

	01	02	03	04	05	06	07	08	09	10	11	12	13	14	15	16	17	18	19	20	21	22	23	24	25	26	27	28	29	30	31	32	33	34	35
Forgetfulness																																			
Headache																																			
Heart pounding																																			
Herpes outbreak																																			
Hives																																			
Hoarseness																																			
Hot flashes																																			
Hunger pangs																																			
Increased sensitivity to alcohol, caffeine, or sugar																																			
Increased sensitivity to noise, light, cold, etc.																																			
Insomnia																																			
Irritability																																			
Itching																																			
Joint pain																																			
Leg cramps																																			
Mood swings																																			
Nausea/vomiting																																			
Nightmares																																			
Panic attacks																																			
Pelvic pain																																			
Poor judgment																																			
Poor self-esteem																																			
Rash																																			
Restlessness																																			

SYMPTOMS   DAY OF CYCLE

SYMPTOMS	01	02	03	04	05	06	07	08	09	10	11	12	13	14	15	16	17	18	19	20	21	22	23	24	25	26	27	28	29	30	31	32	33	34	35
Seizures																																			
Self-criticism																																			
Self-doubt																																			
Sinus disorders																																			
Skin rash																																			
Sleepiness																																			
Sore throat																																			
Stiffness																																			
Suicidal thoughts																																			
Tension																																			
Tingling in hands and/or fingers																																			
Poor coordination																																			
Urinary disorders																																			
Vaginitis																																			
Vision changes																																			
Weight gain																																			
Yeast infection																																			
Other																																			
Other																																			
Other																																			

DOCTORS DIFFER . . . AND SO DO THE TREATMENTS

Here's the rub. Though things have improved over the past two decades, not all health-care providers are convinced that PMS is "real"—that is, that PMS is a condition with an actual identifiable physiological basis. Suffice it to say that if a physician prescribes tranquilizers or diuretics ("water pills") to a client without fully evaluating her regularly recurring physical symptoms, the doctor does not view PMS as something to be taken seriously. Some physicians seem reluctant to view PMS as a "real" (i.e., treatable) condition. Fortunately such health-care providers are growing fewer in number.

Viewing PMS as an inevitable, disabling monthly condition limits a woman's potential for creativity and productivity as a valuable member of her family, church, and community. Health-care providers who hold this outdated view are unable to offer a woman the answers she is seeking. Because PMS is treatable, it need not be a debilitating component of women's lives, detracting from their ability to function at their best—emotionally, physically, and spiritually—from day to day.

If a health-care provider conducts a thorough investigation that includes menstrual and PMS charting *before* offering a wide array of possible treatment options (such as those outlined in this chapter), then it's safe to say that the practitioner is fully informed about PMS and well equipped to treat this condition.

Understanding that health-care providers differ in their approaches to PMS allows us to seek appropriate medical care intelligently. Knowing the range of treatment options enables us to make wise choices about the recommendations we receive.

WHAT ABOUT PROGESTERONE?

Progesterone is a hormone that is only produced during the premenstrual phase of the menstrual cycle following ovulation. It appears to have been designed to be women's dominant postovulatory hormone, whereas estrogen plays a more significant role throughout the entire menstrual cycle.

Progesterone is secreted by the ovaries from a place called the corpus luteum. The corpus luteum is created when an egg is released from its sac, or follicle, within the ovary. It then becomes a temporary gland until it is no longer needed. All of this requires a great deal of hormonal coordination, as you can well imagine, and the system doesn't always work perfectly.

Thinking about PMS as a *progesterone deficiency syndrome* has been helpful to many women in treating PMS. A few have experienced complete relief with progesterone therapy, others experience little, and some experience a marked reduction in PMS signs. Since not all health-care providers prescribe progesterone for PMS symptoms, a woman's careful choice of a health-care provider can make all the difference in this regard.

But, please remember, progesterone is still a controversial treatment for PMS for several reasons:

- The exact cause or causes of PMS are still unknown.
- Studies on the treatment of PMS using progesterone are inconclusive.[21]
- Some health-care providers deny (or cannot accept) that PMS exists due to their professional training and/or personal bias.
- Progesterone may be obtained without a prescription, making some physicians less likely to recommend it.
- Effective progesterone therapy requires proper timing.

What You Should Know Before Starting Progesterone Therapy

How can you work with your health-care provider to determine when to start progesterone therapy and how long it should continue? Remember, progesterone cannot be taken at just any time during the cycle since it's only produced in large quantities *after* ovulation—twelve to sixteen days out of every cycle. Consequently, *taking progesterone when you don't need it will disrupt the delicate balance of hormones required to cycle naturally and normally.* The normal physiology of menstruation and ovulation will dramatically change, actually creating more problems than those it is meant to relieve. (More on this in chapter 9 on contraceptives.)

Because there is no single clinical test that allows health-care providers to diagnose PMS,[22] our providers must work with us individually to make a diagnosis and offer follow-up treatment. This process is most effective if your health-care provider:

- recognizes that progesterone is considered by many health-care professionals to be a legitimate therapy for some women with signs of PMS.
- is thoroughly familiar with menstrual charting as taught by physicians and certified natural family planning (NFP) professionals.
- has an adequate clinical understanding of progesterone deficiency disorders.

- monitors your reaction to progesterone, evaluates your progress, and makes changes in the timing and dosage as needed.

Are there many health-care providers who currently meet this criteria? Unfortunately, the answer is no. But it is my sincere hope that as women become more familiar with PMS and the menstrual cycle, they will seek informed and improved treatment. As the demand for greater expertise in this area becomes more apparent, more health-care providers will want to satisfy the needs of their clients.

When Progesterone May Help

Signs of progesterone deficiency to watch for include these:

Premenstrual spotting. When the progesterone level is too low, it is common for a woman to experience light premenstrual spotting for a day or more prior to the onset of her period. While this doesn't always mean she will also experience PMS, it is one of the signs to look out for. [WARNING: Other conditions can cause premenstrual spotting, so it's a sign that should be discussed with your health-care provider soon.]

Short menstrual cycles. Without enough progesterone, menstruation is likely to occur more frequently. Progesterone therapy happily corrects this condition in most women. Again, since other conditions can also cause short cycles, be sure to consult your health-care provider for a specific diagnosis and advice.

Other progesterone deficiency disorders. Progesterone is the hormone that maintains pregnancy by keeping the uterus quiet and shutting off the menstrual process. Thus, recurrent miscarriages may be a sign of progesterone deficiency. Infertility, or the inability to become pregnant after six months of trying without the use of contraceptives, may also be related to inadequate levels of progesterone.

PMS signs. If PMS signs have been charted successfully, they will support the evidence that progesterone levels are too low when used in combination with menstrual charting.

How to Take It

Most clinics and providers who manage PMS use progesterone by the "Wall Calendar Method." That is, they tell their clients to start progesterone therapy on the fourteenth, fifteenth, or sixteenth day of their cycle. (Or ten days prior to the start of menstruation.) This is based on the assumption that ovulation takes place on the fourteenth day of the menstrual cycle.

The big question here is: How often does ovulation take place on day fourteen? According to Dr. Thomas Hilgers, an infertility specialist who has developed, tested, and refined the Ovulation Method of natural family planning over the past three decades, ovulation occurs on the fourteenth day only *13 percent* of the time. Since Dr. Hilgers believes that human life begins at conception, he warns health-care providers to be careful about the timing of progesterone therapy to avoid interfering with ovulation (see chapters 6 and 7).

Even beyond this consideration, it's much more effective to look at each woman's cycle on an individual basis to obtain the best results from progesterone therapy. Obviously, this can't be done by using the "Wall Calendar Method"—*it requires menstrual charting to pinpoint the exact time of ovulation.* (More details on this in chapter 7.)

"One will see dramatic improvement in the relief of PMS symptoms with the use of progesterone when it is combined with the Ovulation Method and menstrual charting," says Dr. Hilgers. "We see a 90 percent success rate with the use of progesterone during the post-peak phase of the cycle." That is, if the dose of progesterone is timed to coincide with the disappearance of fertile ("peak") cervical mucus following ovulation, the effectiveness of this remedy greatly improves.

This method of natural progesterone supplementation is known as *cooperative progesterone replacement therapy,* or CPRT, because progesterone is given at exactly the same time it is being naturally secreted by the body. *By boosting the body's own supply of progesterone, the premenstrual phase is thus given the hormonal support it needs to alleviate PMS signs and symptoms.*

This concept differs from that used by most health-care providers treating PMS with progesterone today. CPRT is different in three ways because it acknowledges the tremendous variety that exists among women's menstrual cycles, determines when ovulation occurs before starting progesterone therapy, and is geared to one's "body clock" rather than a wall calendar.

If your health-care provider is unfamiliar with this approach to CPRT or with NFP, give her/him a book to read on the subject. (See Resources.)

Further Considerations

If progesterone is used as a remedy for PMS, be sure that it is "pure" progesterone rather than a progesterone-like substance or substitute such as medroxyprogesterone acetate (Provera). Most so-called progesterones given orally are not really progesterone at all; consequently, they don't work the same way and are not as effective in alleviating PMS. These substances are more accurately called *progestins* and *progestogens*. Both are synthetic formulations of progesterone. The names sound alike, but the chemical structure of these drugs—progesterone, progestogen, and progestin—are distinctly different.

Natural progesterone is available in several forms. Oral natural progesterone is the only form available by a health-care provider's prescription. Natural progesterone is also available as a skin cream, oil, under-the-tongue (sublingual) drops, or gelatin capsules that are taken vaginally or rectally. Because pure progesterone has difficulty going through the digestive system without being broken down biochemically, a gelatin capsule containing progesterone powder may be placed in the vagina or rectum just before going to bed at night where it then dissolves and is absorbed into one's blood supply during sleep. Typically, women who use this form of natural progesterone apply two to four 200-milligram suppository capsules per day, though the dosage starts at one capsule and can be as high as six suppositories. If your local druggist or health food store does not carry natural progesterone in the nonprescription form you prefer to try, you may order it by mail.

For many women, natural progesterone works most effectively when taken three days after ovulation (Peak plus 3 according to the Ovulation Method) through the twelfth day after ovulation (Peak plus 12). This schedule coincides most closely with the body's own output of progesterone. If you decide to try natural progesterone, start with one vaginal suppository or 100 milligrams of the oral micronized form. You may adjust the dosage upward by one suppository or 100 milligrams during each of your next few cycles, as needed, until you reach triple the original dosage.

Another form of natural progesterone, available only by prescription, is liquid progesterone. It is applied rectally by syringe according to the schedule described above and is less expensive than the vaginal suppositories; it's also less irritating to the digestive system and isn't as unpleasant to use.

There have been no reported side effects associated with using natural progesterone in small doses (20 to 40 milligrams per day). Larger doses may cause drowsiness. Many women, however, say they experience a sense of calmness rather than feeling sleepy.

Although FDA (Food and Drug Administration) labeling of pure progesterone requires that it be listed as a cause of birth defects, no scientific data supports this conclusion. In fact, a number of different studies in the past decades have shown that pure progesterone does not appear to cause birth defects, and ACOG's (the American College of Obstetricians and Gynecologists) Advisory Committee to the FDA has recommended that the labeling be dropped. Progesterone has been used in this form for about forty years—it isn't "new"—and the clinical evidence thus far shows that it can be taken safely during pregnancy.

While not unusual or harmful in and of itself, vaginal dryness associated with progesterone use can be overcome by inserting one capsule of vitamin E (400 I.U.) into the vagina at night along with the capsule of progesterone. In cases of irritation of the vaginal outlet related to vaginal dryness, vitamin E may also be used as a remedy.

What About the Dose?

The effectiveness of CPRT for treating PMS is definitely dose-dependent, meaning that the degree of relief of PMS symptoms related to CPRT is directly related to the dose needed. Some women experience relief with 400 milligrams per day, whereas others may only need 200 milligrams. Still others may need as much as 600 to 800 milligrams daily, or more. For women using progesterone skin creams, a much lower dose is usually effective.

To arrive at an appropriate dosage, use a three-cycle approach to assess adequate progesterone dosage:

CYCLE #1: Learn a fertility appreciation method. This enables you to understand your menstrual cycle and identify when CPRT will be most effective for you. Knowing when you ovulate is the key to CPRT.

CYCLE #2: Perform a routine hormonal profile during the postovulatory (premenstrual phase) of the menstrual cycle. Also, chart PMS signs. This involves taking a blood sample and analyzing the level of progesterone, estrogen, and beta endorphins present. In some cities saliva testing for progesterone levels is available.

CYCLE # 3: Start CPRT and continue charting PMS signs. The starting dosage will depend on the results of the blood sample test done during Cycle #2. This dosage may need to be raised or lowered, depending on your PMS symptoms and the type of natural progesterone used. Once you reach the dosage of progesterone right for you, it will work with regularity from one cycle to the next.

Progesterone is easy to use once you have established an appropriate regimen. Reaching your goal—the relief of your PMS signs—requires commitment and determination; the dramatic improvement of your symptoms will be the best reward of all.

A RANGE OF SOLUTIONS

Since there is no single answer to this condition, without a currently identifiable "cause-and-effect disease," we are free to choose among a wide range of solutions. If PMS symptoms do not require, or are not alleviated, by progesterone therapy, other solutions are available. Therefore, staying open to new possibilities and not feeling bound by any given product or treatment plan is all part of taking a positive approach to this condition.

Whereas some women experience anywhere from a marked decrease to a complete resolution of PMS symptoms with progesterone treatment, others find their symptoms also improve with dietary changes and exercise. You may want to try the nutritional/lifestyle approach, herbal remedies, or over-the-counter medications (Figure 24) before using natural progesterone. If your symptoms are severe, try a personalized combination of these three approaches.

A Nutritional/Lifestyle Approach to PMS

Eat wisely. Your diet throughout the month, and especially when PMS symptoms are greatest, ideally should be high in complex carbohydrates, moderate in protein (with emphasis on alternatives to red meat), and low in salt, fat, and refined sugar. Some women are also helped by decreasing their intake of dairy products and bleached flour.

Stop smoking.

Reduce or eliminate your intake of alcohol, MSG (commercial name: Accent, used heavily in Chinese cooking), *and caffeine* (coffee, tea, soft drinks, chocolate, and Excedrin). Many women find they are more sensitive to these substances during the premenstrual phase of their cycles, so it may be helpful for you to avoid them either temporarily or throughout the entire month—whichever gives you the most relief. Note: Women with PMS have a substantially reduced ability to tolerate alcohol.[23] This is true for a number of reasons.

First, alcohol causes a quick, dramatic rise in blood sugar. This provokes a surge in the release of insulin, driving blood sugar levels down for a long period. With low blood sugar levels, unpredictable mood swings are more likely to occur. Second, alcohol interferes with a process known as *gluconeogenesis*, the energy-releasing metabolic response that breaks down stored glucose when blood sugar levels are low. Alcohol-induced *hypoglycemia* (low blood sugar) results even with very light alcohol consumption, disrupting available blood sugar for as long as two to three days. Third, hypoglycemia following the ingestion of alcohol can worsen PMS if a woman later drinks more alcohol to deal with the emotional effects of low blood sugar.

Alcohol cravings can be the body's way of getting more available blood sugar, but in the end the hypoglycemia that results will bring about a desire for still more alcohol. If this has been part of your experience, a modified hypoglycemic diet, along with taking additional vitamins and minerals, will be an essential part of your PMS treatment plan.

Try not to go for long periods without food. Eat smaller meals more frequently (six to eight times daily). Prepare foods you enjoy and take time to eat. Hunger sensations, low blood sugar, and food deprivation contribute to the severity of PMS symptoms. Consult a qualified nutritionist, read current books, and/or talk to a PMS support group leader for additional ideas on how to cope with cyclical symptoms related to low blood sugar.

Supplement your diet with ample amounts of B vitamins: B6 (50 milligrams up to three times daily); B12 (200 micrograms twice daily), and pantothenic acid (100 to 200 milligrams daily). In addition, you may also want to try taking a B-complex supplement (100 milligrams three times daily). Caution: Do not exceed this dosage of vitamin B6. Taking 200 milligrams or more a day has caused toxic reactions, including numbness or pain in the hands and feet, awkwardness in walking, general clumsiness, and nerve damage.

Boost your intake of essential fatty acids. Gamma linoleic acid (GLA), for example, effectively aids in relieving a number of PMS symptoms. In addition to easing food cravings, GLA may help reduce emotional irritability and cyclical symptoms of depression. This supplement may be taken in the form of flax seed oil, borage oil, black currant seed oil, or evening primrose oil (trade name: Efamol). The usual recommended dose is 500 milligrams taken two or three times daily or as directed on the bottle. Headaches can occur at high doses; simply take less if you encounter this side effect.

Try vitamin E. Begin with 150 to 200 milligrams, slowly increasing to 300 to 400 milligrams daily (some sources recommend gradually reaching a daily dose of 800 milligrams). This vitamin may be especially helpful if you are experiencing breast discomfort. Gingko biloba extract (120 milligrams daily) has been reported to be an effective remedy for reducing symptoms in the fluid retention group.

Take plenty of vitamin C. Dietary time-released supplements of 500 to 1,000 milligrams (for a total of 2,000 to 6,000 milligrams daily) may significantly strengthen your immune system's ability to fend off infection. Your stools will likely be looser once you begin taking a higher dosage of this vitamin; don't be too concerned if you experience this common side effect unless frequent diarrhea results.

Remember vitamin A. Daily doses of vitamin A (10,000 I.U. daily) and natural beta-carotene (15,000 I.U. daily) will boost your blood levels of antioxidants and guard against vitamin A deficiency, which can increase the severity of PMS.

Don't forget your minerals: Calcium (1,500 milligrams daily), chromium picolinate (200 micrograms daily), and magnesium (1,000 milligrams daily) have been used with success to reduce PMS discomforts, as has zinc (50 milligrams daily, not to exceed a total of 100 milligrams of this mineral from all combined supplements).[24] Consult your nutritional specialist and/or health-care provider for more information, as needed.

Consider using herbal remedies. Follow the expert help of a trained practitioner with whom you feel comfortable. Angelica, for example, has been used by Chinese women for nearly 2,000 years as a treatment for premenstrual symptoms. Also called dong quai or dang gui, it contains considerable amounts of vitamins B12 and E. Other herbs—including ginger root, crampbark, wild yam, dandelion, red raspberry leaf, valerian, kava kava, borage, St. John's-wort, and motherwort—have also been suggested as effective home remedies for relieving the severity of various PMS symptoms. Consult your local Christian herbalist or an up-to-date primer for specific doses. (A brief overview of general suggestions and contraindications follows this section.)

Whenever possible, keep your sense of humor. Laughter is often the best medicine for despair and frustration.

Ask your health-care provider to check your thyroid function. Some women who experience PMS are helped considerably by correcting an undiagnosed thyroid problem.

Eat foods high in magnesium and potassium, such as bananas and oranges. Have high-protein nondairy snacks between meals—nuts, broiled chicken or turkey, and soy products.

Lower your salt intake to reduce fluid retention-related symptoms (bloating, swelling, etc.). Many health-care providers also prescribe a diuretic such as spironolactone (Aldactone) for premenstrual bloating and weight gain. The drug is taken from the time of ovulation to the onset of menstruation. Research has shown mixed results on the efficacy of spironolactone for PMS.[25] Even so, treatment with diuretics has been shown in some studies to reduce the severity of PMS-related fatigue and depression as well as to help women cope with fluid retention.

Drink at least one quart of purified water daily. This is especially important during the week before your period until the week after. Stay well-hydrated, especially when exercising and/or when the temperature rises outdoors. Though it might seem that watering your system will increase premenstrual fluid retention, drinking plenty of water will actually flush extra fluid from your body and reduce bloating before your period starts.

Add amino acids to your diet: DL-phenylalanine (375 milligrams up to four times daily) and L-tyrosine (500 milligrams twice daily, preferably in the early morning and sometime before dinner; take with water or juice—not milk— along with 50 milligrams of vitamin B6 and at least 100 milligrams of vitamin C to aid absorption). L-tryptophan, an excellent PMS aid, is currently banned from commercial sale in the United States due to an outbreak of a rare blood disorder associated with L-tryptophan products sold in New Mexico. Though the disease was later proven to be related to contaminants in the supplements, not the amino acid, L-tryptophan supplements are still unavailable. For now, try tryptophan-rich dietary sources instead—brown rice, cottage cheese, meat, peanuts, and soy protein.

Exercise regularly to reduce stress and improve well-being. Moderate forms of exercise—such as swimming, aerobic walking, cycling, and stretching—are especially effective in reducing PMS-related discomforts.[26] Benefits include increased blood circulation; some relief of pelvic congestion and elimination of toxins from the body; increased sweat production, which helps to decrease fluid build-up; and improved emotional well-being, leading to better sleep and less nervous tension.

Get enough sleep. In the book *The PMS Solution* (see Resources), the author asserts that PMS is a sleep disorder and that PMS sufferers benefit from getting lots and lots of sleep. Check it out for yourself.

Practice stress management for timely PMS relief.[27] Take regular "time outs" for rest and renewal—schedule longer breaks on tense days when possible, listen to music, enjoy a long bath or shower, spend specific periods reading the Psalms or in quiet prayer. (A few practical stress management ideas come later in this chapter.)

Evaluate your emotions. You owe it to yourself—and those you love—to take a closer look. Severe mood swings or chronic depression indicate that something more than your menstrual cycle may be affecting your emotional well-being. Make an appointment now to assess your symptoms with your health-care provider. Numerous studies indicate that antidepressant therapy is often an effective treatment for disabling emotional symptoms associated with PMS.[28]

Stay informed. As new treatments become available, you will want to reevaluate and possibly modify your approach to easing PMS discomforts. Health magazines and newsletters are excellent sources for updating your personal plan as well.

Realize that PMS has hidden benefits. What? Did I really write what you think you just read? Yes. And here's why:

When the volume gets turned up, we're more likely to listen. Perhaps our monthly cycles are a blessing in disguise. As our emotions become amplified prior to menstruation, we can actively choose to "hear" what our feelings may be telling us instead of ignoring our emotional discomfort. Because we are less likely to ignore the daily stresses we may be putting up with during the rest of the month, we can use our increased premenstrual sensitivity as a warning device. We can learn to read the danger signs as a prevention tool—and intervene in healthy ways when needed—rather than become the monthly victims of our too-busy lifestyles.

Increased emotional sensitivity can lead us to greater dependence on God's strength. For ample proof of this phenomenon, peruse the Psalms. Isn't it comforting to know that no matter how gross we feel, God's there with us? From a biblical perspective, we see that human weakness may be supernaturally transformed by Christ's sustaining grace and the Holy Spirit's work within us. When we are weak (and are willing to admit it), we personally discover the magnitude of God's strength revealed to us in new ways.

A woman's cycles bring an added dimension to her sexuality. In my previous book, *The Christian Woman's Guide to Sexuality*, I share a perspective of women's reproductive design: that we were created different from men for a distinct purpose. It's no accident of nature that women, who are capable of six separate sexual functions, tend to experience a greater variation in their desire for sex than do men. Rather than compare my sexuality to a man's, I have sought to understand and appreciate my own uniqueness. Within marriage this has taught me that my own biological rhythms are a gift, not a curse.

Taking time to be quiet can enhance spiritual growth. PMS, even periods, can foster an atmosphere conducive to prayer—for obvious reasons. So why do we tend to look at cyclical challenges as something to be conquered? Certainly, we can do what we can to reduce or eliminate the discomforts, but we'll never do away with our need to slow down, take stock of life stresses, and pay attention to the unhealthy ways we may be choosing to cope month-to-month. Thank you, thank you, thank you, Lord, for our built-in clocks that keep calling us back to YOU as our only sure source of hope and help!

PMS Symptoms and Related Herbal Remedies

As Christians, we believe the Lord made the earth and everything in it, and we joyfully worship our Creator with awe and humility. The fact that many Web sites, herb suppliers, and authors have connections with divination, Wicca, black magic, and so on, does *not* mean the herbs God created for our benefit (Genesis 1:29) are off-limits when employed appropriately. Herbs were given to us to use, not abuse. Use prayer and discretion when seeking and applying God's wisdom to herbal health formulas.

Since I have not thoroughly investigated the many sources I have located in books and catalogues, there are no specific suppliers or authors I can recommend to you with 100 percent confidence at this time. The following brief overview of helpful herbs traditionally used for aiding PMS symptoms is simply a starting point. Since the complexities involved in herbal medicine are beyond the scope of this book, I'm leaving it to you to do the necessary additional research on the specific doses, indications, risks, sources, and available herb products in conjunction with your own health-care provider's advice. (NOTE: Herbal remedies are medicinally powerful. *The suggested list below is not intended to be a prescription for the treatment of any health problem.* Herbs must be used with knowledge and care since individual responses to their use vary.)

Fluid retention—black currant, corn silk, dandelion leaf, juniper, fennel seed, Pellitory-of-the-Wall, stone root, Uva Ursi (bearberry), saw palmetto, heartsease, stinging nettles.

Pelvic Congestion—blue flag, squaw vine, ginger root.

Cramps—red raspberry leaf, ginger root, crampbark, kava kava, black haw bark, evening primrose, prickly ash, squaw vine, pasque flower (warning: the fresh plant is toxic), rosemary, vervain, valerian, yarrow, white willow, penny royal, wormwood, angelica root, rue, and black cohosh also may help relieve uterine cramping, but should be used *only if you are absolutely certain that you aren't pregnant.* (For a list of other herbs that must be avoided during pregnancy and other physical conditions, please see below.)

Hormone balance—chaste berry, fennel seed, squaw vine, false unicorn root, sarsaparilla root, dong quai, blessed thistle, red raspberry leaf, dandelion root.

Progesterone support—chaste berry, wild yam, sarsaparilla root.

Headaches—feverfew, gingko biloba, rosemary, skullcap, thyme, willow, wintergreen, valerian, wood betony.

Mood swings—peppermint, valerian, strawberry leaf, black cohosh, sarsaparilla root, squaw vine.

Yeast infection prevention—Pau d'Arco tea.

Stress/fatigue—green tea, licorice, suma, valerian, gingko biloba, skullcap, sarsaparilla root, nightcap, Gotu Kola, rosemary, vervain, Siberian, ginseng (trade name: Elagen).

Insomnia—chamomile, passion flower, nightcap, melilot, valerian.

Anxiety/Irritability—skullcap, false unicorn root, passion flower, chamomile, red clover, hops, valerian, vervain, lime flowers, dong quai, sage, kava kava, lemon balm, wood betony, linden.

Depression—St. John's-wort, damiana, vervain, licorice, black cohosh, kava kava, rosemary, lavender, licorice, gingko, oat straw, motherwort (during perimenopause), melilot.

Nausea—ginger, peppermint, meadowsweet, red raspberry leaf, bitter orange.

Skin problems—marshmallow, Oregon grape, evening primrose, fennel, red clover, tea tree, yellow dock, stinging nettles.

Cold sores/herpes outbreak—echinacea, Siberian ginseng golden seal, mango, St. John's-wort, red clover, lady's mantle, false unicorn root, thyme, savory, melissa, orange blossom, peppermint, marigold, tea tree.

Liver cleansing (used especially during the first two or three months of herbal PMS treatment to promote liver function)—milk thistle, dandelion root, vervain, barberry, wormwood, red clover, yellow dock, black flag, turmeric, vervain.

Urinary tract disorders—buchu leaf, corn silk, cranberry (if using cranberry juice, buy the pure, unsweetened form; add as little sweetener as possible), yarrow, gravel root, hydrangea (don't consume the leaves: they're toxic), kava kava, shepherd's purse, marshmallow, plantain, thyme, rose hips, slippery elm, Uva Ursi, white deadnettle, saw palmetto.

Bowel disorders—slippery elm, yerba maté, thyme.

WARNING: Most herbalists agree that herbal therapies should *not* be used during the first trimester of pregnancy; many prefer not to treat *any* long-standing illnesses with herbal remedies in pregnancy. The following herbs are *not to be used during pregnancy under any circumstances* because they may cause miscarriage or other problems:

Medicinal and laxative herbs: alder, buckthorn, Chinese angelica (dong quai/dang gui), autumn crocus, barberry, black cohosh*, blood root, blue cohosh*, broom, cascara, cat's claw, comfrey, cotton root, fern (male), fever-few, ginseng (avoid high doses and prolonged use), golden seal*, greater celadine, green tea, juniper, life root, lovage, marjoram, mistletoe, mugwort, nutmeg*, penny royal*, Peruvian bark, passion flower, poke root, rhubarb, rosemary, rye, sage, sassafras, senna, shepherd's purse*, sweet flag, tansy, thyme, Tree of Life, vervain, wild yam*, wood betony, wormwood, yellow dock.

*These herbs are believed to be safe in pregnancy when used during childbirth.

Culinary herbs (small amounts used in cooking to flavor foods are okay, but do not ingest in large quantities): celery seed, cinnamon, fennel, fenugreek, lavender, oregano, parsley, rosemary, sage, and saffron.

Essential oils (do not ingest or use for massage, bath oil, aromatherapy, etc.): anise seed, arnica, basil, birch, cedar wood, chamomile, clove, cinnamon, clary sage, cypress, fennel, hyssop, jasmine, juniper, nutmeg, marjoram, myrrh, oregano, penny royal, peppermint, rosemary, sage, thyme, and wintergreen.

OTHER KNOWN CONTRAINDICATIONS: Do not use these herbs if you have the condition listed beside them. Also, be aware that allergic reactions are possible with the use of herbs, as with any medicine.

Angelica (dong quai, dang gui)—Avoid this herb if you have high blood pressure or an inflammatory condition.

Feverfew—Do not take this herb if you are on an anticlotting drug. When taken fresh, feverfew can cause mouth ulcers; discontinue use if this occurs.

Golden Seal—Do not take this herb if you have high blood pressure.

Licorice—Avoid excessive use if you have high blood pressure or heart disease; do not take if you are currently on a digoxin-based drug.

Meadowsweet—As this herb is rich in salicylates, avoid it if you are allergic to aspirin.

Melilot—Should not be taken if you're on an anticlotting drug.

Peppermint—May reduce milk flow during breastfeeding.

Sage—Do not take medicinally if you have epilepsy.

St. John's-wort—May cause photosensitivity; do not take or apply before exposure to bright sun.

Turmeric—Should not be used in large amounts.

Yarrow, Willow—May interfere with iron and other mineral absorption.

Yellow Dock—High doses may result in diarrhea.

Over-the-Counter Medications
Approved by FDA for Treatment of
PMS and Menstrual Cramps[29]
Figure 24

EFFECTIVE COMBINATIONS
(TAKE RECOMMENDED DOSE OF BOTH DRUGS AT THE SAME TIME):

Analgesic and diuretic
Analgesic, antihistamine, and diuretic
Antihistamine and diuretic
Any two diuretics with varying actions, such as ammonium chloride
    and caffeine

ACTIVE INGREDIENTS TO LOOK FOR
FOR FLUID RETENTION AND BLOATING:

Pyrilamine maleate—an antihistamine that is effective when used in
    one of the combinations listed above
Pamabrom—a diuretic
Caffeine—a stimulant with diuretic properties
Ammonium chloride—a diuretic (NOTE: Do not take if you have impaired
    liver or kidney function, or for longer than four to five days.)

FOR FATIGUE:

Caffeine

FOR MOODINESS:

Pyrilamine maleate—an antihistamine that is effective when used
    in combinations as listed above

FOR PAIN (HEADACHES, CRAMPS, ETC.):

Aspirin and other salicylates—an analgesic
Acetaminophen—an analgesic
Ibuprofen—an analgesic
Naproxen sodium—an analgesic
Caffeine—boosts analgesic properties of a drug when used
    in combination with another pain reliever.
    (NOTE: Excedrin contains caffeine for this reason.)

Quick Tips for Stress Relief

Take a relaxation break. Close your eyes for five minutes. Say "Stop" to whatever you are doing. Now slow down. Breathe slowly and deeply as you silently say the first three verses of Psalm 23. Entrust your body, mind, will, soul, and spirit to the Lord's care as you find "safe pasture" in His comforting, gentle presence. Leave your worries, cares, and concerns outside the Shepherd's protective gate; spend these quiet moments reflecting on Christ's unfailing, never-changing love for you. Surrender your efforts at controlling life's situations—including your PMS symptoms—as you recognize God's sovereign authority over every aspect of your existence.

Use HALT. When tension mounts, apply this handy acronym as you ask yourself: Am I hungry? Angry? Lonely? Tired? Chances are good that you are experiencing at least one of these PMS-aggravating conditions when your nerves make you want to scream, collapse, sob, throw dishes, or escape to Bora Bora. Why not do yourself and everyone else a favor by dealing with what's at hand? Have a high-protein milkshake. Express your anger openly in a "for-my-eyes-only" journal. Pray. Call a friend. Get some sleep (or rest) as soon as possible. Don't just keep going and going and going and going. Be kind to yourself, okay?

Nourish your spirit. Beyond eating good food, you need to feed yourself with God's good things—biblical promises, the psalmists' poetry, scriptural truth, inspiring music, soothing scenery, Creation's wonders.

Move your body. Stretch. Walk. Breathe. Aerobic exercise boosts endorphin levels in the bloodstream, providing natural pain relief and promoting relaxation; oxygen rushes into every cell, reviving tired organs; stamina builds to meet the day's demands.

Get in the water. Soak in a warm, relaxing bath; add a tension-relieving essential oil to the tub: lavender, chamomile, mandarin, marjoram, melissa, neroli (orange blossom), orange, clary sage, ylang ylang. If a long bath is unappealing to you, take a long shower or go for a leisurely swim.

Forget the scales. Weigh yourself once every month, two or three days after your period is over. Avoid weighing yourself during the last two weeks of your cycle and during menstruation. It's a set-up for disappointment and may make you want to miss meals, impose PMS-worsening dietary restrictions, and/or engage in other unhealthy food-related practices (bingeing and purging, self-starvation, skipping a high-protein snack after eating too much chocolate, etc.). Just because our culture endlessly promotes unrealistic beauty standards, causing millions of women to dislike—and even despise—their bodies, this does not mean that we have to hate and harm our bodies, too.

PMS Relief Strategies Review
Figure 25

1. *Chart your symptoms.*
2. *Make necessary dietary changes.*
3. *Manage stress.*
4. *Get enough exercise.*
5. *Maintain a steady blood sugar level.*
6. *Seek medical help when needed.*
7. *Try a variety of remedies; use those that work best for you.*

HOW FAMILY AND FRIENDS CAN HELP

PMS is often identified, not only by the woman herself, but by her family and friends—those people with whom she has the most frequent contact. For this reason, it is important that, whenever possible, those who are closest to her be well informed about this condition to enable them to be supportive.

This chapter contains many ideas about how to relieve PMS that your friend/sister/mother/daughter/wife may not know about. Perhaps you could talk with her about them sometime. Then neither of you has to suffer. You can help her cope by:

Treating the woman suffering from PMS according to her age. That means like an adult, unless she's only twelve. But since most twelve-year-olds don't have PMS, you're probably safe if you avoid having a parental type of attitude about this problem.

Do practical things to help out. Do the dishes, the laundry, some grocery shopping, or fix a few meals. (If it's Saturday, how about breakfast, lunch, *and* dinner?) What if you work full time outside the home and she doesn't? Then she probably will be especially grateful for some practical help, as well as for time out (in the tub, at the library, out for a walk, kids away for the evening, etc.).

Avoid PMS jokes. For obvious reasons. Instead, listen actively to her concerns and complaints.

Assist and aid her in implementing the lifestyle and nutritional ideas outlined above. Hint: back rubs are a big favorite with most women.

Support her exercise schedule. Encourage her to get lots of sleep, rest, and relaxation. Find ways to ease at-home stress. And try not to take PMS-related mood swings personally.

Primary Dysmenorrhea and Other Types of Pelvic Pain— Determining the Difference

We are all familiar with the secret code word for menstruation, and the word is . . . (a steady drumroll here, please) . . . *cramps!*

Did you know that up to 80 percent of all women have some degree of discomfort during their menstrual periods?[1] That painful menstruation, called *dysmenorrhea*, is the most common symptom requiring women to take time off work or school?[2] Or—and this is the good news—that "cramps" can be effectively treated in *most* of these cases?[3]

Like PMS, menstrual cramps are a fact of life for many, if not most, women. Painful periods are *not* a figment of women's imaginations or a plea for sympathy—they're real. (Believe me, we wish they weren't.) And also, like PMS, the exact cause of menstrual cramps is not fully understood.

Misinformation about menstruation abounds. That's why it's helpful to compare fact with fiction before looking at specific ways to cope with cramps. Discovering what we already know about menstrual pain and then replacing any misinformation with up-to-date data is a good place to start. (See Figure 26.)

A Self-Check Quiz on Painful Periods
Figure 26

STATEMENT	TRUE	FALSE
1. A "tilted" or "tipped" uterus can cause painful periods.	—	—
2. Alcohol is a good remedy for relieving menstrual cramps.	—	—
3. Painful periods are a sign of a hormone imbalance and infertility.	—	—
4. Ibuprofen (Advil, Motrin, Nuprin) is as good or better than other non-narcotic painkillers in treating painful menstruation.	—	—
5. Contraceptives have little effect on menstrual cramps.	—	—
6. Painful periods that are not relieved by antiprostaglandins may indicate that another physical condition is responsible.	—	—

ANSWERS AND COMMENTS

1. *False.* A tilted, tipped, retroverted, or retroflexed uterus only causes painful periods if it has been displaced by surgery or disease, such as endometriosis, pelvic adhesions, adenomyosis, or fibroids. More on these conditions later.

2. *False.* Alcohol relaxes the uterus only slightly, is of limited benefit, poses the potential for abuse, and should not be used for this purpose. You're better off with a heating pad, some red raspberry leaf tea, and two aspirin (if you're not allergic to it).

3. *False.* Painful periods are a normal part of fertility. They are associated with *regular* cycles and normal ovulation *unless* the pain develops after adolescence, gets worse over time, or occurs at other times during the menstrual cycle.

4. *True.* Because of its prostaglandin-inhibiting action, ibuprofen and other antiprostaglandins are currently the most effective non-narcotic pain relievers for menstrual cramps.

5. *False.* Devices such as the IUD and diaphragm, when in place, can make cramps much more severe. However, oral contraceptives (OCs) often do relieve cramps. Refer to chapter 9 for reasons why women should *not* simultaneously use OCs as a remedy for normal menstrual cramps and a birth control method.

6. *True.* A medical diagnosis is needed to determine the cause of pelvic pain. This is especially true if you have not previously had painful periods.

SO WHAT CAUSES THOSE AWFUL CRAMPS ANYWAY?

Powerful hormones called *prostaglandins* are currently believed to be the primary culprit. Found in the menstrual blood and uterine wall in greater amounts in women who have painful periods, prostaglandins cause increased uterine contractions that interfere with blood supply to the uterus, producing cramping sensations called *ischemia*.

Prostaglandins also stimulate the intestines—hence the nausea, loose stools, and/or diarrhea many women experience when menstruating, especially on days when the menstrual flow is heaviest. Stretching of the cervix, caused by the passage of blood clots during menstrual bleeding, contributes to painful periods as well.

Mild discomfort often accompanies the onset of the menstrual flow and is perfectly normal. Lower back pain, tenderness in the lower abdomen, digestive upset, and cramping of the uterus are very common during the first twenty-four hours. The line between "normal/not needing treatment" and "normal/needing treatment," discussed briefly in chapter 2, will depend upon *your own opinion* about the degree of discomfort you are experiencing *rather than on a clinical measurement of your symptoms.* The information included here will help you to know what your options are.

First of all, keep in mind that there are two different types of cramps. *Primary dysmenorrhea*, or "normal" menstrual pain, initially occurs in young women who have just begun to menstruate. As many of us know, this can be a very severe—even incapacitating—condition. Often accompanied by nausea, diarrhea, and weakness or fainting, primary dysmenorrhea is most common during adolescence and then subsides almost completely by the time a woman reaches her late twenties. This aggravating problem may persist, however, until the first pregnancy, occur intermittently throughout the reproductive years, or occasionally continue until menopause.

While pregnancy can help to alleviate primary dysmenorrhea (especially during the nine months one is pregnant!), it is not necessarily a reliable "cure." Giving birth dramatically alleviates this condition in some, but not all, women. The relief is possibly due to the stretching of the cervix during labor or the enlarging of blood vessels in the uterus during pregnancy.

Since the most common type of pelvic pain in women is primary dysmenorrhea, it makes sense that we should go beyond treating cramps with Pamprin or Midol—unless these remedies alone sufficiently alleviate monthly cramping discomfort.

TREATMENTS FOR MENSTRUAL CRAMPS

Here are several different approaches to dealing with menstrual pain, only one of which involves taking medications. By avoiding risk factors (see Figure 27) and using a combination of natural and pharmaceutical approaches, most women can see menstrual cramps become a thing of the past.

Menstrual Cramp Risk Factors
Figure 27

Do any of the following risk factors apply to you? If so, you are at higher risk for menstrual cramps. By reducing your number of risk factors, you may also decrease your level of menstrual discomfort.

Use of tampons	Chronic or recurrent bladder infections
Use of IUD, cervical cap, or diaphragm	Chronic or recurrent yeast infections
Irregular or inadequate exercise	Chronic stress
Poor posture resulting in pelvic misalignment	Pelvic inflammatory disease
Sitting for long periods without stretch breaks	Uterine fibroids
Excessive intake of alcohol, sugar, dairy foods, salt, animal fats, processed food products*	Endometriosis, constipation
Vitamin and mineral imbalances	Irritable bowel syndrome
Nutritional deficiencies (low levels of essential fatty acids, for example)	Immune system dysfunction, diabetes

*Use of alcohol and other substances (e.g., MSG, sugar, nitrates, and nitrites) may affect pain sensitivity; excessive intake of high-fat, high-protein foods (dairy products, poultry, meat, and eggs) boosts the production of prostaglandins.

Antiprostaglandin Therapy

Medications that inhibit the release of prostaglandins in the body may eliminate or reduce the severity of cramps related to menstruation. To be most effective, antiprostaglandins should be started *before* the cramps begin. Once your period starts, the prostaglandins are released into your bloodstream, making it more difficult to stop the cramps quickly. This is where keeping a menstrual diary can be a real bonus. By knowing when your period is ready to start, you can take the medication early enough to prevent severe or sudden cramping, say, in the middle of your birthday party or an important meeting with your boss.

A variety of prostaglandin-inhibiting drugs besides aspirin are now available for menstrual cramp relief. (See Figure 28.) Ask your health-care provider for more information on specific medications. Many require a prescription; none are completely risk-free. Your local pharmacist may also be of assistance in explaining the comparative costs and possible adverse effects of each drug.

Prostaglandin-Inhibiting Drugs Used to Treat Painful Periods
Figure 28

GENERIC (TRADE) NAMES

ibuprofen (Motrin-IB, Advil, Nuprin)

naproxen sodium (Anaprox, Anaprox DS, Aleve)

naproxen (Naprosyn)

mefanemic acid (Ponstel)

fenoprophen calcium (Nalfon)

Contraindications to use: Do not use any of these drugs if you have ever had an allergic reaction to aspirin or have been told not to take a non-steroidal anti-inflammatory drug (NSAID). Antiprostaglandins do not contain aspirin, but are likely to produce an allergic response in those who are also allergic to aspirin. Also, Naprosyn (naproxen) should not be used at the same time as Anaprox (naproxen sodium). *If you develop an allergic or adverse reaction while taking one of these medications, contact your physician immediately.* Do not take any of these medications if you are younger than fifteen or have gastritis, peptic ulcer, enteritis, ileitis, ulcerative colitis, asthma, heart failure, high blood pressure, or bleeding problems.

Signs of overdose. You may possibly have accumulated too much of this drug in your system if you begin to experience drowsiness, heartburn, indigestion, nausea, and vomiting. Contact your health-care provider for further advice.

NOTE: Women who are experiencing menstrual cramping due to other disorders—such as endometriosis, uterine fibroids, or ovarian cysts—may find that these drugs afford limited relief. Consult your health-care provider for further diagnosis and treatment.

Nutritional Therapy

As with PMS, vitamin and mineral supplements, amino acids, and dietary changes can be very effective in contributing to the relief of menstrual pain. Supplements of vitamin B6, vitamin C, vitamin E, magnesium, zinc, calcium, and essential fatty acids (see chapter 3 for commonly used daily dosages) have been reported to be especially useful.

Vitamin B6 helps the body break down *catecholamines* (substances that regulate the transmission of nerve impulses) and may make a difference if you experience anxiety or depression after ovulating.[4] Be careful, however: A maximum daily dose of 100 to 150 milligrams (divided into smaller amounts of 25 to 50 milligrams, taken with meals) can be beneficial, but it is possible to overdose on B6.[5] During your period, you may want to try taking more magnesium (100 milligrams every two to three hours during the days you're menstruating) to ease discomfort. The amino acid DL-phenylalanine (375 milligrams, three to four times daily) may also be effective in treating chronic pelvic pain, including discomfort caused by endometriosis.[6] But do not take this supplement if you have any of the following conditions—high blood pressure, PKU, diabetes, or panic attacks.

The dietary recommendations for PMS apply here as well—plenty of high-fiber complex carbohydrates, low-fat foods, and little meat. (Fats and meat products can boost prostaglandin production.) Some women find that eliminating dairy products from their diet can help relieve menstrual cramps as they turn to other calcium-rich foods—green leafy vegetables (broccoli, collard greens, kale), grains, beans, legumes, canned sardines and salmon (with bones), sea vegetables (kelp, hijiki, dulse, agar-agar), herbs, nuts and seeds, mineral water, and calcium-fortified orange juice.

Herbal Therapy

The following recipes have been reported to be quite effective in relieving normal menstrual discomfort (Figure 29). Be sure to strain the mixtures before use. For specific suggestions and contraindications regarding the use of herbal medicine for menstrual pain, consult your local Christian herbalist or a detailed instruction manual. (NOTE: *Recipes for the teas and tonics listed here are not intended to be a prescription for the treatment of any health problem.*)

Herbal Teas and Tonics for
Easing Menstrual Discomfort
Figure 29

Red Raspberry Leaf Tea

Steep 1 oz. red raspberry leaves in 2 cups water for 15 minutes. Take two cups daily.

Blind Nettle Tonic

Use 2 tsp. plant or flowers with 1 cup water. Take one to one and a half cups a day, unsweetened, a mouthful at a time.

Milfoil Tea

Use 1 Tbsp. dried herb with 1 cup water. Parboil and steep for five minutes. Take one cup a day.

Lady's Mantle Tonic

Mix equal parts of lady's mantle, blind nettle, and milfoil together. Steep 1 tsp. in 1/2 cup boiling water. Take one to one and a half cups a day, unsweetened, in mouthful doses. If you make a large batch, store the surplus in a covered container in the refrigerator.

Herbal Bath

Mix together equal parts of lady's mantle, oak bark, shave grass, and oat straw. Boil 8 to 9 oz. of this mixture in 5 qt. water briefly; remove from stove and steep for 10 minutes. Use warm for a sitz bath. To take a sitz bath, fill the tub with about four inches of water and keep your knees up. Wrap the upper part of your body in a large towel or blanket, staying in the tub for 10 to 20 minutes. Splash the water on your abdomen, or cover yourself with a warm washcloth soaked in tub water. Add extra hot water as needed.

Heat Therapy

Hot water bottles, heating pads, eucalyptus oil, and warm baths all aid in relieving menstrual pain by promoting the circulation of oxygen in the pelvic area. An added plus—while laying down or in the tub, you are partaking in a quiet time of rest that will also do you good. Put on some soft music and drink a cup of herbal tea for a particularly refreshing few moments alone. When lying flat, keep your legs elevated with a pillow under your knees; if lying on your side, bring your knees comfortably up toward your chest.

Exercise Therapy

The same types of exercise listed in the last chapter on PMS are also excellent ways of relieving menstrual pain and pelvic congestion. Relief results from increased oxygen circulation and the release of those naturally secreted painkillers, beta-endorphins, that act to inhibit prostaglandins. Stretching exercises may help to relieve pelvic pain as well. Here are some basic principles for exercise.

- *Exercise shouldn't hurt*. Pain during exercise is a sign that something is wrong. Slow down or change what you are doing. The "no-pain, no-gain" approach has been proven to be detrimental to your health.
- *Exercise should feel good*. Especially when you are finished. If you exercise enough to get your circulation going but avoid overdoing it, you will feel exhilarated and refreshed afterwards. Plus, there's an added benefit to avoiding exercise extremes. When you keep your heart rate from going too high, exercise burns fat more effectively.
- *Exercise should be fun*. That is, enjoyable—before, during, and after.
- *Exercise should be regular*. As much as possible, try exercising three to five times weekly—or at least every other day—to obtain the best benefits.
- *Exercise shouldn't be boring or overly repetitious*. In other words, the best kinds of exercise are the most interesting and varied.
- *Exercise is best fueled by complex carbohydrates*. Fruits, whole grains, rice, pasta, legumes—these are the high-energy foods that will keep your blood sugar up while boosting your ability to burn body fat. And, interestingly enough, they're the same foods that help ease menstrual discomfort.
- *Exercise and eat sensibly, not faddishly*. While exercise and dieting fads come and go, stick with the basics to stay healthy. Don't take foolish risks with extreme diets and workouts that can endanger your well-being.

When in doubt, walk! Did you know that walking is turning out to be the easiest, cheapest, least stressful, and most accessible physical activity there is (Figure 30)?

"You don't have to have sweat pouring down your brow to achieve benefit from aerobic exercise," points out Dr. James Rippe, cardiologist and medical director for the University of Massachusetts Medical School's Center for Health, Fitness and Human Performance. "Both a high-class athlete and the average person can achieve enough exercise from walking to derive the maximum benefit to their hearts. Very simply, fitness walking is the best exercise for conditioning the vast majority of Americans."

Calories Burned in One Hour of Walking
Figure 30

BODY WEIGHT	125	140	155	170	195	220
PACE (SLOW TO FAST)						
2 m.p.h.	120	135	149	163	187	211
3 m.p.h.	247	277	307	337	386	436
4 m.p.h.	353	445	493	540	620	700

Work up to walking briskly—about three to four miles per hour (m.p.h.) for sixty minutes three to four days weekly or forty-five minutes five to six days a week. For a free booklet on the "how-to's" of fitness walking, see Resources at the end of the book.

Swing your arms to increase lung capacity. The more movement the upper body makes, the greater the aerobic benefit.

Walk uphill and downhill, if your knees are strong enough. Walking on a fourteen-degree incline requires four times the effort of walking on level ground! Walking downhill requires more energy as well.

Don't wait—walk. The next time you find yourself waiting for your doctor or dentist, tell the receptionist you'll be out walking. Check in at times indicated.

Don't shop—walk. Mall-walking, the modern version of window-shopping, is a viable substitute for the great outdoors in inclement weather. Take a friend—talking helps pass the time. Leave your wallet at home. If the mall has more than one level, use the stairs at each end to vary your route back and forth.

Walk, don't run. Unless you prefer running, that is. Walking at a speed of greater than 4.5 miles per hour isn't walking—it's jogging. Slow down and give your joints a break.

Walk, don't join. Why spend money on a fitness club membership when walking is free? Why go out for lunch for social interaction when you can burn calories and visit at the same time? Save money and take a friend! A two-to-three-mile walk can be completed in under an hour, and you can do an awful lot of talking in that time.

Vary your routine with swimming, cycling, tennis, and housecleaning as desired to make life more interesting. Remember, exercise benefits our cardiovascular system, muscles, bones, and overall sense of well-being. (Why is this so easy to forget?) And it not only can increase our life span but also the harmony and efficiency of our cycles.

ABNORMAL PELVIC PAIN: SECONDARY DYSMENORRHEA

If the onset of menstrual cramps *occurs after adolescence*, if the pain *is not limited to menstruation*, or if *their severity increases over time*, a physical examination by your health-care provider is necessary to determine the cause. Called *secondary dysmenorrhea*, this type of menstrual pain develops in women who had little or no cramping with their periods previously. It is much less common than the primary form of dysmenorrhea and is often associated with some type of physical abnormality of the reproductive organs. You need to take it seriously.

A number of female reproductive disorders can be responsible for causing "crampy" pain in the lower abdomen (Figure 31). These include endometriosis, adenomyosis, pelvic inflammatory disease (PID), ovarian cysts, endometrial and ovarian cancer, sexually transmitted diseases, intrauterine devices (IUDs) and diaphragms, nonmalignant tumors such as fibroids or polyps, and pregnancy problems (tubal, or ectopic, pregnancy; miscarriage; or retained portions of the placenta following childbirth).

As a general rule of thumb, *any change in a normal body function that becomes chronic needs immediate medical evaluation.* Figure 31 will help you distinguish between some of the types of pelvic pain women experience and their possible causes. The chart also indicates when to contact your health-care provider if you are experiencing any of these symptoms. NOTE: If the symptoms you are experiencing require you to "contact your health-care provider now," it is possibly an emergency—please don't wait. Detailed information about many of these conditions and a discussion of their appropriate treatments will follow in later chapters.

One final word of caution: If the cause of your pain cannot be determined, and if ultrasound and/or laparoscopy results are normal, having further surgery probably will not get rid of the pain. (See discussion on pelvic pain in chapter 17.) The pain is real regardless of what is causing it. *If you have pelvic pain, you need appropriate diagnosis and treatment.*

Check out all possibilities thoroughly, and if nothing turns up, don't be shy about evaluating your lifestyle and sexual history closely. Psychological, spiritual, social, and/or physical stress has multiple effects on the human body—including causing pain. In such cases, a variety of pain-management strategies, including counseling, may be your best bet.

Some Causes of Pelvic Pain in Women: Distinguishing the Difference
Figure 31

SIGNS AND SYMPTOMS	POSSIBLE CAUSE / TREATMENT
Cramps accompanying the onset of menstruation.	Prostaglandins. *Consult health-care provider and/or apply home treatment.*
Pelvic discomfort lasting for several hours in the middle part of the menstrual cycle.	Ovulation. *Consult health-care provider and/or apply home treatment.*
"Crampy" pain starting two to seven days before the onset of menstruation. May also occur around the time of ovulation.	Endometriosis. *Consult health care provider.*
Forceful uterine contractions during menstruation; periods may become heavier as well.	Benign growths inside the uterus (fibroids or polyps); endometriosis, adenomyosis. *Make appointment with health care provider.*
Crampy pain after menstrual bleeding has begun, accompanied by fever and continuing after menstruation.	Tubal or pelvic infection (such as PID, gonorrhea, or chlamydia), but may also be caused by a forgotten tampon, so check first. If no tampon is present, *make appointment with health-care provider now.*
Deep pelvic pain during intercourse.	Pelvic, cervical or bladder infection; ovarian cysts; scar tissue; endometriosis; fibroid tumors; cancer; or changes in the vagina (shorter or narrower) after hysterectomy. Also: appendicitis or an inflammatory intestinal disease. *Consult health care provider.*

SIGNS AND SYMPTOMS	POSSIBLE CAUSE / TREATMENT
Menstrual pain after insertion of an IUD that continues for more than several cycles.	Uterine infection or infection caused by the IUD; partially expelled IUD. *Make appointment with health-care provider.* (See chapter 5 for reasons to have the IUD removed.)
Cramps accompanying use of a diaphragm.	Pelvic pressure; possible irritation or infection. *Consult with health-care provider.*
Strong, periodic uterine cramping during pregnancy, possibly accompanied by spotting, changing to heavier bleeding.	Labor; miscarriage. *Contact health-care provider now.*
Cramps immediately following childbirth.	"After pains" associated with the uterus closing the placental site. *Consult with health care provider if accompanied by fever, unusual odor or excessive bleeding.*
Continued or sudden cramping after the first few days following childbirth.	Infection or retained placental fragments, especially if accompanied by fever, prolonged bleeding, or foul-smelling discharge. *Contact health-care provider now.*
Sudden, severe pelvic pain following a missed period.	Tubal pregnancy. *Contact health-care provider now.*
Onset of menstrual pain after tubal ligation.	Post-Tubal Ligation Syndrome. *Consult with health-care provider.*
Vague pressure in the pelvis or abdomen accompanied by stomach bloating and abnormal vaginal bleeding.	Ovarian cysts or pelvic cancer. *Make appointment with physician now. Consult health-care provider and/or apply home treatment.*

5

Variations on a Theme: Heavy, Long, Late, Light, and Missed Periods

The key question related to menstrual patterns seems to be: *How do I know if my periods are normal?* Because each of us is totally unique in our changing cyclical patterns, menstruation isn't necessarily the same from year to year (or month to month) even in the same woman, much less for different women.

Many things can be responsible for this—sleeping, eating, and exercise habits; weight changes; work, school, and/or family stress; prescription and over-the-counter medications; food and environmental toxins; smoking; birth control technologies; substance abuse; aging; childbearing; breastfeeding; emotional or physical trauma; surgery; reproductive illness; chronic disease; and hormonal fluctuations (caused by any of the preceding factors).[1]

Since menstrual patterns change over time and are influenced by so many factors, it helps to have some general guidelines to follow in determining the answer to this concern.

ESTABLISHING MENSTRUAL PATTERNS

First, it's essential to become familiar with a few basic terms. Some of these terms are already quite familiar to us, while others are completely new and unfamiliar (see Figure 32). (I especially like the word *menometrorrhagia*—a tongue twister in any language, wouldn't you say?)

Uterine Bleeding
Figure 32

NONSPECIFIC TERMS	DESCRIPTION
Normal uterine bleeding (menstruation)	Uterine bleeding lasting anywhere between three to seven days, typically occurring at twenty-four to thirty-two day intervals. This is counted from the first day of your period to the first day of your next period. It includes all phases of the menstrual cycle, including days when bleeding doesn't take place. The menstrual flow normally measures four to five tablespoons of fluid; only one-third is blood.
Abnormal uterine bleeding	Any variation from your normal menstrual pattern, including all abnormal bleeding from the vagina which may or may not be related to a specific cause
Spotting	Light, irregular bleeding which may or may not be prolonged
Amenorrhea	Absence of menstrual flow
Menopause	Cessation of menstruation which normally accompanies aging
Cryptomenorrhea	Blocked flow due to an abnormality in the reproductive system
Hypomenorrhea	Light flow during regular menstrual periods
Oligomenorrhea	Long intervals between cycles, which often occur at irregular intervals, resulting in less frequent bleeding
Polymenorrhea	Short intervals between cycles, resulting in more frequent bleeding
Menorrhagia	Prolonged menstrual flow
Metrorrhagia	Irregular flow; frequent menstruation
Menometrorrhagia	Prolonged, irregular menstruation

How can anyone possibly say there is such a thing as regular menstrual periods? I prefer the term normal myself. It's much more accurate and thus less worrisome when I'm trying to decide if my body is just off-schedule or acting strangely for a reason—and whether I should be concerned about it or not.

Heavy Bleeding: Emergency or Not?

While some bleeding changes require medical treatment, most bleeding patterns are *not dangerous* and therefore *do not* require treatment. The following will help you to determine whether you need immediate medical evaluation or not. If you do not, take time to find a health-care provider who will listen to your concerns carefully and evaluate your symptoms thoroughly. Many things can cause changes in your periods and bleeding patterns.

Warning Signs: Abnormal Uterine Bleeding

Call your health-care provider for an appointment if you experience:

- Any bleeding or spotting from the vagina after menopause that is not related to hormone replacement therapy.
- Any bleeding after intercourse that is not related to menstruation.

Contact your health-care provider immediately if you experience:

- Any bleeding that soaks four or five pads within two hours.
- Any bleeding during pregnancy, *especially* if accompanied by period-like cramps or backache.

See your health-care provider immediately or have someone take you to an emergency room right away if you experience:

- Any sudden *heavy* blood loss that makes you feel dizzy, faint, weak, or excessively drowsy. These are warning signs of shock.

Normal Versus "Regular" Menstrual Bleeding

Did you know that few women have perfectly regular periods? That most of us vary on the exact interval, length, and amount of menstruation from one cycle to the next? That it isn't all that unusual to vary up to a week in cycle length, to bleed longer, or to have a lighter (or heavier) flow at times? And that most of us worry about these irregularities even when they're normal? (See Figure 33.)

Normal Versus Abnormal Menstrual Patterns
Figure 33

MENSTRUAL PATTERN	EVALUATION NEEDED?	POSSIBLE DIAGNOSIS
Periods don't start exactly the same day.	No	Variation is probably normal if no other unusual symptoms are present.
Skipping a period.	No	Variation is probably normal if no other symptoms are present. If pregnancy is a possibility, take a test.
Chronically heavy periods (this is your usual pattern, not a change for you).	No	Treatment is usually unnecessary aside from periodic checkups, a blood count every six months, and iron supplements. If you have fibroids, avoid birth control pills and estrogen.
Scant menstrual flow (if not a change for you).	No	Unless this represents a change, it is not likely to be due to any health problems.
Blood clots in the menstrual flow.	No	Blood clots are the result of heavier bleeding and a healthy blood-clotting system. If other symptoms concern you, seek medical evaluation.
Slight spotting around the time of ovulation for one day or less (called *ovulatory bleeding*).	No	Hormone changes during ovulation can cause spotting.
Periods consistently start every three weeks (called *polymenorrhea*).	No	As long as this pattern isn't new or unusual, don't worry about it.
Menstrual patterns disrupted for three to six months after going off birth control pills.	No	Menstrual irregularities after taking an OC are very common.
Increased space between periods after the age of forty.	No	Declining hormone production results in fewer periods.

MENSTRUAL PATTERN	EVALUATION NEEDED?	POSSIBLE DIAGNOSIS
Periods start every five weeks, with some variation (*oligomenorrhea*).	Yes	Possibly caused by ovarian dysfunction or hormonal imbalance. Treatment with hormones may reestablish normal function, especially if pregnancy is desired.
Bleeding lasting more than seven days.	Yes	Possibly caused by fibroids, IUD, polyps, uterine infection, or (*menorrhagia*). If anemia or enlarged uterus exists, an endometrial biopsy or D&C may be necessary.
Spotting after intercourse.	Yes	Possibly due to cervical infection or inflammation. If so, the cervix may be treated directly in-office and/or antibiotics may be prescribed.
Light bleeding or spotting lasting several days before each period (*premenstrual spotting*).	Yes	Possibly due to low progesterone levels. If so, CPRT (*cooperative progesterone replacement therapy*) may help, but rule out pregnancy and other concerns first.
Spotting lasting more than a week if under forty years old (*menometrorrhagia*).	Yes	Possibly due to insufficient progesterone levels. If so, CPRT may help, but rule out pregnancy and other concerns first.
Spotting lasting more than a week if over forty years old (*menometrorrhagia*).	Yes	For a complete diagnosis, an endometrial biopsy or D&C may be needed for tissue analysis.
Any bleeding after menopause not related to hormone replacement therapy (*postmenopausal bleeding*)	Yes	For a complete diagnosis, a biopsy or D&C may be needed for tissue analysis.

Note: Rest, stress reduction strategies, recreation, and good nutrition habits are important for all women, especially when menstrual problems persist. Medical treatment and drug therapy alone are inadequate remedies.

Rather than worrying needlessly (which never helps anyway), it's best to evaluate menstrual changes calmly and wisely—that is, without jumping to what I call extreme conclusions.

If our bleeding patterns change, they've done so for a reason certainly, but that reason is highly unlikely to be something as extreme as uterine cancer. It's much more likely to be due to our sleeping/eating/exercise/work habits, an emotional upset, medication, or a simple illness such as a recent upper respiratory infection.

Self-Check Assessment for Menstrual Irregularities

Most of us know this to be true, yet we continue to be alarmed when our periods don't show up on time or become heavier (or lighter or earlier or crampier) than usual. The following questions help to alleviate concern in such situations:

Has anything unusual been going on in my life this month? This can include anything from a new boss at work, final exams, marital stress, moving, or starting a reduced-calorie diet or heavy-duty exercise program. It can also include having unplanned intercourse without using a contraceptive, having an abortion, being sexually assaulted, getting (and being treated for) a sexually transmitted disease, starting to smoke again, drinking too much, or abusing drugs—any drugs.

It would be good if we could say that as Christian women, these things never happen in our lives, but sometimes they do. It helps to be honest about this.

One of the greatest lies the enemy manages to lay on us is that we "deserve" to suffer for our sins—and keep suffering for them over and over again, even after our heavenly Father has forgiven us. The problem is that many of us keep paying (and paying) on debts we no longer owe, and consequently we end up abusing ourselves—through sexual sin, chronic dieting, overeating, overworking, trying to be perfect, and other compulsive behaviors.

The good news is that Jesus has paid the price for our sin already. Through Him we can be forgiven and set free—truly free—from self-abusive, self-hating behaviors. *We need to seek appropriate medical and spiritual support in times of need.* Let's not buy into the enemy's opinion of us. We deserve so much more!

How much rest, recreation, and sleep have I been getting? Believe it or not, our grandparents' generation knew the basics of wellness. They knew that it was important to sleep at least eight hours each night and to stay on a regular schedule, to eat a good breakfast (with lots of fiber) and go for long walks outdoors (for fresh air), to avoid alcohol and tobacco smoke, and to give and receive love.

Think about your own lifestyle habits lately. How much sleep have you been getting? Do you take time for yourself to rest and "recreate" every day? What things have you done "just for fun" this week?

It's quite possible that your life is too busy. If so, slow it down. What are you trying to prove by "overfunctioning"? Did the world come to an end when Jesus left the Twelve to retreat into the mountains to spend time alone with His Father? Do we really think He spent the entire time agonizing in prayer—or might He have actually watched sunsets, listened to birds sing, and looked at the flowers blooming?

Be kind to yourself. For a change of pace, try something different. Do three or four things you enjoy today. Then see what happens. Then do this again tomorrow—and every day thereafter. Sleep nine hours if you feel the need to, or sleep less if you wish. *Decide not to neglect yourself at the expense of others.* Believe me, they'll really thank you for it later.

What have I been eating? More than any other culture on earth, Americans are obsessed with food, fat, diet, and weight. We all know this, yet most of us continue to focus on these things. It's been estimated that up to 80 percent of the women in our country have some degree of eating disorder, that at least half of us are dieting at any given moment. Do you fit into this familiar picture?

If you aren't sure, ask yourself: Do I think about food even when I'm not hungry? Do I notice what other people eat (and how much and how often) they eat? When do I get hungry during the day? Do I eat when I'm hungry and stop eating when I'm not? Do I worry about my weight? Do I continually count calories and/or fat grams? Do I diet frequently? Do I criticize others for their eating habits—silently or out loud? Do I usually notice what size people are before I notice other things about them? Do I see women with the kind of body I'd like to have and try to emulate them (or constantly wish I could look like them)? Do I exercise for reasons other than for fitness and because I enjoy it?

I doubt that there are very many of us who can answer no to every single question. Isn't it amazing how controlled we are by food and body weight concerns? And this way of thinking about food certainly isn't good for us: It actually ends up doing us far more harm than good in the long run.

I'm learning to eat when I'm hungry and stop when I'm not—it's surprising what a revolutionary concept this can be to someone who is a former chronic dieter/overeater/dieter. Best of all, I'm finding how much healthier I can be *without* dieting or overeating. Someday, I may lose weight. But it's not the top priority issue it used to be with me. I've discovered there are plenty of other things more important to think about and invest my energy in than food or dieting.

Note: If this kind of reasoning sounds abhorrent or stupid to you, watch out! You probably haven't come to terms with your own eating disorder yet. For more insight read: *Overcoming Overeating* by Jane R. Hirschmann and Carol H. Munter (New York: Fawcett Columbine/Ballantine Books, 1988), and *Don't Diet* by Dale M. Artens (New York: William Morrow and Company, Inc., 1988), excellent guides for overeaters and undereaters alike. Books like these are loaded with sound information.

Do I exercise appropriately? As with other types of stress, exercise-related stress can throw off our biological clocks—or keep them running. Too much exercise, and women often stop ovulating. Too little, and we're more at risk for things like endometriosis. Menstrual changes are an excellent "stress indicator" in this regard; our bodies have a powerful way of telling us that both overexertion and a sedentary existence are not what our Creator had in mind for us.

If you notice changes in menstrual patterns related to your fitness program (or lack of one), make adjustments as necessary. You may need to tone things down or liven things up, depending on what your ovaries and uterus tell you.

As with overfunctioning and overeating/undereating, overexertion and underexertion have the potential to become self-abusive behaviors (and disruptive to menstruation).

In what ways do I take care of myself and see that my needs are met? List ten things you have done for fun this week. If you can't list ten, make a list of ten things that you enjoy that you will commit yourself to doing this week.

Your list might include: a back rub; a long bath; lunch with your best friend; going to the symphony; going to the library; going to the beach; going to the movies; going shopping; going out to lunch; playing in the sprinkler; playing with your kids; playing with your dog; taking a hike; taking a mini-vacation; taking yourself to the zoo; staying home to sew, reflect, remember, bake bread, wallpaper, listen to music, plant a garden; and taking time out to keep a journal, read a novel, sip some homemade lemonade, pick a bouquet, swing in a hammock, savor a sunrise, sleep, or pray.

It's too bad that medical history forms and annual women's wellness visits don't routinely cover the five questions listed above. I think it would eliminate many menstrual irregularities without the expense and risks associated with drugs and unnecessary surgery.

Heavy periods that aren't a change from your normal menstruating pattern don't usually require any treatment other than self-care and these commonsense coping strategies: Get as much rest as you can while your period's the heaviest; have a blood count done to check your iron every six months (this doesn't require a regular office visit, just an order from your health-care provider and a lab fee); take iron supplements as needed; eat nutritious, high-energy, high-fiber, low-fat meals and snacks; drink lots of liquids as your thirst dictates—especially mineral water; and avoid estrogen, excessive weight gain, and birth control pills if you know you have fibroids—to avoid stimulating their growth.

ABNORMAL BLEEDING

Due to not understanding what causes abnormal uterine bleeding, many women have hysterectomies to deal with this aggravating and often debilitating problem. "Dysfunctional uterine bleeding has been a common wastebasket diagnosis for many conditions in which the true anatomic cause has not been detected, and many unnecessary hysterectomies may be performed because of persistent uterine bleeding without pathologic findings," reads a statement that appeared ten years ago in the medical journal *Surgery, Gynecology & Obstetrics*.[2] Shouldn't we try something a bit less radical first?

A Possible Warning Sign That's Probably Not Serious

Obviously, things other than dieting, stress, and overexertion can cause abnormal uterine bleeding patterns. In fact, there is a long list of things that do (Figure 34). Consequently, it's smart to tell your health-care provider about *any vaginal bleeding that does not fit the average, normal pattern*: twenty-four to thirty-two day cycles, periods lasting three to seven days, and a menstrual flow of up to four to five tablespoons.

Abnormal bleeding is a very common problem in women at the beginning and end of their reproductive years. For women between the ages of fourteen and twenty-five, ovulation isn't likely to take place on a regular, recurring basis until menstrual patterns are well-established. When it comes to abnormal bleeding, pelvic infection and unplanned pregnancy are the primary targets of medical concern for this age group—not cancer.

For women thirty-five to fifty, irregular ovulation and menstrual patterns are not unusual. Polyps, fibroids, and endometriosis seem to be reported and diagnosed with increasing frequency these days. None are life-threatening diseases; in most cases, hysterectomy isn't necessary to cope with these common reproductive problems. (See chapters 15 and 17.)

Because abnormal bleeding is associated with pelvic cancer in a few cases, however, it is especially important if you're over thirty to have any abnormal bleeding medically evaluated—even if your periods aren't unusually heavy. After menopause *any bleeding not related to hormone replacement therapy*—no matter how light in amount or color—should be reported promptly to your physician.

If you're under thirty, the risk of cancer is extremely rare, so unless your bleeding becomes excessively heavy, you have signs of infection, your periods become painful, you're trying to become pregnant, and/or the problem(s) persist, extensive exams and testing may not be necessary.

Possible Causes of Abnormal Bleeding
Figure 34

A NORMAL REPRODUCTIVE EVENT

> physiologic ovarian cysts
> corpus luteum activity
> ovulation

A REPRODUCTIVE DISORDER

> uterine polyps
> uterine fibroids
> endometrial hyperplasia
> endometriosis
> andenomyosis
> polycystic ovarian disease
> benign ovarian tumors
> functioning ovarian tumors
> cervical polyps
> cervical warts
> vaginal warts
> vaginal injury
> foreign body in vagina (a forgotten tampon, for example)
> thinning of the vaginal wall due to low estrogen levels

A CIRCULATORY DISORDER

severe anemia

blood-clotting disorders

leukemia

platelet disorders

A HORMONAL DISORDER

thyroid deficiency

hormone imbalances

adrenal gland tumor

removal of the ovaries

AN INFECTION OF THE REPRODUCTIVE TRACT

pelvic inflammatory disease (PID)

vaginitis

uterine infection

cervical infection

herpes

syphilis

A CANCER OF THE REPRODUCTIVE TRACT

cervical cancer

uterine cancer

ovarian cancer

vaginal or tubal cancer

A CHRONIC DISEASE

kidney disease

liver disease

thyroid disease

diabetes

A PRESCRIBED OR OTC DRUG TAKEN REGULARLY

oral contraceptives

progestin-only contraceptives

aspirin

anticoagulant drugs

antiprostaglandin drugs

anti-inflammatory drugs

hormone treatments

antidepressants and other psychotropics

A BIRTH CONTROL DEVICE

IUD

diaphragm or cervical cap

SPECIAL SITUATIONS

1. During pregnancy, *any bleeding* should be reported to your health-care provider at once for medical evaluation.

Harm to the pregnancy is *unlikely* if light spotting is associated with any of these normal physiological events:

- implantation of the embryo
- shift in location of hormone production (from corpus luteum to placenta)
- dilation of cervix during full-term labor

Bleeding associated with these conditions indicates a *possible* pregnancy loss.

- progesterone deficiency
- premature dilation of cervix
- placenta previa (placenta on or near cervix)
- placenta abruption attached (premature separation of the placenta)

Bleeding associated with these conditions indicates an *inevitable* pregnancy loss.

- miscarriage
- tubal pregnancy
- abnormal pregnancy
- intrauterine fetal death

2. After menopause, *any bleeding not related to hormone replacement therapy* should be reported to your health-care provider.

Diagnosis of Abnormal Bleeding: What to Expect

You can expect certain procedures from your health-care provider when you tell her that you've been experiencing abnormal bleeding. These include:

- a complete review of your medical history and your symptoms;
- a pelvic exam;
- basic lab tests to rule out (or confirm) pregnancy, cervical/vaginal abnormalities, and infection of the reproductive tract;
- a blood workup to check your iron level, thyroid function, hormone levels, or anything else your doctor may be concerned about.

In addition, your health-care provider may also recommend further diagnostic tests and medical services. (See chapters 16 and 18 for more information on specific tests.) If you are over thirty years old, it is especially important to eliminate cancer as a possible cause of abnormal bleeding. Additional tests and treatment may include:

- keeping a detailed menstrual diary for at least one month prior to additional treatment;
- a sonogram (ultrasound examination);
- an endometrial biopsy or D&C;
- a laparoscopy;
- referral to a hormone specialist (an endocrinologist or a reproductive endocrinologist) for expert analysis of unusual hormone patterns;

- hormone therapy;
- endometrial ablation; and/or
- hysterectomy.

Missed Periods and Amenorrhea

Missed periods always cause us concern. That's because we know that the only time it's *normal* to have an extended break from menstruating is during pregnancy, while totally breastfeeding, and after menopause. At any other time our periods generally continue once they have begun.

It's natural to wonder what's up—especially if an unplanned pregnancy or a reproductive disorder may be the cause. After ruling out pregnancy as a possibility, we still need to find out what's disrupting our cycles. While a break from monthly bleeding is rather appealing, the longer we wait to obtain a diagnosis, the more serious the problem could become.

Diagnosis of Amenorrhea

Amenorrhea—the complete absence of menstrual bleeding—can be caused by a variety of different conditions. *Primary amenorrhea* is the term used to describe the absence of menstruation in a woman under the age of eighteen, whereas *secondary amenorrhea* refers to menstrual periods occurring three months or more apart (see Figure 35) .

If missed period(s) have been caused by stress, a short-term illness, or other temporary factors, menstruation will probably resume within a couple of months. *This is not uncommon.*

In fact, any ongoing physical stress such as excessive weight loss (related to anorexia nervosa, an eating disorder), malnutrition, or intensive athletic training may cause a woman's periods to stop for six months or more. However, *all* abnormal cycling patterns—regardless of the cause—should be reviewed by your health-care provider. Early intervention can help you to prevent reproductive disability later.

A complete medical evaluation is especially important if:

- you miss more than three consecutive periods.
- you're at least sixteen years old and haven't had a period yet.
- you're at least fourteen years old and haven't had any breast development, pubic hair growth, or periods.

- you have any of these symptoms in addition to the absence of menstruation—headaches, vision changes, difficulty in coordination.
- you are experiencing signs of abnormal hormone patterns as well as amenorrhea—growth of body hair, acne, breast milk secretions, and occasionally deepening of the voice, enlargement of the clitoris, and increased sex drive.

Regular exams, blood tests to check hormone levels, and hormone treatment may be necessary if you are experiencing any of these symptoms. Don't panic—most conditions that cause amenorrhea are treatable today.

Possible Causes of Prolonged or Absent Menstruation
Figure 35

A NORMAL REPRODUCTIVE EVENT

pregnancy
childbirth
breastfeeding
menopause

A PERSONAL HEALTH CONCERN

chronic stress
change in the diet
emotional shock
rigorous athletic training
malnutrition
serious illness
tubal pregnancy
excessive weight gain or loss
psychiatric disturbances
alcohol or drug abuse
anorexia nervosa
excessive carotene intake
vegetarian, low-calorie diet
prescription drugs (Compazine, Stelazine, Thorazine, Temaril, and Reserpine, for example)

AN ABNORMALITY OF THE REPRODUCTIVE SYSTEM

closed (imperforate) hymen
blocked cervix (cervical stenosis)
uterine scar tissue buildup
     (Asherman's syndrome)
blocked vagina (vaginal stenosis)

A CONGENITAL (PRESENT-AT-BIRTH) ABNORMALITY

anatomical abnormalities of the uterus, cervix,
     ovaries, or vagina
absence of the uterus
absence of the vagina
developmental defects of the ovaries
genetic conditions

AN OVARIAN CONDITION

ovarian cysts
polycystic ovarian syndrome
surgical removal of the ovaries (ovariectomy)
ovarian cancer
premature menopause
ovarian tumors
chromosomal abnormality

A CHRONIC CONDITION OR LIFE-THREATENING DISEASE

chronic disease—tuberculosis, nephritis (kidney disease), hepatitis,
     cirrhosis of the liver
cancer
diabetes
adrenal problems—congenital adrenal hyperplasia, Cushing's
     disease or syndrome, Addison's disease
pituitary problems—Sheehan's syndrome, Simmond's disease, pituitary tumors,
     congenitally dysfunctional pituitary gland
thyroid problems—hypothyroidism, hyperthyroidism, thyroid tumors
colitis
organic brain disease
hypothalamic insufficiency
cystic fibrosis

Medical Evaluation and Treatment for Amenorrhea

Depending on your symptoms, your medical evaluation may include any-thing from a pelvic exam and a couple of basic blood tests to a full-blown diagnostic workup, including extensive blood tests, chromosomal analysis, and a CAT scan. A "stair-step approach" to discovering what's causing your amenorrhea is advisable if you want to avoid unnecessary drugs and medi-cal treatments. By taking your diagnosis one step at a time, you also reap an added benefit—not missing an obvious or less complicated solution to what-ever may be causing you to skip your menses.

A *progesterone challenge test* (PCT) is commonly used as an initial step in diagnosing a woman with primary or secondary amenorrhea if her uterus, breasts, and secondary sexual characteristics appear to be normal. This involves taking progestin tablets orally for five days or receiving a single injec-tion intramuscularly and then waiting to see if any bleeding occurs—usually within two to seven days. Any bleeding at all indicates that your ovaries are producing estrogen and that your pituitary gland, hypothalamus, and uterus are also working normally. This means that you probably aren't ovulating. *Additional unnecessary tests may be avoided if this test is done and if your pelvic exam and basic blood work don't turn up anything.*

If you have menstruated normally in the past, you may want to wait for three months or longer before undergoing a PCT to avoid the risks associated with the test. Many women start menstruating again spontaneously—that is, without drugs, tests, or surgery. Remember, infrequent or missed periods aren't uncom-mon and rarely indicate something serious unless the problem persists over time.

Treatment of Abnormal Bleeding and Amenorrhea

Treatment, as always, should be aimed at the exact cause(s) of your symp-toms. If your health-care provider can't find a cause, be careful about any rec-ommended treatments and consider seeking a second opinion. If the cause of your abnormal bleeding patterns is determined, examine your options and go with the least invasive alternative necessary to reduce risk.

Let's say that your periods have become much heavier recently and your gynecologist locates fibroid growths in the lining of your uterus. Is a hysterec-tomy necessary at this point in time—or would another approach be preferable?

What if you've skipped two periods in the past six months and your doc-tor recommends that you start taking birth control pills but hasn't asked you about lifestyle issues yet? Then by all means bring them up first. Since the persistent absence of ovulation can lead to serious problems (including infertility) later, has your doctor determined whether you are actually ovulating or not? If not, this will also be an important initial step in your treatment. Has she checked your various hormone levels at different times of the month before placing you on steroids (birth control pills) to treat your bleeding symptoms?

I realize that all of this seems rather complicated, but you won't regret avoiding the risk and expense of unnecessary drugs and surgery in the long run. Furthermore, medical abuse becomes more likely when the diagnosis is incomplete, missed, or poorly performed. Don't become the victim of someone's gynecological inexpertness or inexperience. You deserve better.

First, it's important to understand that many tests have revolutionized the diagnosis of gynecological diseases since 1970. These include sonograms, colposcopy, cervicography, endocervical curettage, endometrial biopsy, hysteroscopy, D&C, laparoscopy, and laser surgery. Has your gynecologist received additional training in new or updated diagnostic technologies? If so, how often does she perform these procedures? Does she readily refer to other well-respected specialists when needed? It is your privilege—and your right—to know this information.

Second, if a hysterectomy is mentioned during the first phase of your diagnostic testing, proceed with caution. As cited earlier, abnormal bleeding is sometimes used as a "wastebasket diagnosis" to justify hysterectomy before other alternatives are explored. (More on this later, in chapter 17.) I believe that it is inappropriate for physicians to mention hysterectomy as a possible treatment strategy until a complete and thorough diagnosis has been performed. Even then, it is usually one of several options available to women unless the diagnosis is cancer.

Third, don't be afraid to seek a second opinion if you feel a lack of peace about your physician's explanation of the cause of your abnormal bleeding or amenorrhea. God often redirects our health care in creative ways when we place our trust in Him for answers. This is one of the ways God comes to our aid at an unexpected time, in an unexpected way. One moment everything sounds fine. Then suddenly there's a growing discomfort—even a compelling urgency—to delay acting on what we're being told until we gather more facts from a different source.

Last, when we pray before, during, and after all health-care decision-making, it helps us to make the best choices possible. Once we've decided, we can leave it in God's hands, asking our Maker to bless and guide our doctors' endeavors, skills, and thinking processes.

Part II

FAMILY

PLANNING

6

Everything You Ever Wanted to Know About Ovulation

I don't know about you, but I never thought about ovulation until I wanted to have a baby. Beyond the fact that I assumed I ovulated every month, what did it matter really?

Along life's way—I can't remember when exactly—I began noticing that ovulation was, in and of itself, a Big Moment. It marked the midway point in my menstrual cycle. It was a regularly recurring event with its own set of signs and symptoms that were every bit as remarkable (and perplexing) as PMS. It regularly engaged me—physiologically, emotionally, and spiritually—with God's grand design for the perpetuation of human life. Month by month my body reminded me through ovulation of nature's strange blend of magnificent and tragic themes—life, death, bleeding, healing.

To speak of ovulation only scientifically denies its special significance. The human egg is loaded with tremendous potential as it is propelled toward the womb through the fallopian tube.

Whereas men are designed to release hundreds of millions of sperm with each ejaculation, women were created to offer only one egg, usually once per cycle, around the middle of the month. Whereas men are normally fertile twenty-four hours a day, we are only fertile for a few days out of each cycle.

Whereas men send their life-giving seed away from their bodies, we carry ours within our bodies on a wait-and-see basis. Ovulation, after all is said and done, was made to take place behind closed doors.

THE LINK BETWEEN OVULATION AND CONCEPTION: ASK ANY WOMAN

In a healthy woman, the release of an egg from one of her ovaries is the precursor to pregnancy. Obviously, if a woman knows when she ovulates, she also knows when she is fertile.

How she uses this information will depend upon whether she is married (or not), if she wants to become pregnant (or not), and whether she believes that family planning is okay (or not). These are some of life's major issues and are not to be regarded lightly or frivolously.

The remaining chapters in this section of the book will explore these issues in depth. I don't expect that you'll agree with me on everything. (Besides being major issues, they are also some of today's most controversial as well.)

I'm not going to pull any punches with you. Fertility isn't a game or a dogma—it's a God-given gift and an awesome responsibility, one of the greatest responsibilities and gifts God bestows upon us. Ask any woman who has experienced infertility. She'll tell you never to take this gift for granted. Ask any woman who has chosen adoption for the placement of her child. She'll tell you that there is a time and a place to receive this gift. Ask any woman who has six children and wants to have more. She'll tell you that her children are gifts she couldn't refuse. Ask any woman facing an unwanted pregnancy. She'll tell you that fertility is a gift that is sometimes possible to deny because rearing children is such an awesome, day-in-and-day-out, lifelong responsibility.

We are living in a time when we can decide how we will live with this responsibility and how to reach for the gift if it hasn't been given to us naturally. Recent advances in reproductive medicine have brought us here. And, like it or not, our lives are no longer the same.

MAKING YOURSELF MORE COMFORTABLE MID-MONTH

If we can become adept at detecting the signs and symptoms of PMS and menstruation, then we can also learn how to anticipate and understand ovulation—and how to live with our fertility without drugs or devices. Whether a woman is single or married, teenaged or middle-aged, the release of an egg from one of her ovaries involves four things:

1. A seismic shift in reproductive hormones.
2. A noticeable change in vaginal secretions.
3. A measurable rise in resting body temperature.
4. A cervix with a pout instead of a smile.

Before I explain these symptoms any further, I'd like to add that along with these signs—some directly observable, some not—we can have a wide variety of accompanying symptoms, just as with PMS.

Abdominal tenderness, sharp pelvic pain, cramps, mood swings, water retention, temporary weight gain, change in sex drive, complexion changes, food cravings, headaches, fatigue—*all* of these things and more have been reported by women at or around the time of ovulation. So you see, it's probably worth understanding, more than you might have ever thought it was, whether family planning is an issue for you right now or not.

For instance, when my endometriosis first began, ovulation suddenly became quite uncomfortable. I knew that something wasn't right. At first, my doctor suspected a pelvic infection. Later, laparoscopy revealed that a change in fact had taken place inside my body—but it was during ovulation, and not menstruation, that I really distinguished the difference.

Understanding the signs and symptoms of ovulation also can enable us to better cope with the normal changes our bodies undergo every month. We can get more rest, eat nutritiously, exercise regularly and manage stress appropriately. As with the pre-menstrual phase of each cycle, you may discover that you are more sensitive to caffeine around the time of ovulation, that you may need to take naps, that you feel better if you go for a long walk, that a nice warm bath or a heating pad effectively decreases pelvic discomfort.

Once you familiarize yourself with your own ovulatory patterns, refer to the coping strategies listed in chapter 3. Try a variety of relief measures at ovulation as well as during PMS or your period. You might be pleasantly surprised at the results.

WHAT HAPPENS WHEN WE OVULATE?

If you're gotten a little rusty on your facts of menstrual physiology since reading chapter 1, here's a quick review. The main hormones involved in the menstrual cycle and ovulation are FSH (follicle stimulating hormone), LH (luteinizing hormone), estrogen, and progesterone (Figure 36). The pituitary gland secretes FSH and LH; the ovaries secrete estrogen and progesterone. Following menstruation at the beginning of the cycle, FSH stimulates one or more egg follicles in the ovary to develop. As the follicles develop, estrogen production increases.

Hormonal Process of Pre-ovulatory Phase
Figure 36

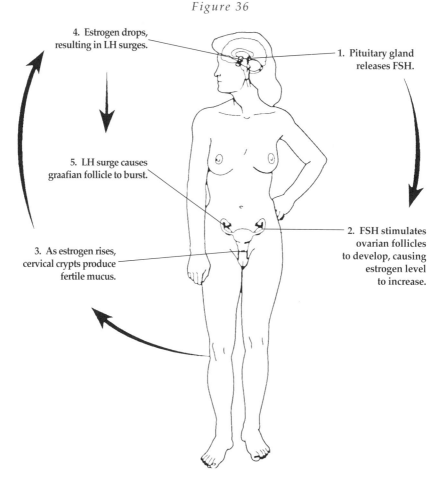

4. Estrogen drops, resulting in LH surges.

1. Pituitary gland releases FSH.

5. LH surge causes graafian follicle to burst.

2. FSH stimulates ovarian follicles to develop, causing estrogen level to increase.

3. As estrogen rises, cervical crypts produce fertile mucus.

Now for a few new amazing facts to add to your rapidly expanding knowledge base. When the estrogen level rises, the cervix is stimulated to produce fertile mucus. The estrogen level reaches a peak about one day prior to ovulation. The estrogen level then drops, causing a surge of LH to enter the bloodstream. The LH surge directly affects the ovarian follicle, causing it to contract and rupture about twenty-four hours following the surge.

When the follicle bursts, an egg is released (Figure 37). This is called *ovulation*. Ovulation commonly takes place between the ninth and eighteenth day after the beginning of menstruation, although it can also occur outside this time frame.

Ovulation

Figure 37

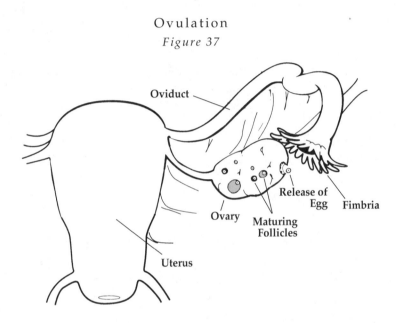

As ovulation takes place, a blood clot forms on the abandoned follicle, and the cells inside the follicle undergo a change. This is called *luteinization*. One of the results of luteinization is the production of progesterone from the follicle, which is now called the *corpus luteum*.

After ovulation, progesterone is the predominant hormone in the cycle until the corpus luteum degenerates. Although there is typically a second rise in estrogen after ovulation, the secretion of progesterone inhibits the secretion of estrogen overall, resulting in the return of infertile cervical mucus. The uterine lining is stimulated to thicken by progesterone and estrogen for the possible implantation of an embryo six to ten days following conception.

After ten to twelve days, the corpus luteum becomes biologically inactive, causing a dramatic decrease in levels of progesterone and estrogen. Progesterone and estrogen are essential to the support of the uterine lining (endometrium). As levels of these hormones fall, the endometrium is shed during menstruation. This drop in estrogen and progesterone levels triggers the pituitary gland to start secreting FSH again, initiating the cycle all over again.

The menstrual cycle varies in length mostly because of differences between women in the length of the *pre-ovulatory phase*—the time between menstruation and ovulation.[1] Following ovulation, the *post-ovulatory phase* tends to be fairly stable, averaging thirteen days in length, plus or minus four days.

KNOW THYSELF

Perhaps you experience no signs or symptoms of ovulation whatsoever, and yet you ovulate right on schedule every month. If ovulation doesn't get your attention by producing discomfort, you still can know when you ovulate by observing other signs—recurring, cyclical changes in your vaginal secretions (cervical mucus), resting body temperature (called the basal body temperature or BBT), and the opening of your cervix. These symptoms are called the *biological correlates of ovulation* and are presented in detail in the next chapter.[2]

In summary, you can use the signs and symptoms of ovulation to help you:

- To know yourself better.
- To know why you experience the things you do and feel the way you do at certain times of the month.
- To know what comfort measures to apply when you experience ovulation-related discomforts.
- To know when something is wrong.
- To know when you're fertile and when you're not.

7

Cycling Naturally in a High-Tech World

Pretend for a moment that you've never heard about birth control. If you're already married, I realize this may be quite challenging, but try it anyway. After all, there once was a time in your life when you didn't have to worry about such fun and perplexing things—remember?

Let's say you're planning to be married in just a few months, so you schedule an appointment with your health-care provider for a premarital exam. During your office visit, you hear about the Pill, Norplant, condoms (in designer colors, no less), diaphragms, foam, cervical caps, contraceptive sponges, and IUDs for the first time. Of these, oral contraceptives, Norplant, and the two leading barrier methods, the condom and the diaphragm, top your physician's "recommended" list for newlyweds.

Which will you use? How do you both feel about the methods your health-care provider has suggested? Were any alternative family planning methods mentioned? How were the risks, benefits, and costs associated with each method described? Did you feel any pressure to use one kind of birth control over another—a combined oral contraceptive rather than a diaphragm, for example?

You leave the office thoughtfully considering your options. When you arrive at home, it suddenly hits you: In order to avoid having a baby after you get married, according to your doctor you must use a drug or device that will completely alter your body's hormone levels or mechanically interfere with lovemaking or cost hundreds of dollars in doctor's and pharmacy fees or increase your risk of stroke, heart disease, and cancer.

Naturally, the next obvious question enters your mind: *Is this what God really has in mind for us if we plan to wait before starting a family?*

None of the methods sounds particularly appealing. You find yourself longing for a *real* alternative to the incredibly wide assortment of "plugs, drugs, jams, and jellies" you've just heard about, wondering if there might be a way to sensibly space your children without altering the act of lovemaking or changing your normal physiology.

THERE IS ANOTHER CHOICE

If you've ever wondered if such an alternative actually exists, there's good news: A natural and effective way to plan your family size and space your children according to God's leading *does* exist—one that doesn't require you to take any drugs, pay exorbitant physician's fees, insert or apply any plastic to your sexual anatomy, or cut into your body.

Sounds too good to be true, right? Yet that's exactly what natural family planning is. It's a way of responding to the God-given design—and reality—of your fertility without drugs, devices, or surgery. What's even better, NFP is as effective as almost all other methods of family planning, including oral contraceptives, when used correctly.[1]

Now just because NFP is "natural" doesn't mean it's "easy." It definitely requires clear, caring communication between spouses and a mutual commitment to the unique dimensions and demands NFP brings to a marriage.

Connie and Loren Navratil say this enhanced level of communication and commitment between them regarding their sexuality has brought the greatest rewards in their practice of natural family planning. They emphasize that NFP isn't only a method of family planning—it's a way of life.

"Through natural family planning, the process of sharing our sexuality and knowing about our fertility was amazing to us," says Connie, the mother of two children ages one and five. "What NFP did was challenge Loren and me at the very center of our souls where we had to question our sexuality, our spirituality, and just about every aspect of our being."

"The path we are walking on is not the path that the world or society takes," adds Loren. "It is the path the Lord has shown us, but we've had to look for it, and I mean *really* look for it. We don't know how we're perceived by other couples. Often we feel that we're like a three-headed monster preaching something totally foreign to most couples in a world that promotes contraceptives and abortion and divorce."

Because most health-care providers have never been trained to teach NFP, it's unusual for them to offer NFP instruction or services to their clients. A possible additional factor in this regard is that NFP doesn't generate income for physicians compared to OCs and other contraceptive technologies. Since NFP doesn't require an office visit, a doctor's prescription, or surgery, the medical system doesn't derive any economic benefit from its use.

"To allow new life to begin is intimate cooperation with God, a sacred trust coupled with personal responsibility," wrote Walter Trobisch. "Here there is no room for superficiality. It is a matter of earnest and exacting precision, for we are dealing with the affirmation of one's own physical body. Beyond this step of self-acceptance lies a renewed reverence for one's own creatureliness, as well as a new love and awareness of the Creator."[2]

QUESTIONS TO CONSIDER

Currently, there are four approaches to teaching natural family planning across the United States. These include the *Ovulation Method* developed by Doctors John and Evelyn Billings (also called "the Billings Method"); the *Creighton Model of the Ovulation Method*, a standardized NFP program created by Dr. Thomas Hilgers that is similar to the Billingses' technique; the *Sympto-Thermal Method*, developed by Dr. Konald Prem and promoted by John and Sheila Kippley through the Couple to Couple League; and the *Fertility Awareness Method*, offered primarily through health education classes and community-based women's health groups (Figure 38).

In selecting which method to use, you may want to consider the following questions:

- Where is this particular method of NFP taught?
- Who teaches this method and what does their training involve?
- How and where are follow-ups and charting evaluations provided? What is the fee for this service?
- Does this method stress a strong denominational viewpoint, and, if so, are we comfortable with this perspective? If this method is not taught from a Christian perspective, what spiritual emphasis is it being taught from?

- Is periodic abstinence from intercourse and/or genital contact an essential component of this method? Are we both comfortable with that? (Not all NFP methods place equal emphasis on avoiding genital contact during a woman's fertile time.)
- Are we both willing to commit ourselves to practicing NFP and seeing what the Lord has to teach us about our sexuality minus contraceptives?

In the sixties, Dr. Evelyn Billings, with her husband Dr. John Billings, performed extensive groundbreaking research in the Ovulation Method of natural family planning. She pointed out that couples in a stable relationship usually find it easier to accept a method that involves some days without intercourse during the month than do couples experiencing marital difficulties.

"The [ovulation] method requires commitment," admitted Dr. Billings honestly. "It appeals most to couples who are motivated to use a natural method and who are willing to take joint responsibility for fertility control. It helps to generate love. In the absence of loving concern, it will not work."

NFP Methods Offered in the U.S.
Figure 38

OVULATION METHOD OF NATURAL FAMILY PLANNING (OM/NFP)—DRS. JOHN AND EVELYN BILLINGS	
Where taught	Through books and at natural family planning centers across the country.
Who teaches	Often taught by women to women due to the intimacy of the subject matter involved; instructors are often RNs in a hospital or doctor's office. OM is also taught by couples, nuns, and physicians in various locations across the country. The beauty of this method is that it is being taught around the world to illiterate women by use of simple cartoons and line drawings. Mucus observation is much simpler than many women think it is!
Key texts	Dr. Evelyn Billings and Ann Westmore, *The Billings Method: Controlling Fertility without Drugs or Devices* (New York: Random House, 1980). Dr. John J. Billings, *Natural Family Planning: The Ovulation Method* (Collegeville, Minn.: The Liturgical Press, 1972).

Effectiveness rates	The *method-effectiveness rate* for the Ovulation Method when used to avoid pregnancy is between 97.1 and 99.5 percent. (0.5 to 2.9 pregnancies per 100 couples using the method according to instructions over a twelve-month period.) OM's *teaching-related effectiveness rate* is 94 and 100 percent. (0 to 6 pregnancies per 100 couples during twelve months of us as effected by instructor error.) The *use-effectiveness rate* is between 75 and 86 percent, as determined by women employing this method for one year. (14 to 25 pregnancies per 100 couples over a twelve-month period.) Obviously, *how a couple uses the Ovulation Method makes all the difference in how effective it is in preventing—or achieving—pregnancy.*
Method	Success of this method depends on understanding instructions, accurate observation, accurate charting, mutual motivation, and loving cooperation. Complete abstinence for one cycle (or one month, whichever is shorter) is necessary until initial chart is reviewed by an instructor. (Billings, *Natural Family Planning*, p. 2)
Method emphasis	Enables all pregnancies to be planned. Based on sound scientific knowledge. Can assist many infertile couples to achieve pregnancy. Natural and therefore completely harmless. Morally acceptable. Does not require regularity of cycles. Does not require pill-taking of any kind. Helps to establish physical and mental harmony in marriage. Able to be used successfully by any woman who wishes to do so. (Billings, ibid., cover.)
Method requirements	Personal knowledge, understanding, and application of the method as taught by the Billingses through their books and associated NFP centers.
Advantages	Freedom from system-wide steroids and the messiness of barrier methods of birth control. Recognition of the reality of fertile times. Learning to live in harmony with one's physical body on a day-to-day basis. Increased appreciation of the various nuances of the menstrual cycle. Enlarged communication between spouses regarding wife's physical and emotional changes throughout the month. Woman-centered. Encouragement of alternatives to intercourse on fertile days.

Disadvantages	Lack of standardized evaluation and follow-up care may contribute to this method's poor use-effectiveness rate (good instruction and ongoing support seem crucial for most couples). A woman-centered approach leaves husband less informed (and consequently less motivated in many cases). Likely to be unsuitable in troubled marital relationships if both partners aren't committed to using this method or if couple is ambivalent about having a baby.

OVULATION METHOD OF NATURAL FAMILY PLANNING CREIGHTON MODEL (OM-C/NFP)—DR. THOMAS W. HILGERS

Where taught	Through a network of service programs developed and operated by the Pope Paul VI Institute for the Study of Human Reproduction located in Omaha, Nebraska.
Who teaches	Certified physicians, practitioners, and instructors who have received extensive on-site training at the Institute.
Key texts	Dr. Thomas W. Hilgers, *The Ovulation Method of Natural Family Planning*. Dr. Thomas W. Hilgers, Ann M. Prebil, K. Diane Daly, and Susan K. Hilgers, *The Picture Dictionary of the Ovulation Method*. (Available from the Pope Paul VI Institute, 6901 Mercy Rd., Omaha, NE 68106.)
Effectiveness rates	The *method-effectiveness rate* for the Creighton Model of NFP when used to avoid pregnancy is 99.6 percent. (0.4 pregnancies per 100 couples using the method according to instructions over a twelve-month period.) The *use-effectiveness rate* is 94.8 percent. (5.2 pregnancies per 100 couples during twelve months of use as effected by teacher/user-related error.) Both the method-effectiveness and use-effectiveness rates to achieve pregnancy are much higher.
Method instructions	1) Faithfully record daily observations. 2) Chart symptoms at the end of every day, recording the most fertile sign of the day. 3) Avoid genital contact during initial instruction in order to make accurate observations of the mucus sign. Couples are also told that they are free to use this method as a means of either achieving or avoiding pregnancy.
Method emphasis	Detailed, standardized analysis of the mucus sign. Openness to the procreation of new life through rejection of a contraceptive mentality toward sex. Shared responsibility between married partners.

Method requirements	Loving cooperation between spouses, enhanced marital communication through the SPICE approach (spiritual, physical, intellectual, creative, and emotional) to lovemaking.
	Observation and charting of the mucus sign.
	Abstinence from intercourse and genital contact during woman's fertile period.
	Follow-up visits with certified NFP instructor or practitioner every six to twelve months after initial learning phase.

Advantages	Medically safe.
	Highly reliable.
	Morally acceptable to all Christians.
	Easy to learn.
	Inexpensive.
	Highly versatile.
	Precisely identifies fertile and infertile days in a woman's ovulatory cycle.
	An invaluable aid for infertile couples desiring to become pregnant. (Hilgers, *The Ovulation Method of NFP*, p. 3.)

Disadvantages	Periodic abstinence required to practice method as taught (unacceptable to some couples).
	Instruction by certified NFP instructor or practitioner necessary (couples can't learn OM-C at home on their own).
	Difficult to use with ambiguous signs of fertility (during weaning from breastfeeding or a vaginal infection, for example).
	Strong denominational emphasis (some may not agree with Roman Catholic interpretation of biblical teaching on marital sexuality, etc.).
	Lack of spontaneity in lovemaking (although some note that genuine self-control in this area can actually deepen intimacy and that the reality of one's fertility shouldn't be separated from intercourse).

SYMPTO-THERMAL METHOD OF NATURAL FAMILY PLANNING (STM/NFP)—JOHN AND SHEILA KIPPLEY

Where taught	Through an extensive organization of local Couple to Couple League chapters around the country. Contact CCL directly for the group or instructor nearest you. CCL also offers a home study course and evaluation of monthly charts by mail.

Who teaches	Married couples, trained through CCL, who have used STM for at least six months themselves.

Key texts	John Kippley, *The Art of Natural Family Planning*, CCL's *Practical Applications Workbook*, *The Effectiveness of Natural Family Planning*, *Birth Control and Christian Discipleship*, *Birth Control and the Marriage Covenant*; Sheila Kippley, *Breastfeeding and Natural Child Spacing*. All are available from CCL, P.O. Box 11084, Cincinnati, Ohio 45211.
Effectiveness rates	Kippley cites many significant studies in *The Art of Natural Family Planning* to substantiate the effectiveness of the STM rather than relying on a single source. These reports show a very high rate of effectiveness—higher than even the Pill. Kippley also is careful to state that each couple's motivation is the determining factor as to how effective the use of STM will be.
Method	The Sympto-Thermal Method utilizes all four signs of fertility—observation of *emphasis* cervical mucus, basal body temperature recordings, ovulation pain, and manual cervical assessments—instead of one. Ecological breastfeeding is also emphasized, providing an important means of natural child spacing to modern American couples that families have used throughout history.
Method requirements	Make love during the post-ovulatory phase of the menstrual cycle only, until familiar with this method. Record accurate observations of fertile symptoms daily. Love one another regardless of whether you are having intercourse or not. Talk together frequently about how it's going. Obtain technical and personal support from CCL as often as needed.
Advantages	Ecological, aesthetic, and inexpensive to use. Highly effective. Promotes ongoing openness to new life. Values personal autonomy. Numerous health benefits. Avoidance of sterilization. Total reversibility. (Kippley, *The Art of Natural Family Planning* , pp. 9-31.)
Disadvantages	Similar to the disadvantages associated with the Ovulation Method.

FERTILITY AWARENESS (FAM)

Where taught	Health education classes, feminist health centers, holistic health programs, Planned Parenthood offices, university-based clinics, churches, and birthing centers.
Who teaches	Health educators, midwives, nurses, physicians, and self-taught instructors.

Key texts	Nona Aguilar, *The New No-Pill, No-Risk Birth Control* (New York: Rawson Associates, 1986). Toni Weschler, *Taking Charge of Your Fertility* (New York: Harper Perennial, 1997). Federation of Feminist Women's Health Centers, *A New View of a Woman's Body* (New York: Simon and Schuster, 1981). Merryl Winstein, *Your Fertility Signals: Using Them to Avoid or Achieve Pregnancy Naturally* (St. Louis: Smooth Stone Press, 1989). Barbara Kass-Annese and Dr. Hal Danzer, *The Fertility Awareness Handbook* (Alameda, CA: Hunter House, 1992).
Effectiveness rates	Reported to be as high as with other NFP methods, though Dr. Hilgers and the Billingses found that genital contact during a woman's peak fertility substantially affects the pregnancy rate.
Method emphasis	A woman's right to control her own body and to better understand her fertility by living with it naturally.
Method requirements	Varies with book, program, and instructor because FAM programs are not standardized. Available for married and unmarried couples alike in most places.
Advantages	Does not stress abstinence during a woman's fertile period, though some couples mention that their "courtship time" each month is what makes NFP uniquely enriching. Widely available.
Disadvantages	Some FAM programs and texts contain viewpoints that conflict with Judeo-Christian perspectives of human sexuality. Because a wide variety of FAM programs are available, it's important to consider the spiritual beliefs of instructors and authors when selecting an NFP method.

NATURAL FAMILY PLANNING BASICS:
AN INTRODUCTORY OVERVIEW

If natural family planning is a new concept for you, here's a quick look at what it involves. For more information, contact a national NFP group for a copy of their catalog, resource lists, and recommended instructors.

The Benefits of NFP

- Freedom from messy and meddlesome contraceptives—and their significant side effects.
- Greater understanding of your menstrual cycle and how ovulation fits into your own unique biological pattern.

- Deepened appreciation for the gift of fertility (and your potential children!), based upon an ongoing openness to the Holy Spirit and God's creative design for your family.
- Mutual cooperation and enhanced communication within marriage regarding lovemaking and sexuality.

How NFP Works

- Ovulation occurs on only one day during each menstrual cycle in most cases.
- A healthy male is always fertile, i.e., twenty-four hours a day, seven days a week, 365 days a year (366 in leap years); whereas a healthy woman is only periodically fertile for a brief time each month.
- A woman's egg dies after twelve to twenty-four hours unless it's fertilized.
- With sufficient cervical mucus, sperm may live as long as three to five days. The cervix contains tiny storage areas, called *cervical crypts*, where the sperm are nourished and continually circulate (Figure 39).

Cervical Crypts
Figure 39

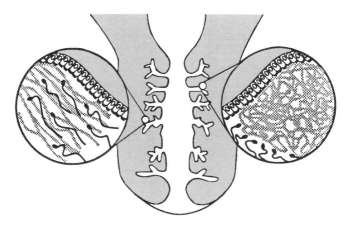

Sperm require fertile cervical mucus to survive long enough to complete their trip. There are three basic patterns of cervical mucus—infertile, fertile, and extremely fertile. The microscopic view of the most fertile mucus reveals a channel-like pattern through which the sperm can "swim" to their final destination—the farthest reaches of a woman's fallopian tubes. Healthy sperm simply *love* eggs and, like wee bits of steel drawn in unison to a very powerful magnet, indefatigably and inexorably make the journey God designed them for.

Pregnancy can result from genital contact without penetration (or, in very rare cases, ejaculation) on fertile days. This very thing happened to one of my friends, further proving the point that sperm are one of the most amazing— and tenacious—cells of the (male) human body.

The primary and most reliable sign that a woman is fertile is the presence of fertile mucus. It is normally distinguishable from *infertile* mucus by its color, texture, smell, and stretchiness. Above all, fertile mucus is usually highly lubricative/slippery; abundant (up to ten times more fertile mucus is produced than infertile mucus); and very, very stretchy—up to an inch or more when placed between the thumb and index finger (Figure 40).

Testing Cervical Mucus
Figure 40

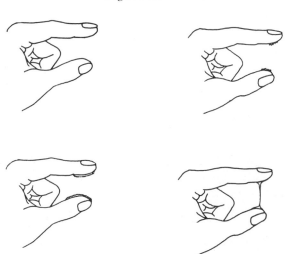

Other possible signs of ovulation include:

- A rise in resting body temperature.
- A sharp pain or dull ache in the abdomen lasting several hours that recurs monthly.
- A slight opening of the cervix.

These signs *are not as reliable* when used alone to plan pregnancy but can help to confirm that you're fertile. The Ovulation Method of NFP relies on the mucus sign to determine days of fertility; the Sympto-Thermal Method of NFP uses all these signs to enable couples to designate fertile days.

Daily observations of a woman's fertile signs can help to determine when she is likely to conceive a baby. These observations can be effectively used to either achieve or avoid pregnancy each month. Many different types of charting methods can be used, although most NFP programs offer their own charts for their clients' use. An example of one charting technique is provided here as an example only and should not be substituted for individualized NFP teaching and follow-up reviews (Figures 41, 42).

Sample NFP 28-Day Chart
Figure 41

DAY	PERIOD	CERVICAL MUCUS	TEMP.	SEXUAL EXPRESSIONS	OTHER
1					
2					
3					
4					
5					
6					
7					
8					
9					
10					
11					
12					
13					
14					

DAY	PERIOD	CERVICAL MUCUS	TEMP.	SEXUAL EXPRESSIONS	OTHER
15					
16					
17					
18					
19					
20					
21					
22					
23					
24					
25					
26					
27					
28					

NFP Charting Terms
(With Symbols)

Figure 42

Cervical mucus and associated events (sexual expressions, menstruation, mid-cycle pain, temperature shifts, spotting, cervical assessments, and PMS) are observed and recorded daily. The following simple symbols may be used:

CERVICAL MUCUS—SENSATION ON FINGERS
OR TOILET TISSUE

A: Absent/dry
D: Damp/not slippery
W: Wet/not slippery

CERVICAL MUCUS—SENSATION ON FINGERS OR TOILET TISSUE

S:	Shiny/not slippery
D+:	Damp/slippery
W+:	Wet/slippery
S+:	Shiny/slippery

CERVICAL MUCUS—STRETCHINESS

1/4:	stretches about one-quarter inch
1/2:	stretches about half an inch
3/4:	stretches about three-quarters inch
1:	stretches one inch or more

CERVICAL MUCUS—COLOR

C:	Clear
K:	Cloudy
Y:	Yellow
W:	White

CERVICAL MUCUS—CHARACTERISTICS

G:	Gummy
TS:	Tacky/Sticky
CP:	Creamy/Pasty

CERVICAL MUCUS—PEAK

PEAK:	The last day of any mucus
1:	*First* full day after PEAK
2:	*Second* full day after PEAK
3:	*Third* full day after PEAK

MID-CYCLE PAIN

M:	*mittelschmerz*

TEMPERATURE SHIFTS

+°	Elevated
−°	Lowered

SEXUAL EXPRESSIONS

I:	Intercourse
P:	Pleasuring

MENSTRUATION

H:	Heavy
M:	Medium
L:	Light
EL:	Extra Light

SPOTTING

B:	Brownish bleeding
R:	Red spotting

CERVIX

CO:	Cervix open
CS:	Cervix shut

PMS

PMS:	PMS present

(NOTE: These symbols are to illustrate charting styles *only*; refer to your NFP texts and/or instructor for more information. Some programs use highly standardized symbols, which are then necessary for accurate chart evaluation within that program. *The information contained in this book about NFP is not intended to replace individual instruction in an NFP method if you wish to achieve or avoid pregnancy.*)

Daily Temperature Chart
Figure 43

Month **March** thru **April**

Date of Cycle	12	13	14	15	16	17	18	19	20	21	22	23	24	25	26	27	28	29	30	31	32	1	2	3	4	5	6	7	8	9	10	11
Date of Month	01	02	03	④	⑤	06	⑦	08	09	10	11	12	13	14	15	⑯	⑰	18	19	20	㉑	㉒	23	㉔	㉕	㉖	㉗	28	29	30	31	32

TEMPERATURE IN TENTHS OF DEGREES

days of higher temperatures

6 days before the rise began

.5 / .4 / .3 / .2 / .1 / 99 / .9 / .8 / .7 / .6 / .5 / .4 / .3 / .2 / .1 / 98 / .9 / .8 / .7 / .6 / .5 / .4 / .3 / .2 / .1 / 97

Types of Thermometers
Figure 44

Basal thermometer

Digital thermometer—unbreakable

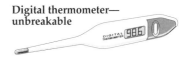

Cervical Changes During the Menstrual Cycle
Figure 45

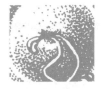 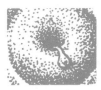 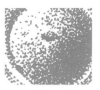

MENSTRUATION	DRY DAYS low, firm, pointed, closed cervix	FERTILE slippery mucus high, soft, open cervix	DRY DAYS low, firm, pointed, closed cervix

Practicing NFP

The following rules apply to *all* NFP methods:

- After beginning to chart signs of fertility, avoid genital contact for one cycle to allow accurate recording of symptoms.
- Record daily observations of fertility signs and symptoms diligently.
- At the end of the first recorded cycle, have your chart reviewed and interpreted by an experienced NFP instructor or practitioner. Repeat these evaluations as needed. (CCL and the Pope Paul VI Institute will review charts by mail if necessary.) With each month, you will become more sure of yourself and more comfortable with the process of NFP.
- Continue observing and charting as you enter this new adventure together—learning to make love without drugs and devices. It's bound to seem scary at first. Practicing NFP, remember, is a way of life—not simply a pill you can swallow once each morning. It takes much more thought and commitment than that to work. (Sad to say, some couples give up on NFP too early, before giving themselves time to grow into it.) Compared to the alternatives, however, NFP seems almost miraculous.
- Realize that ovulation can occur early or be delayed due to stressors such as:

Illness	Travel	Grief
Moving	Final exams	Anxiety
Worry	New job	Weight gain/loss
Overexertion	Holidays	Family stress

Marital problems	Substance abuse	Crash dieting
Sleep disruption	Emotional shock	Work/school

As discussed in the chapters on menstruation and PMS, apply stress management and nutritional strategies to minimize daily strain on your reproductive system. One of the beauties of NFP is that it takes stress into account; NFP programs all address the inevitability of "special situations" and dealing with them.

- With each day, watch your dependence on the Lord grow as you relinquish "control" of this area in exchange for trust.
- Listen to the still, small voice of God in a cooperative, creative Christian approach to determining the size of your family and the spacing of your offspring.

Female Cycle of Fertility/Infertility
Figure 46

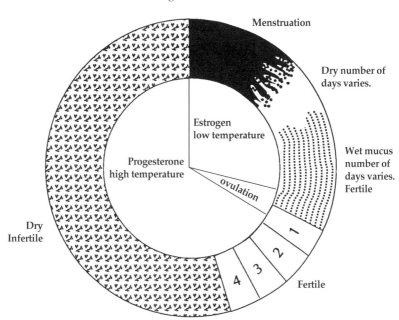

MAINTAIN YOUR SPIRITUAL SUPPORT SYSTEM

Please, never forget that you are living in a society that thinks OCs, Norplant, Depo-Provera, IUDs, surgical sterilization—and even abortion—are "better" than NFP. We need to pray often for a reversal of this eternally significant situation.

When you become discouraged by the daily demands of your fertility and NFP, remember who made you and why. If in doubt about the validity of your reasoning about natural family planning, attend NFP meetings and seminars regularly; subscribe to NFP newsletters; form your own women's or couples' support group so that you may pray for and encourage one another; find an older woman who has used NFP to "mother" you in your pilgrimage while inspiring you with real-life, on-the-road success stories. Most important, ask the Lord for patience and perseverance, depending on His Word and Holy Spirit for help and direction.

"In its broad outlines, nothing could be much simpler to understand than natural family planning," says John Kippley, who cofounded the Couple to Couple League in 1971 with his wife, Sheila. "A woman learns to observe a few simple bodily signs which indicate when she is fertile or infertile, and the couple conducts their sexual conduct according to whether they are trying to achieve or avoid having a baby." (See Figure 46.) Truly amazing, isn't it, when one considers how complicated many have made this process for all these years?

8

$\mathcal{A}$ True Story
About Love, Life, and Fertility

"It is not good to have zeal without knowledge,
nor to be hasty and miss the way."

PROVERBS 19:2

There's been a great deal of interest in some Christian circles lately about an issue close to the hearts of all married couples—birth control and family planning. A variety of different arguments have emerged, challenging our previous notions about the impact of contraception on the wide use of abortion.

One can find plenty of convincing and knowledgeable Christians at both ends of the spectrum regarding family planning—from those advocating a "childless-by-choice" position (to better fulfill their calling and mission) to a "no-birth-control-for-believers" perspective (trusting God to send only the children a couple is intended to have). Both extremes offer convincing support for their positions, from ancient Hebrew texts to the writings of Martin Luther.

Not surprisingly, everyone seems to have an opinion regarding this timely topic. That's good! When it comes to contraception, many of us have been quite content not to rock the boat—or the cradle—since the Pill introduced the concept of "choice" to our generation in the sixties. But many questions about contraception still remain unanswered. Is it possible to find a biblical balance between the two extremes of the family planning pendulum these days?

As you might imagine from what you've read of this book thus far, I'm not inclined to judge any Christian for what he or she may believe about family planning; I don't accept anyone's judgment of my husband and me on this topic either. If you're interested in reading my opinion (and Francis Schaeffer's and Dietrich Bonhoeffer's) on this fascinating subject, you won't want to miss what comes next. And, of course, there's a long story behind all of this.

NEW QUESTIONS

It began ten years ago with the birth of our youngest son, Jon. Jon taught me a valuable lesson about the blessing of "letting God choose" the size of one's family. He also taught me a lot about the reality of living in the kind of world in which women's bodies break down due to repeated childbearing.

Complications during Jon's birth left a significant part of my perineum thin. Two physicians told me that a fifth baby's passage would likely damage the area irreparably. Lovemaking might be unpleasant and uncomfortable for the remainder of my life. A third opinion confirmed that even reconstructive surgery could not guarantee repair of any further debilitating injury. FACT: Some women are stronger than others when it comes to having babies.

Naturally concerned, Dave and I started asking God to direct us concerning the size of our family. We also prayed that my tissue would eventually rebuild and strengthen itself. It was difficult to accept that I would never again experience the joys and challenges of childbearing. After all, I had spent the previous twelve years of my life continuously pregnant or nursing my babies. Now what? Did God want me to risk permanent impairment for the sake of bearing more children?

Suddenly I was forced to ask myself questions I had never considered: What was more important—having additional children or maintaining marital intimacy with my husband over a lifetime? How did my husband feel about it? (He responded—unequivocally—by offering to have a vasectomy.) Should I trust the Lord to heal me or take reasonable measures to enable me to live with the reality of my body? (We prayed. We waited for five years. Nothing changed.)

I thought about my friend Ginny's fourteen pregnancies in seventeen years (including two miscarriages) and wondered what it might be like to have ten more of my own—perhaps by C-section. Or was it all right to accept my physical limitations? In addition to my vaginal weakness, in 1983 I developed a chronic pain condition called fibromyalgia syndrome (FMS) that I could not take medication for during pregnancy. Did God want me to endure extra pain for the sake of enlarging our family—or be thankful for the children He had already blessed us with?

These are just a few of the questions my husband and I wrestled with. We had used ecological breastfeeding, natural family planning, and barrier methods of contraception to space our four children over fourteen years. It was great being able to understand the rhythms and patterns of my body while periodically responding to the Holy Spirit's promptings to participate in the procreation of new life. Now we asked ourselves if we should continue to rely on fertility awareness to prevent further conception or consider a permanent means if it was truly time to stop.

TWO THEOLOGIANS' VIEWS ON FAMILY PLANNING

We searched through the Scriptures—and you know what we found? We discovered that the Bible *does not* condemn family planning, contrary to what some claim. Later we also were comforted by Francis Schaeffer's and Dietrich Bonhoeffer's well-considered, compassionate opinions on the subject. Besides these two isolated references, written at least thirty years apart, we could find no recent reference to family planning from a prolife evangelical theologian.

Interestingly, Dr. Schaeffer believed that women's unique pattern of fertility is a result of the Fall (though some scholars dispute this interpretation). He writes:

> I think there is nothing in Scripture which would in any way lead against the use of contraception. How many children a couple should have should be between them and God. I do feel that for a Christian couple to decide to have no children would be wrong—for this is a part of what God means it to mean to come together [*sic*]. I could well visualize some couples not wanting to cut off the number [of children they will have] by their own choice; and after they had a certain number, to let the Lord set the final number. On the other hand, this too [not using contraception] would be an individual decision before the Lord Himself.[1]
>
> I do not think the Bible is against birth control as such. As I see it, the Bible says that one result of the Fall was increased conception. [Since increased conception is a result of the Fall and therefore abnormal, the use of] birth control in offsetting conception would then be the same as [the use of] medicine [in treating disease, which, of course, is another abnormal consequence of the Fall]. The difficulty is, of course, that in the relativistic world in which we live, birth control is then used not only in

sexual relationships in marriage, but to make easy promiscuous relationships. But this does not make birth control wrong in itself.

Christianity should give us a fullness of life in which the whole person is free before God. The idea that anything that is pleasurable is wrong really misses the point that God made the whole person and God means for the whole person to be fulfilled—not only in heaven but in the present life. Thus the Biblical teaching of morality is to be our standard. We are not to add to it, and anyone who binds us with legalism beyond the Bible is really doing Satan's work and not God's.[2]

Seeing this perspective, Dave and I relaxed a bit as we realized that women's monthly cycles of ovulation and experience of childbirth are actually quite different from all other creatures in God's creation. Considering that most healthy women are fertile about once every four weeks (when not pregnant or breastfeeding) during their reproductive years, human fertility is quite different from other species—strikingly so, as a matter of fact. Also, women aren't normally fertile during menstruation. (Odd, when you think about how easy that is to detect in other species.) Therefore, Schaeffer's argument carries substantial weight.

Closely related to Dr. Schaeffer's argument is a point of view held by Dietrich Bonhoeffer in his excellent, thought-provoking book *Ethics*:

> Marriage involves acknowledgment of the right to life that is to come into being, a right which is not subject to the disposal of the married couple. Unless this right is acknowledged as a matter of principle, marriage ceases to be marriage and becomes a mere liaison. Acknowledgment of this right means making way for the creative power of God which can cause new life to proceed from this marriage according to His will. Destruction of the embryo in the mother's womb is a violation of the right to live which God has bestowed upon this nascent life.[3]
>
> The right of nascent life is violated also in the case of a marriage in which the emergence of new life is consistently prevented, a marriage in which the desire for a child is consistently excluded. Such an attitude is in contradiction to the meaning of marriage itself and to the blessing which God has bestowed upon marriage through the birth of the child. Certainly a distinction is to be drawn between the consistent refusal to allow children to come of a marriage and the concrete responsible control of births.

Human reproduction is the matter of the will to have a child of one's own, and for precisely this reason it would not be right for blind impulse to simply run its course as it pleases and then go on to claim to be particularly pleasing in the eyes of God; responsible reason must also have a share in the decision. There can, in fact, be weighty reasons which in a particular concrete instance will call for a limitation in the number of children.

If precisely during the past hundred years birth control has become such a burning question, and if very wide circles of men of all religious denominations have expressed agreement with the principle of birth control, this is not to be interpreted simply as a falling away from the faith or a lack of trust in God. It is undoubtedly connected with the increasing mastery of nature which has been achieved by technology in all fields of life and with the incontestable triumphs of technical science in the widest sense over the facts of nature, for example, in the reduction of infant mortality. . . .[4]

In this situation it is of the highest importance that men's consciences should not be weighed down and oppressed. Certainly, for the sake of God's commandment, it may be necessary to impose extremely hard requirements. But in the present case the facts are not so clear. Scope must therefore be allowed for the free action of a conscience which renders account to God. In this sphere, more than in any other, a false rigorism of any kind may entail the most disastrous consequences, ranging from pharisaism to a complete turning away from God.[5]

These are strong, balanced words from two of the twentieth century's foremost Christian thinkers. We can learn much from their perspective in the midst of today's heated debates.

MORE QUESTIONS

After a great deal of searching, Dave and I saw that using family planning to deal with the difficulties caused by frequent conception is not immoral, just as using reproductive medicine to relieve other aspects of the Fall on reproduction is not immoral (using anesthesia for unbearable childbirth pain or taking fertility drugs to promote conception or employing surgical treatment of endometriosis to treat infertility). For those who assert that it is God alone who opens and closes the womb, neither family planning nor these medical interventions are acceptable.

John 1:12 and 13 offer scriptural support that seems to have been overlooked. Here the Bible clearly states that Jesus was the only child ever to be uniquely conceived by God. It also states that any other child ever born has been created as a result of natural God-created biological laws—*genetic inheritance, sexual desire, and a husband's will*—working in conjunction with God's will.

This text clarifies what Dietrich Bonhoeffer writes. It is not God alone who causes new life to spring into being. We extraordinarily ordinary human beings play a key role in procreation through our decisions and actions—by either choosing to engage in or abstain from intercourse at particular times of the month or by using contraceptives.

Engaging in intercourse at a fertile time of the month favors conception between fertile people. By consciously choosing to engage in intercourse at times that decidedly favor conception, doesn't this also place people in a position of planning their family? Because our bodies work according to God-created laws, our decisions and actions directly impact the number of children we bear. It is not God alone who chooses the children we have, but God working in conjunction with the natural laws He created—in addition to our decisions and actions.

HOW WE RESPONDED

Like Francis Schaeffer and Dietrich Bonhoeffer, Dave and I are now firmly convinced that the issue of family planning is a matter of faith, stewardship, and personal conviction before the Lord. Making the choice to say, "Send us the children You would have for us," to God and not practicing natural family planning or contraception is a tremendous proclamation of faith. We wholeheartedly commend men and women who are applying their faith to this area of their lives. But we also make the important distinction that family planning is an issue of personal conviction rather than scriptural doctrine.

We also agree with Dr. Schaeffer's and Dr. Bonhoeffer's recommendations that we should be cautious when someone proclaims "as one of God's commands what Scripture is silent about," and we should "thought"-fully and prayerfully reflect on matters of conscience as believers redeemed in Christ.

There is room for disagreement within the body of Christ about family planning, and as individuals we can ask the Holy Spirit to guide our decision-making for the glory of God. Let's be honest about this—repeated childbirth and closely spaced children can damage a woman's health. My body is living proof.

For each family and each couple, the number of children they are capable of bearing and/or caring for will be different. For Dave and me, having four children has been a blessing; we are thankful for our good-sized brood. We are also very much at peace with the size of our family as it is now.

FERTILITY: HANDLE WITH CARE

Preventing new life from entering the world is a serious decision, with eternal consequences that must be weighed along with our physical and emotional ability to adequately love and care for our children. It involves difficult decision-making that reaches right to the center of our marriages, into the heart of our calling and identity as husbands and wives and as Christians.

I am deeply concerned that many followers of Christ use birth control with so little thought and prayer. But I am just as concerned about the growing popularity of the view that all family planning is sin. Perhaps it is the proverbial swinging of the pendulum: What goes too far one way is bound to swing way back to the other side. I believe the time has come for a balance between the two positions.

I continued to have children until I could hear the Lord saying, "Stop." It was a matter of faith and conscience. I rest in the knowledge that I will be held accountable for my decisions before God when I meet Him face to face. I believe that Christ's love will cover any error I might have made, one way or the other.

This is the place we have arrived at after much prayer, study of Scripture, and honest discussion. It hasn't been an easy or comfortable process, but we are now fully convinced in our own minds that this is what the Lord would have for our marriage and family. We are content knowing that God's grace is sufficient for us.

POSTSCRIPT

In 1991 I was asked to participate on a panel at the Christianity Today Institute, in part because I had written several books—*The Mystery of Womanhood, Without Moral Limits,* and *The Woman's Complete Guide to Personal Health Care*—that provoked some discussion among evangelicals about fertility and family planning issues. I would like to share with you several excerpts from articles written by two Institute participants as a result of this meeting.

Raymond C. Van Leeuwen, professor of religion and theology at Calvin College in Grand Rapids, Michigan, wrote:

> The Bible is quite clear on God's basic will for sexual behavior; adultery, for example, is prohibited, and sex is seen to belong within marriage. Does the Bible also forbid birth control, as some Christians argue?
>
> Evangelical home-schooling advocate Mary Pride has stirred up controversy by claiming in books like *The Way Home* that it does. She

notes that God *commands* humans to "be fruitful and multiply, and fill the earth" (Gen. 1:28). She and a handful of other writers have argued that any practice of birth control goes against this biblical "commandment."

There are many things that can be said in response, but only one comment is essential, because it is utterly decisive: *Genesis 1:28 is not a commandment, but a blessing.* Thus it does not refer to what humans must do to please God, but what God does for and through humankind. The text says, "God blessed them, and God said to them, 'Be fruitful and multiply.'" Blessing is something that God does: "I will indeed *bless* you, and I will multiply your descendants" (Gen. 22:17). Fertility is an essential aspect of God's blessing to animals, as we see in Genesis 1:22, and to humans alike; it is his gift to his creatures. . . .

We must beware of confusing matters. God gave this *blessing* to the human race as a whole. He does not direct it to everyone. Some couples are barren, and their earnest prayers for a child are not fulfilled. Others, like the apostle Paul, are called to life without marriage. If Genesis were a blessing (or a command!) to be applied to every individual, then Paul would have been disobedient in his apostolic singleness. Everyone would be obligated to pursue marriage and to order their marriage in a way that would produce many offspring.

This issue has to do with more than how we interpret specific passages in Scripture, however. Many who categorically prohibit birth control seem to have fallen prey to legalism, to imposing on believers burdens never intended in Scripture. . . .

God's sovereignty works in and through human actions and, if necessary, in spite of them. To suggest that birth control is evil or perverse *because* it undermines God's sovereignty is to underestimate God's sovereignty. Of course, human choice ought to be made in the realm of freedom set within the limits of God's law. But where there is no law, our choices are free (Gal. 5). They can neither defeat God's purposes nor subvert or usurp his sovereignty.

Within the limits of faithful marriage, sex is one of the good gifts of God's creation, whether or not it seeks in every instance to be fruitful in a procreative sense. Within the appropriate boundaries God has set for sex, there is much room for responsible Christian freedom, for what God has made is very good indeed.[6]

In addition, George K. Brushaber, a senior editor of *Christianity Today*, offered the following six-point summary of the Institute's daylong discussion:

Birth control and family planning are full of ethical issues and pitfalls. What conclusions should Christians draw?

First, *birth control relates to the much larger issue of family planning.* This is why we need a theology of the family grounded in what the Scriptures teach about marriage, sex, children and parenthood. . . .

Second, *Scripture does not dictate the number of children, but does expect husbands and wives to be good stewards of their fertility.* The Bible assumes that openness to children is part of the marriage commitment of spouses to each other and to God. We should scrutinize any exceptions. . . .

Third, *we can clearly say that Scripture does not categorically prohibit birth control.* It does, however, give us some guidance about the appropriateness of various methods. Some are morally reprehensible (such as those that cause the death of an unborn child). Abortion, of course, is never an acceptable method of birth control. Others (such as those that prevent fertilization and thus block conception) are morally neutral, though subject to certain common-sense considerations. . . .

Fourth, *Scripture gives us guidance on when birth control is inappropriate and immoral.* Birth control should not be used, for example, to justify or facilitate illicit sexual union. Contraceptive practices are wrong when they permit the degradation and devaluation of one spouse by another. Contraceptives are also unacceptable if their use simply makes it more convenient for husband and wife to indulge themselves, pursuing materialistic values at the expense of the spiritual growth in parenthood and obedience to the divine will. . . .

Fifth, *there clearly are situations when some form of birth control will be acceptable—even preferable.* Take a couple whose marriage is seriously threatened and the basic relationship between the spouses is in jeopardy. . . . A couple that has received genetic counseling and finds itself at high risk of bearing children with debilitating diseases, such as Tay-Sachs, may quite responsibly opt not to have children. Additionally, we should not forbid the use of contraceptives when a pregnancy would put the health and well-being of the wife at grave risk, physically or psychologically. Similarly, an ill or weak child perhaps should not be asked to compete with a new sibling for a time.

Finally, *the nature of marital love calls for a regular sexual relationship, a goal for which birth control may be responsibly used.* Paul the apostle urged married believers not to "deprive each other except by mutual consent for a time" (1 Cor. 7:5 NIV). Sexual intimacy can be a regular high point in the ongoing relationship, a tasting of exalted joy that has roots in the receiving and expressing of deep affection. This aspect does not depend on the sex act's procreative dimension to be valid. Our freedom in

Christ will permit us to use that which is not forbidden or immoral, as we seek to be obedient and faithful in service.[7]

Come to me, all you who are weary and burdened, and I will give you rest. Take my yoke upon you and learn from me, for I am gentle and humble in heart, and you will find rest for your souls. For my yoke is easy and my burden is light.

—MATTHEW 11:28-30

9

*L*ife-Affirming Answers to Contraceptive Questions

As I have traveled around the country speaking about women's health care, I have found that the majority of people who participate in my classes and seminars do not clearly comprehend how various birth control methods work to prevent birth. Perhaps this is partly because most of us rely on our health-care providers to tell us everything we need to know about birth control.

When it gets right down to it, a surprisingly high number of people—including many of our health-care providers—don't fully understand or acknowledge the possible range of actions that OCs, IUDs, and progestin-only products (such as skin implants, called Norplant) use to prevent birth. And among those who do understand I've found a certain amount of denial.

Many women have written to me, have called on the phone, or have pulled me aside at conference breaks to tell me what their doctors have said when asked about OCs, in particular. Typically, what I hear is this: After learning about the possible abortive effects of OCs from one of my books, classes, or radio interviews, women ask their doctors if the Pill can, in fact, abort pregnancy once it has begun. The doctors' answers are invariably the same. They tell their clients, "This is merely a theoretical risk given everything we know about how today's oral contraceptives work. OCs primarily act to make the cervical mucus infertile and stop ovulation, so conception is unlikely."

Although this reply sounds good, it avoids giving a complete explanation, as you will see from the text and footnotes below. *As long as a birth control technology acts upon the uterus to render it incapable of nurturing new life, it* can *also act as an abortive drug or device.* And there is no absolute proof to the contrary at this point. Period.

I don't believe ignorance is bliss when it comes to contraceptive technologies. If my health-care provider prescribed something for me with the potential to harm me or my developing baby, I would definitely want to know about it. Wouldn't you?

HOW *DO* TODAY'S BIRTH CONTROL TECHNOLOGIES WORK?

I have gathered some data together for this book for you to consider as you examine today's most popular birth control methods. What I would like you to do as you read the following pages is imagine that you're sitting in a jury box inside one of those large marble and mahogany courtrooms replete with a wise judge dressed in flowing robes. The judge will ask you, a member of the jury, to recommend a verdict based on evidence presented by several expert witnesses.

A complete summary of the most relevant excerpts of the defendants' testimonies is given below. Since you have already heard ample testimony from the defense through wide media coverage of its beliefs and viewpoints, only evidence obtained during the prosecuting attorney's cross-examination of the witnesses is included for the record below.

The Evidence Against the Pill

Prosecuting Attorney: "Is it possible for women using combined oral contraceptives to ovulate? If so, can the egg be fertilized?"

Witness—Official Representative, U.S. Department of Health and Human Services: "... Though rare, it is possible for women using combined pills [estrogen and progestogen or progestin] to ovulate. Then other methods work to prevent pregnancy [i.e., implantation]. Both kinds of pills make the cervical mucus thick and 'inhospitable' to sperm, discouraging any entry to the uterus. In addition, they make it difficult for a fertilized egg [i.e., embryo] to implant by causing changes in fallopian tube contractions and in the uterine lining. These actions explain why the mini-pill works, as it generally does not suppress ovulation."[1]

Prosecuting Attorney: "If a woman's egg should become fertilized while she is taking combined oral contraceptives, what prevents the embryo from implanting in the uterus?"

Witness—Dr. J. Richard Crout, Director of the Food and Drug Administration's Bureau of Drugs: ". . . Fundamentally, these pills take over the menstrual cycle from the normal endocrine [hormonal] mechanisms. And in so doing they inhibit ovulation and change the characteristics of the uterus so that it is not receptive to a fertilized egg."[2]

Second Witness—Dr. Alan Guttmacher, former Director of Planned Parenthood, commenting on the effect of combined OCs on the uterine lining: "The appearance of the endometrium [uterine lining] differs so markedly from a normal premenstrual endometrium that one doubts it could support implantation of a fertilized egg."[3]

Prosecuting Attorney: "Doctor, is there any additional specific evidence you can cite regarding why an embryo cannot survive in the womb if the mother is taking this medication?"

Witness—Dr. Daniel R. Mishell, M.D., University of Southern California School of Medicine: ". . . They [combined OCs] alter the endometrium so that glandular production of glycogen is diminished and less energy is available for the blastocyst [early embryo] to survive in the uterine cavity."[4]

Prosecuting Attorney: "As a representative of a company that manufactures and markets combined oral contraceptives, what is your opinion as to how these drugs prevent an embryo from surviving in the uterus?"

Witness—Spokesperson, Ortho Pharmaceutical Corporation: "The progestogen changes the mucus in the cervix and helps prevent the sperm from reaching the egg. Also the lining of the uterus does not become fully developed so that even if an egg does ripen and is fertilized, there is little likelihood that it would become implanted."[5]

Prosecuting Attorney: "Based on your recent research, is it possible for women taking combined oral contraceptives to ovulate?"

Witness—Dr. Stephen R. Killich, M.D., University Hospital of South Manchester, Manchester, Great Britain: "It is concluded that follicles developing during oral contraceptive cycles have the potential for ovulation, but this is of doubtful clinical significance [i.e., the development of an actual viable, unwanted pregnancy] for the vast majority of women."[6]

Prosecuting Attorney: "How would you define the term 'birth control pill?'"

Witness—Contributor, Random House College Dictionary: "Birth control pill: an oral contraceptive for women that inhibits ovulation, fertilization, or implantation of a fertilized ovum, causing temporary infertility."[7]

Prosecuting Attorney: "Which pills claim to prevent implantation of an early embryo should fertilization occur in spite of an OCs other 'mechanisms of action'"?

Witness—Editor, Physician's Desk Reference '96: "Clearly, every available brand of combined oral contraceptive has the capacity to act against the implantation of an early embryo. If fertilization takes place, the embryo will likely reach the uterus about seven days after conception. But all OCs are designed to prevent the embryo from embedding in the endometrium due to the drugs' hormonal impact on diminishing buildup of the uterine lining."[8]

The Evidence Against Progestin-Only Products

Prosecuting Attorney: "Can the mini-pill be guaranteed to prevent ovulation, and, if not, what other mechanism does it employ to destroy any early embryos which may be conceived as a result?"

Witness—Russ Wilks, Spokesman for Syntex Laboratories, manufacturer of the first mini-pill, upon its release in 1973: "[The progestin-only mini-pill does not] interfere with ovulation. . . . It seems to affect the endometrium so that a fertilized egg cannot be implanted."[9]

Prosecuting Attorney: "Do all progestin-only birth control products act in a similar manner to the mini-pill?"

Witness—Official Representative, Food and Drug Administration: "Progestin-only contraceptives [mini-pills, Norplant, vaginal rings, Depo-Provera] are known to alter the cervical mucus, exert a progestational effect on the endometrium [uterine lining], interfering with implantation and, in some cases, suppress ovulation."[10]

Prosecuting Attorney: "What is the federal government's opinion on how the mini-pill functions to prevent birth?"

Witness—Official Representative, U.S. Department of Health, Education, and Welfare: "[The mini-pill] may prevent an egg's release from a woman's ovaries, makes cervical mucus thicker and changes lining of the uterus, making it harder for a fertilized egg to start growing there."[11]

Prosecuting Attorney: "According to the American Medical Association and the American College of Obstetricians and Gynecologists, how does the mini-pill—which contains only progestogen—act?"

Witness—Spokesperson for the American Medical Association, acting in cooperation with the American College of Obstetricians and Gynecologists: "The mini-pill acts primarily by alerting the cervical mucus rather than by suppressing ovulation, as does the pill."[12]

Prosecuting Attorney: "As one of the authors of a nurse's handbook on drugs, can you tell me how progestogen—a synthetic hormone similar to progestin—works?"

Witness—Author, Nursing '85 Drug Handbook: "Progestogen . . . causes endometrial changes that prevent implantation of the fertilized ovum."[13]

Prosecuting Attorney: "How often is it possible for a woman to ovulate when taking the mini-pill?"

Witness—Authors, Contraceptive Technology, 1988-1989: "Research on mini-pill users has shown that ovulation is prevented in only 15-40 percent of cycles. [The ovulation rate is 60 percent to 85 percent.] The contraceptive effect of mini-pills, therefore, depends substantially on factors other than suppressed ovulation."[14]

Prosecuting Attorney: "In your interview with the director of a clinical trial of Norplant at San Francisco General Hospital, what did he say about how the new progestin skin implants work?"

Witness—Writer, Self magazine: "According to Dr. Philip Darney, M.D., . . . the minute doses of progestin released into the bloodstream are believed to block [a viable] pregnancy in three ways—by preventing the release of an egg in, on average, half of a woman's menstrual cycles, by causing a thickening of the cervical mucus that impedes sperm's ability to reach an egg, and by preventing implantation within the uterine wall of any eggs that are fertilized."[15]

Prosecuting Attorney: "Is the uterine lining not capable of supporting human life after conception takes place if a woman uses a progestogen-only birth control method?"

Witness—Editor, Physician's Desk Reference '96: "No, it is not. For Micronor (Ortho), a progestogen-only OC, the mechanism of action statement in the *PDR '96* reads as follows: 'The primary mechanism of action through which Micronor prevents conception is not known, but progestogen-only contraceptives are known to alter the cervical mucus, exert a progestational effect on the endometrium, and, in some patients, suppress ovulation."[16]

The Evidence Against IUDs

Prosecuting Attorney: "As the manufacturer of the Lippes Loop, what is your company's opinion on how the device functions?"

Witness—Spokesperson, Ortho Pharmaceutical Corporation: "How the IUD prevents pregnancy is not completely understood. Some believe that the presence of the IUD may speed up the normal contractions of the fallopian tubes so that when a fertilized egg [i.e., early embryo] reaches the uterus, the endometrium is not ready to receive it, and the egg is discharged with the next menstrual flow. It is also possible that the IUD simply causes changes in the uterus that prevent a fertilized egg from implanting."[17]

Prosecuting Attorney: "Does the IUD prevent ovulation?"

Witness—Official Representative, Department of Health, Education, and Welfare: "How the IUD prevents pregnancy is not completely understood. Several theories have been suggested. IUDs seem to interfere in some manner with the implantation of the fertilized egg in the uterine cavity. The IUD does not prevent ovulation."[18]

Prosecuting Attorney: "Can you describe several mechanisms by which an IUD may act to destroy the embryo?"

Witness —Authors, Contraceptive Technology, 1988-1989: "Several mechanisms of action of IUDs have been suggested: 1) Local foreign body inflammatory response causing lysis [breakdown] of the blastocyst [early embryo] and sperm, and/or prevention of implantation. 2) Increased local production of prostaglandins that inhibit implantation. 3) Competition of copper with zinc, inhibiting carbonic anhydrase and possibly alkaline phosphatase activity. Copper may also interfere with estrogen uptake and its intercellular effects on the endometrium. 4) Disruption of proliferative-secretory maturation process by progestin-elaborating IUDs, thereby causing endometrial suppression and impairing implantation. 5) Disruption of implanted blastocyst from the endometrium."[19]

Prosecuting Attorney: "As a manufacturer of an IUD device, what is your company's opinion on how it works?"

Witness—Spokesperson, GynoPharma Inc., manufacturer of the ParaGard IUD: "There are many different ideas on how the ParaGard IUD prevents pregnancy after it is placed in the uterus. . . . Some people think that the copper on the IUD changes the environment of the uterus (womb) and tubes; therefore, it may prevent the implantation of a fertilized egg [early embryo]."[20]

Prosecuting Attorney: "When do most scientists believe the effects of the IUD are exerted—before conception or at implantation?"

Witness—Dr. Robert G. Edwards, geneticist and IVF (in vitro fertilization) researcher: "Most scientists would now accept that the effect [of the IUD] in most species, including man, is exerted at implantation."[21]

Prosecuting Attorney: "From what you understand about how the IUD works, would you classify its effects as contraceptive or abortifacient?"

Witness—Dr. Thomas W. Hilgers, M.D., specialist in human fertility, Omaha, Nebraska: ". . . In light of current accepted medical definitions of contraception, abortifacient, pregnancy, conception, and abortion, the conclusion is that the primary action of the IUD must be classified as abortifacient."[22]

Prosecuting Attorney: "As the maker of an IUD device, what is your company's opinion on how it works?"

Witness—Spokesperson, Searle Laboratories, manufacturer of the Cu-7 IUD: "IUDs seem to interfere in some manner with the implantation of the fertilized egg [early embryo] in the lining of the uterus."[23]

Prosecuting Attorney's Concluding Statements

"Your Honor, members of the jury, on the basis of the evidence presented in this courtroom today, it is clear that many of the birth control products women have been using to prevent pregnancy cannot be guaranteed to prevent the conception of human life. Therefore, the defendants are guilty of using confusing language to mislead consumers about the specific actions by which the products they promote work to prevent birth. These three family planning methods—OCs, progestin-only products, and IUDs—cannot be guaranteed to solely act to prevent conception. Clearly, they carry the postconception potential to act against birth by abortive means as well.

"By using evasive terms such as 'fertilized egg' to represent human life in its earliest stages of prenatal development, the manufacturers and prescribers of these products lead their customers and clients to believe these technologies do not induce abortion. However, the evidence in this case reveals that these technologies are capable of inducing abortion by chemical and mechanical means. Consequently, all birth control products' mechanisms of action should henceforth be labeled in precise, easy-to-understand language to allow consumers to make a fully informed choice regarding family planning. The prosecution rests its case."

Rendering a Verdict

Now that you've heard nearly two dozen testimonies from key witnesses supporting the prosecution's indictment of the language used to promote modern birth control technologies, what is your verdict?

Are these methods—combined oral contraceptives, IUDs, mini-pills, Norplant, and other progestin-only technologies—guaranteed to prevent fertilization 100 percent of the time? Given the historical record of evidence, they are not.

If there is even a shadow of a doubt that a given birth control product allows conception to take place and "prevents pregnancy" by denying embryo sanctuary in the womb, neither physicians nor their patients who oppose abortion should endorse, prescribe, or use it.

DEFENDING LIFE AT THE DRUGSTORE LEVEL

To better identify the technologies capable of inducing abortion, I propose we create new words to describe different categories of birth control methods according to what they act against. *The word* contraceptive *is inaccurate if it is used to describe a birth control technology that does more than prevent conception.* The term *contraception* should only be used to describe those methods that are, in fact, designed to prevent fertilization 100 percent of the time.

By using appropriate and "method-specific" terms to describe birth control technologies, we can avoid applying misleading labels to products that do more than act against conception (Figure 47).

Method-Specific Descriptions of
Birth Control Technologies
Figure 47

Contraceptive	If a method acts against fertilization, it should be called a contraceptive (contra-against; ception-conception).
Contranidational	If a method acts against the implantation of an early embryo, i.e., a "fertilized egg," it should be called contranidational (contra-against; nidation-implantation).
Contragestive	If the method acts against pregnancy—defined here as the post-implantation phase of prenatal development—it should be called a contragestive (contra-against; gestive-gestation, or pregnancy).
Contrafetal	If the method acts against the developing human person in the womb, it should be called contrafetal (contra-against; fetal-fetus).

As you can see from the following chart, only a few birth control technologies are designed to oppose only fertilization (Figure 48). Only barrier methods of contraception, vaginal spermicides, and surgical sterilization are designed to prevent fertilization without a backup mechanism to prevent implantation or pregnancy. All other currently available forms of birth control carry the potential to destroy developing human beings after conception by rendering the womb incapable of sustaining nascent life.

The *Physician's Desk Reference '96* clearly explains the way all combination oral contraceptives work to prevent births. In each product's "mechanism of action" description, the same explanation is used. It simply says: "Combination oral contraceptives act by suppression of gonadotropins [e.g., sex hormones]. Although the primary mechanism is inhibition of ovulation, other alterations include changes in the cervical mucus, which increase the difficulty of sperm entry into the uterus and the endometrium [uterine lining], which reduce the likelihood of implantation." (NOTE: This statement has been changed in later *PDR* editions.)

The term *implantation* here refers to the embedding of an early embryo in the womb, because only a fertilized egg can implant in the uterine lining, not an unfertilized ovum. In other words, *since combination oral contraceptives do not stop a woman's ovaries from releasing eggs 100 percent of the time, they are also*

Birth Control Technologies
Figure 48

	CONTRAFETAL	CONTRAGESTIVE	CONTRANIDATIONAL	CONTRACEPTIVE
Acts against:	Fetus	Pregnancy	Implantation	Fertilization
Designed to induce abortion:	Always	Always	Always (if conception occurs)	Never
Availability:	Upon doctor's orders as elective surgery	By prescription or through women's health groups or from midwives herbalists, homeo-pathic doctors	By prescription	By prescription or over the counter or upon physician's orders as elective surgery
Specific techniques:	Vacuum aspiration D&C D&E Saline induction Prostaglandin induction	Epostane (RU486) Anti-HCG vaccine Menstrual extraction Abortifacient plants and herbs	Morning-after pill IUDs Progestin skin implants (Norplant) Progestin-loaded vaginal rings Mini-pills Low-estrogen OCs	*Reversible:* Condom Diaphragm Cervical cap Cervical sponge Spermicidal agents *Irreversible:* Vasectomy Tubal Ligation *Special class** OCs Mini-pills IUDs Norplant Vaginal rings
	ABORTION-INDUCING TECHNOLOGIES			CONCEPTION BLOCKING TECHNOLOGIES

*Note: These products belong to a special class of birth control methods that may act as both contraceptive and contranidational technologies. It is not currently known how often each specific method prevents conception. Research studies clearly indicate that it is not possible at this time to precisely identify fertilization rates in users of these methods.

designed to work to prevent birth in two other important ways: by changing the cervical mucus to discourage the movement of sperm toward an egg that may be traveling through the fallopian tube, and by making the uterine lining (endometrium) incapable of supporting a new life if an egg is fertilized and the early embryo—a developing person in the first week of his or her development—then seeks shelter and sustenance after reaching the inside of the womb.

Normally the uterine lining significantly thickens and develops a rich blood supply by the time a woman ovulates. Oral contraceptives dramatically alter this natural physiological feature by acting to make the endometrium too thin and blood-deprived to be capable of nourishing life. *Thus, the pregnancy will be aborted by chemically-induced means if an egg is fertilized following the failure of an OC's other mechanisms of action* (hormonal suppression of ovulation and interference with sperm mobility). In other words, by the time the early embryo reaches the womb seven to ten days after conception, implantation will be unlikely to occur, and the new life will be unable to survive (Figure 49).

For your information, I've included a list of combination oral contraceptives that contain the "mechanism of action" statement given above, as indicated by brand name and manufacturer (Figure 50) with the applicable page numbers from the *PDR '96* for the combined OCs. Check out the specific details for yourself in the latest *PDR* located in your library's reference section.

If you would like more information, here are a couple of questions you might ask your pharmacist as you start discussing today's birth control products: Is there an oral contraceptive on the market that does *not* change the lin-

The Embryo's Journey
Figure 49

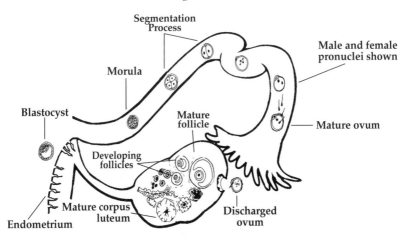

ing of the uterus—or do all available OCs include this as a mechanism of action? What birth control products would you recommend that act to prevent conception by completely stopping ovulation or without altering the uterine lining?

In addition, the uterine lining is not capable of supporting human life after conception takes place if a woman uses a progestogen-only birth control method, due to hormonally caused irregularities in the endometrium. Any woman using a progestogen-only birth control product should be clearly informed that ovulation has been shown to take place as much as 80 percent of the time in women using this method, potentially increasing the likelihood that the product's abortive backup mechanisms will prevent birth from taking place.

Pharmaceutical Products with Abortion-Inducing Potential
Figure 50

COMBINED OCS

TRI-LEVELEN (Berlex), p. 652

OVCON (Bristol-Meyers Squibb), p. 760

DESOGEN (Organon), p. 1817

MODLICON (Ortho), p. 1872

ORTHO-CEPT (Ortho), p. 1851

ORTHO-CYCLEN (Ortho), p. 1858

ORTHO TRI-CYCLEN (Ortho), p. 1858

ORTHO-NOVUM 1/35 (Ortho), p. 1872

ORTHO-NOVUM 1/50 (Ortho), p. 1872

ORTHO-NOVUM 10/11 (Ortho), p. 1872

ORTHO-NOVUM 7/7/7 (Ortho), p. 1872

BREVICON (Roche), p. 2134

NORINYL 1+35 (Roche), p. 2134

NORINYL 1+50 (Roche), p. 2134

TRI-NORINYL (Roche), p. 2164

NOR-QD (Roche), p. 2135

LO/OVRAL (Wyeth-Ayerst), p. 274

LO/OVRAL 28 (Wyeth-Ayerst), p. 2751

NORDETTE 21 (Wyeth-Ayerst), p. 2755

NORDETTE 28 (Wyeth-Ayerst), p. 2758

TRIPHASIL-21 (Wyeth-Ayerst), p. 2814

TRIPHASIL-28 (Wyeth-Ayerst), p. 2819

PROGESTIN-ONLY PRODUCTS

NORPLANT skin implant system (Population Council)

DEPO-PROVERA contraceptive injection (Upjohn)

IUDs

PARAGARD T 380A (Ortho) copper intrauterine contraceptive

HCG ANTAGONISTS (CONTRAGESTIVES)

(These drugs induce abortion by acting against the hormone secreted by the embryo that sustains pregnancy—human chorinic gonadotropin, or HCG. Availability in the U.S. is currently limited to experimental use; none are listed in the *PDR*.)

ANTI-HCG VACCINE

EPOSTANE

MIFEPRISTONE (RU486)

ABORTION-INDUCING PROSTAGLANDINS (CONTRAGESTIVES)

(These drugs induce abortion by stimulating uterine contractions.)

CYTOTEC (Searle)
PROSTIN E-2 Vaginal Suppository (Pharmacia & Upjohn)

HOW WILL WE RESPOND?

With the use of some methods—oral contraceptives, progestin skin implants (Norplant), for example—abortion is always a possibility.[24] With other technologies—such as RU486, anti-HCG vaccine, and prostaglandins—the method itself is specifically designed to induce abortion as its primary goal.

Recent publicity generated by RU486 alerted health-care consumers to the reality and availability of abortion-inducing drugs abroad. Now that we have identified other drugs and devices capable of inducing abortion, how will we respond?

Surviving Infertility Treatment Without Sacrificing Your Dignity

A proverb of Solomon portrays the yearning to bear a child as an unquenchable desire, comparing the barren womb to drought-stricken earth and raging fire (Proverbs 30:16). But until this century, folk remedies were the only possible solution medicine could offer.

More than two million American couples—about 7.1 percent of married couples—who want to have a baby are currently unable to conceive a child. They purchase a costly array of infertility treatments and services, including diagnostic tests and drug therapy, surrogacy arrangements, *artificial insemination* (AI), and newer *assisted reproductive technologies* (ARTs) such as *in vitro fertilization* and *embryo transfer* (IVF/ET), *gamete intrafallopian transfer* (GIFT), and *surrogate embryo transfer* (SET).

In the months following an infertility diagnosis, visits to physicians and clinics become a regular part of one's monthly schedule, turning testing, treatment, and the timing of intercourse into a way of life (Figure 51). Entering this unexplored territory can be disorienting and disheartening, with no clearly marked road maps to follow.

Since the diagnosis of infertility doesn't necessarily mean the inability to ever have children but rather difficulty in conceiving, the path leading to pregnancy can quickly become expensive and emotionally exhausting. Compounding this situation is the fact that medical and social choices facing infertile couples have escalated dramatically in recent years. Available options have created new problems as well as new opportunities. Most importantly, couples face the difficulty of deciding when to stop trying every new treatment and whether to pursue high-tech or third-party solutions to achieving one's primary goal: parenthood.

INFERTILITY TESTS AND TREATMENTS

Couple's history and physical exam: A complete health history may be the single most important diagnostic tool a physician can employ. It should include information on the couple's education, employment, personality, stimulant and substance use, medications and treatments, nutrition and diet, exercise, immunizations, surgical history, family health history, psychological history, and sexual history. The physical exam seeks possible physiological and anatomical causes of infertility.

Semen analysis: Basic characteristics of sperm and seminal fluid are examined, including the quantity and activity of the sperm.

Resting body temperature and other menstrual cycle mapping: Since the resting, or basal body temperature, changes during the menstrual cycle, charting these changes may help to pinpoint ovulation. The woman performs this procedure herself, so the cost involves only the price of the thermometer.

Cervical mucus evaluation: Another method of ovulation prediction relies upon examination of cervical mucus. Microscopic analysis of these secretions reveals hormone-related changes in the mucus.

Measurements of hormone levels: A patient's blood and urine are tested for levels of hormones related to ovulation.

Post-coital test: One to two days before ovulation, the couple has intercourse two to four hours before arriving at their physician's office; one to three samples of the deposited discharge is then taken from different areas along the length of the cervical canal and analyzed.

Infection screening: Tests for sexually transmitted diseases are included to determine whether reproductive loss may be associated with infection.

Sperm antibody test: Antibodies to sperm may be present in a woman's vaginal secretions; this test examines the sperm-mucus interaction.

Ultrasonography: High-frequency sound waves are used to obtain detailed outlines of the reproductive system, especially changes in the ovaries related to ovulation.

Endometrial biopsy: A hollow tube is passed through the cervix for removing a small amount of the uterine lining for microscopic examination. This is used to date the menstrual cycle.

Hysterosalpingogram: Radio-opaque dyes are slowly injected into the uterus while X-rays are taken to determine the condition of the fallopian tubes.

Laparoscopy: Direct visualization of the female reproductive tract through a long, narrow, illuminated instrument. Minor surgery can also be done during this procedure.

Hysteroscopy: Direct visualization of the interior of the uterus through a long, narrow, illuminated instrument inserted through the cervix; also allows minor surgery to be conducted.

Hamster-egg penetration assay: The husband's sperm are incubated with hamster eggs and watched for signs of fertilization.

Vaginal and/or cervical insemination: Semen is injected into the vagina or at the opening of the womb and left to swim up to the fallopian tubes.

Intrauterine insemination: Semen is placed directly into the uterus to bypass the vagina and cervix when vaginal abnormalities, cervical mucus deficiencies, and sperm motility problems exist.

Superovulation: Fertility drugs are given to induce multiple ovulation prior to insemination or egg retrieval (for use in IVF or GIFT). An Atlanta couple's actual drug costs between September 1989 and August 1990 were:

Lupron injection	$282
Pergonal shots	$914
Progesterone shots	$275
HCG shots	$230
FSH shots	$552
Approximate lab monitoring costs	$3,415
Total	**$5,668**

Source: *Atlanta Journal-Constitution*, 10/27/91

THREE COUPLES' EXPERIENCES

Few Christian couples remain childless by choice. The Bible and traditional church teaching celebrate children as a gift of God, a heritage to be openly embraced by all believers. Most couples marry with the expectation that a child will come into their lives as a result of their sexual union. When the time seems right to start a family, they discontinue using contraceptives, duly noting the time of the next expected menstrual period on the calendar.

Because couples now have the ability to prevent the births they do not want, most assume they will conceive quickly and easily once they start "trying" to have a baby. Susan and Rod were typical newlyweds in this regard.[1]

"We had decided to wait about two years before starting our family," says Susan. "About eighteen months after we were married, I went off the Pill so my system could get cleaned out before I became pregnant."

"We were busy the next few years with church activities, several moves, and numerous other things, so we were pleasantly surprised when I found out I was pregnant," she continues. "Our joy quickly turned to sadness when I miscarried at seven weeks. Some people told me I'd be pregnant again in no time (one of those thoughtless things people say at difficult times)."

But Susan didn't get pregnant again right away. "Not long afterwards, I began thinking that maybe there was something wrong, that maybe there was a reason I wasn't getting pregnant as easily as my friends were," she remembers. "I managed to keep pushing these thoughts aside. My worries became a reality when our new pastor and his wife spoke of their years of pain in struggling with infertility. They voiced my own experience exactly—but *infertility* was such a scary sounding word."

Fortunately, Susan's story ended happily: She conceived a child six months after starting on Clomid, an infertility drug that induces ovulation. Benjamin was born in March 1989, nearly eight years after Rod and Susan were married. Medical treatment, while costly and time-consuming, proved to be an effective remedy in their situation.

Tom and Susie share a different story about their search for parenthood.[2] After six years of marriage and fifteen months without using contraceptives, medical tests revealed that Tom would never be able to produce sperm.

"We were totally in shock," Susie explains. "We could not imagine why that would have happened to us. It was devastating to Tom."

Yet the Lord provided Susie the grace to accept the difficult diagnosis of her husband's involuntary sterility. "I truly thank God for providing me with an incredible amount of understanding," she says, "because *it didn't matter to me*. I had loved Tom for who he was, not because I thought he had sperm! I wanted to be understanding and didn't want him to blame himself."

In today's world of high-tech infertility treatment, however, Tom's diagnosis did not preclude a possible pregnancy for Susie. Her physician could have performed artificial insemination using sperm from an anonymous "father" that would have enabled her to conceive and carry a baby of her own. A relatively inexpensive and easy to perform procedure, this technique is now used by an estimated 30,000 couples each year in the United States.

After the diagnosis, Susie and Tom found themselves facing questions about whether or not they planned to use artificial insemination by donor (AID). "Many of our friends wondered why we didn't try other methods of having children. Some suggested donor insemination, but we just didn't feel that was a natural way to have children," she points out. "It's not in keeping with God's design for procreation. I know a lot of people who have considered it, but we knew this wasn't the way God wanted us to have our family."

Tom and Susie knew when to say "STOP" to medical treatment. The ready availability of AID was not reason enough for them to use it. Instead, they decided to enter the next phase of their life and thus chose adoption. They are now the parents of two young children named Catherine and Clark.

Debbie and Kevin decided to continue pursuing the medical route to pregnancy even after they had spent over $35,000 and ninety-two grueling months in treatment. "To not go through this," asserts Debbie, "would make me feel like it was my fault, because I wasn't willing to try. No one, not even I, can look at me today and say, 'If you really wanted a biological child you could have one.'"[3]

Debbie offers the following description of the initial phase of her infertility treatment:

> I [took] my basal body temperature approximately 1,260 times for forty-five consecutive months. . . . And that is the easy part. During the diagnostic phase, I had three endometrial biopsies—which consists of taking tissue from the inside of the uterus to determine hormone levels—and two postcoital tests—removal of the cervical mucus [following intercourse] to analyze sperm activity. . . . I have also had two diagnostic laparoscopies—the navel surgery done with general anesthesia to look at the ovaries, tubes, and uterus. The second of these surgeries included a hysteroscopy—examination of the inside of the uterus—and a D&C. . . . All of that comprised the diagnostic workup. My diagnosis was unexplained infertility.[4]

Debbie has also endured three miscarriages, six months of artificial insemination, one year of hormonal treatment, several additional surgeries, in vitro fertilization, and many weeks of daily drug injections to stimulate ovulation. When last interviewed, she and her husband Kevin were attempting to achieve another pregnancy via sperm washing.

"As you can see, this type of care requires a great deal of time off work, not to mention money," Debbie explains. "My husband is a D.C. Police Detective, and his federal insurance does not cover infertility. Luckily, I was able to extend my Maryland insurance on an individual basis, but not everything is covered. Most insurance companies don't cover these procedures.

"Considering the present state of medical technology and research in infertility, I will probably never have a biological child," she concludes. "I won't be able to produce a child who will have my husband's smile and his wonderful eyes. And that thought is devastating to me and my family."[5]

BEFORE BEGINNING TREATMENT

Each year infertile couples spend ever-increasing amounts of time, money, and energy on medical treatment and infertility services.[6] Perhaps you've already discovered that the possibilities appear to be almost endless—and how difficult it is to decide what treatments to use and when to use them.

The appeal of new reproductive technologies to infertile couples is understandably irresistible. But in light of the high costs and low success rates associated with many ARTs, it's doubtful couples completely understand what's involved before electing to embark on their procreative journey.

There are five basic questions to consider *before* entering today's complex maze of infertility diagnosis and treatment. Whether you are just thinking about scheduling an appointment with a physician or are currently in the care of a reproductive health specialist, prayerfully discussing your replies to these questions may enable you to avoid getting lost along the way.

1. Is prolonged medical treatment worth the pain, expense, and disruption to our lives?
2. Might adoption or remaining childless be what the Lord would have for our lives right now?
3. Would treatment be so expensive that our financial stewardship might be jeopardized?
4. Are there any reproductive technologies I should avoid, and why?
5. If it isn't time to stop treatment now, when would it be?

Joni Eareckson Tada and her husband, Ken, decided to put a time limit on their pursuit of pregnancy to avoid years of tests and treatment. "I did want a child very desperately," Joni said in an interview for *Today's Christian Woman*. "We went through all the tests couples go through, and it was very frustrating and demeaning. But we said we would only try to have a child until I reached forty."[7]

Joni's birthday signaled the end point of her struggle. "I turned forty in October, and basically we have decided we will not have children," she stated. "It was very difficult for me early in our marriage, but God has helped me deal with it and has taken away the desire."

Given all of the options now available, waiting on the Lord for answers runs counter to the current trend to plunge ahead with a we'll-try-anything approach to infertility. Either way, there are no guarantees. And no matter what the outcome, it's clear that Christian couples facing infertility benefit from ongoing emotional and prayer support while considering how to cope with this difficult diagnosis.

Current Questions and Concerns

Surprisingly, many infertility treatment techniques portrayed as no longer experimental have yet to be successful in many mammals, including primates. Not until 1988 did the federal government take the first step to determine the long-term safety of laboratory conception.

Besides serious risks linked to the high rate of multiple pregnancies associated with IVF (increased incidence of premature birth, low-birth-weight babies, and a higher cesarean section rate), researchers and consumer groups cite concerns about cancer, birth defects, and other long-term health questions related to ARTs.

"I have become very concerned that the fertility drugs of the 1980s and 1990s will become the next DES story," Lucinda Finley, an expert on reproductive health law at the State University of New York, explained in an interview with the *Atlanta Journal-Constitution*. "DES . . . was supposedly going to help reduce miscarriages and make babies bigger and healthier.

"Now it is the drugs that help people get pregnant that are being greeted with such enthusiasm," says Finley. "Women are being pumped up about these [drugs] without really knowing the long-term effects. I get very sobered by how little the pharmaceutical industry learns from each of its disasters."

Notably, widespread application of most ART procedures take place without governmental regulation in regard to safety and effectiveness. There are no licensing requirements for practitioners and no federal or state guidelines for training, and there is no regulation of embryo laboratories or uniform reporting of treatments and outcomes. Yet anyone who donates blood or submits a urine sample to any licensed medical facility is protected by these standard safeguards. To attract business, it's not uncommon for clinics to minimize the risks of the procedure to potential clients, quote success rates from other programs, or give confusing statistics that don't tell how many live births have resulted from their services.

"Reproductive technologies are not all that good," says Dr. Ed Payne, M.D., professor of family medicine at Augusta Medical College and the author of *Biblical Medical Ethics*: "The current average for IVF is that one in eight procedures results in a live birth, or 12 percent. So if a couple is spending $5,000 to $8,000 or more per procedure, they're going to pay an average of $40,000 to $60,000 to continue through until they may get a baby." (GIFT is even more costly—over $14,000 per attempt.)

"They are expensive procedures apart from the moral problems," he points out, adding that it's also "very common for women who undergo fertilization procedures to become pregnant [without technical intervention] in the process."

In a follow-up study of 1,145 infertile couples reported by the *New England Journal of Medicine*, 41 percent of the treated couples conceived—but so did 35 percent of the *untreated* couples. Researchers concluded that the spontaneous cure rate of infertility is high. Stating that pregnancy occurs frequently in couples diagnosed as infertile but who have received no treatment or have stopped all treatment, they found that for many infertile couples, the potential for conception without treatment is at least as high as with treatment.

ART programs currently operating in the United States generate approximately $2 billion in business per year at an estimated 300 clinics. *Forbes* magazine claims IVF programs represent a lucrative market, largely due to the rise in pelvic inflammatory disease and age-related infertility.

"IVF is essentially the end of the road," says Dr. Linda Giudice, Associate Professor of Gynecology and Obstetrics at Stanford University in Palo Alto, California. "It becomes apparent that if this is not going to work, there aren't too many options left."

Where insurance coverage for infertility treatment is mandated by state government and the high cost of IVF is no longer a barrier, ART clinics and programs are more popular and plentiful than in states that do not require third-party reimbursement.

"Some new IVF clinics seem more interested in selling stock than in actually serving customers," concludes *Forbes*. "Such facilities are mushrooming throughout the country—all targeted at the growing number of infertile couples' quest for conception."

"These clinics, although operating as businesses, may be better described as ongoing privately funded research projects, with no overseeing regulatory body," says Carol Peters, president of the deMiranda Institute for Infertility and Modern Parenting. "The medical community, which enjoys a special status in society, is not regulating itself."

Thinking It Through

For couples waging an emotional battle on the front lines of infertility, ethical questions associated with ARTs pale in comparison to the promise each new possibility offers—the chance of taking home a baby born or biologically produced from one's own body. The overwhelming desire to bear a child can affect the way couples deal with the theological questions.

"I guess there's a contradiction with using technology to conceive a child, but I believe it's God-given technology," says former infertility patient Suzie Chapin. "However, there's always the question, 'Is this His will?' I figured, if it wasn't, then I wouldn't have been able to do it."

Former barriers to pregnancy—sterility, age, virginity, menopause, family status, infertility, and sexual preference—no longer limit a woman's ability to attempt conception. Given the menu of ARTs now available (Figure 51), couples can choose to proceed cautiously, running counter to the trend of plunging ahead with a we'll-try-anything approach.

The ART Menu
Figure 51

ART (assisted reproductive technology): Any treatment, technique, or procedure that involves the manipulation of human eggs and sperm for the purpose of establishing a pregnancy.

Embryo freezing: A technique for preserving developing human beings through freezing, or cryopreservation, to allow embryos to be placed in storage until they are thawed at a later date for the purpose of transfer to a woman's womb. If the woman and man who donated their gametes (eggs and sperm) for laboratory fertilization decide they do not want to use or donate the embryo(s) to another couple, the embryos are either destroyed or used for ART experimentation, by the couple's prearranged consent (given in writing before IVF is performed).

GIFT (gamete intrafallopian transfer): The placement of sperm and oocytes into an unblocked fallopian tube through a laparoscope for fertilization inside the body. As a result, this ART does not involve any laboratory handling of human embryos.

IVF (in vitro fertilization): Conception occurring in laboratory apparatus; name literally means "in glass" fertilization.

SART (surrogate embryo transfer): The transfer of an embryo from an IVF laboratory or from the womb of a fertile donor to the uterus of an infertile recipient who will attempt to carry the embryo to term.

ZIFT (zygote intrafallopian transfer): A technique in which eggs are collected from a woman's ovary and fertilized in the laboratory via IVF; the fertilized egg (zygote) is then placed inside a woman's fallopian tubes through a small abdominal incision.

Complicating this scenario is the fact that choices facing infertile couples have escalated dramatically in the last ten years. Couples now face the difficulty of deciding when to stop trying the next available treatment.

"I would stress that before a couple gets involved in these procedures, they talk to their pastor or someone knowledgeable to get a biblical perspective and understand what the moral issues are before they go blindly into it," Dr. Payne says. "They should understand the pitfalls that the physicians involved in the procedure may or may not point out."

Given the enormous emotional and financial investment involved, infertile couples need to carefully think through their options when they are offered treatment. With fertility clinics proliferating across the country, a realistic understanding of current options can help couples make wise decisions about which direction to take.

Ethical Issues

Reproductive technologies are evolving faster than our ability to form a consensus on limits; new ARTs are developed, researched, and implemented before social scrutiny guides or restricts a technique's application. Without moral or legal limits to use as a compass, new directions in infertility treatment are negotiated by consumers—couples who are often willing to try anything as a possible route to pregnancy. Ethical guidelines, where they do exist, are selected and voted upon by the same health-care providers who perform the ART procedures.

"While we don't have mandates, our position is that we offer *guidance* to our members," explains Joyce Zeitz, public relations coordinator for the American Fertility Society (AFS) in Birmingham, Alabama. "We came out with our first ethics report back in 1986. We now have two ethics committees working independently. Our newest report, 1994, covers such areas as the use of donated eggs for menopausal women and preimplantation genetic diagnosis." Concerning these techniques and other artificial conception methods such as embryo splitting, Zeitz says the AFS's official position is that "research should continue in these areas."

In Europe legislative bodies are considering or have already implemented a wide range of restrictions. French officials recently proposed prohibiting IVF in postmenopausal women; Italy has announced plans to limit artificial conception; and commercial surrogacy has been outlawed in Great Britain. In West Germany, where memories of the Nazi experiments still trouble a new generation of scientists, embryo experimentation and fertilization by donors has been banned.

Until recently in the United States, federal funding for embryo research was withdrawn under the Reagan and Bush administrations. As testing was conducted with government monies elsewhere—primarily in Great Britain and France—studies remained privately funded here. In January 1993, on the twentieth anniversary of the Supreme Court's *Roe v. Wade* decision, President Clinton lifted the previous restrictions.

With current widely-used prenatal diagnostic techniques such as chorionic villus sampling and amniocentesis, parents wait ten to fifteen weeks until discovering whether their baby has a genetic disability, with second-trimester abortion offered as a solution. Embryo diagnosis offers an attractive alternative. After a woman's egg is fertilized in a Petri dish and develops to the eight-cell stage three days later, one cell is removed for DNA testing. If a defective gene is found, the embryo is discarded rather than transferred to the mother's womb. The test adds about $2,000 per IVF cycle. At least 200 genetically linked traits, including gender, have already been identified for possible diagnosis using this technique.

"You have to accept that you're doing an abortion when you use IVF, if you believe that life begins at conception. But I don't believe life begins at conception," says Dr. Geoffrey Sher, a founder of the Pacific Fertility Medical Center in San Francisco. "We're doing all these things already by amniocentesis, etc. It's nothing new—it's just better and earlier."

New Possibilities, New Problems

Robert G. Edwards, a British geneticist, first achieved IVF in his Cambridge laboratory in 1968. Using eggs obtained from surgically removed ovaries, he and another researcher used their own sperm to inseminate ova in hopes that an embryo would develop. Edwards spent the next nine years experimenting with human embryos, including testing them for growth in the reproductive tracts of rabbits.

According to Edwards, the aim of IVF was not solely to treat infertility but to conduct genetic research. In his book, *A Matter of Life*, Edwards explains, "It had occurred to me that, once the problem of *in vitro* fertilization was solved, the sex of embryos could be identified at a very early stage by examination of their chromosomes, and that it would be possible therefore to choose whether the mother gave birth to a girl or a boy . . . certain diseases could perhaps be reduced."

Not everyone agrees with Edwards that such powerful knowledge is necessary or desirable. "I worry about the possibility of making a child into a product we consume, about whether we are turning ourselves into products to be manipulated at our own whim," says Dr. Paul Lewis, Ph.D., Assistant Professor of Religion at St. Olaf College in Northfield, Minnesota. "We can select for certain traits or not, and the possibility of making a child exactly in our image—whatever hair color, eye color, and IQ we want. It seems to me that we're in many ways a consumer society where everything becomes a product that has to be hawked and sold to the consumer market."

In the most comprehensive moral analysis of ARTs to date, the Vatican's "Instruction on Respect for Human Life and the Dignity of Procreation" condemns all types of prenatal genetic screening for the purpose of aborting genetically disabled embryos and fetuses. Released in 1987, the statement declares that research using human embryos "constitutes a crime against their dignity as human beings" and questions the morality of IVF as a practice that "has required innumerable fertilizations and destruction of human embryos."

"The human being must be respected—as a person—from the very first instant of his existence," it affirms. "A diagnosis which shows the existence of a malformation or a hereditary illness must not be the equivalent of a death sentence."

THINKING THROUGH THE ISSUES: IVF AND AID

Is in vitro fertilization (IVF) a morally acceptable choice for Christians? And what about artificial insemination by donor (AID)? Both technologies offer possible answers to infertile couples confronting specific reproductive disabilities, such as male sterility or blocked fallopian tubes. If a couple coping with this kind of diagnosis can't have children without using one of these techniques, why would it be wrong?

While these techniques seem superficially appealing, it's essential to take a closer look at both before answering this question. The appeal of new reproductive technologies to infertile couples is understandable, but do most people fully understand the ethical concerns associated with these procedures?

Unfortunately, this issue is amazingly similar to what's happened regarding postconception birth control methods. The medical establishment has done a remarkably successful sales job promoting new experimental treatments through confusing and unclear language. I'd like to see signs out in front of every infertility clinic with a warning printed in bright, bold letters: PROCEED WITH CAUTION.

Before trying either IVF or AID, try to think with your head as well as follow your heart. Your intense desire to have a baby is powerful and understandably real, but it may make you especially vulnerable to medical exploitation. If you are a Christian who values the sanctity of human life, there are a number of serious concerns to think through regarding IVF and AID before choosing either of these options.

A summary of ethical concerns about specific reproductive technologies follows for your prayerful consideration. I encourage you to utilize the endnotes section also to do your own research.

Points to Consider: In Vitro Fertilization (IVF)

IVF is not possible without extensive embryo research.[8] In fact, the first successful laboratory conception took place at Cambridge University in England when Robert G. Edwards, a geneticist, and a colleague used their own sperm to create embryos from eggs taken from a woman's surgically removed ovaries. Edwards spent the next nine years experimenting with human embryos, including testing them for growth in the reproductive tracts of rabbits.

Dr. Georgeanna Jones, the reproductive endocrinologist at Eastern Virginia Medical School, which was responsible for the first "test-tube" baby's birth in the United States, admits that *Roe v. Wade* was a "fortuitous" decision that allowed IVF research to proceed. Life in the lab is clearly expendable. How else do IVF technicians learn this procedure than to experiment on the offspring of infertile couples?

IVF is a highly profitable technique that commercializes human reproduction.[9] One in every three IVF clinics in the United States is owned by venture capital investors and operated on a for-profit basis. In states where IVF is paid for by health insurance companies due to legislative mandate, IVF clinics are more plentiful. About one-quarter of all IVF clinics have never had a live birth, and the overall failure rate for the procedure is greater than 90 percent. With the average cost for a single IVF attempt close to $5,000, this technique benefits the health-care system much more than it does consumers.

IVF allows for preimplantation diagnosis and disposal of unwanted human embryos.[10] New technologies can detect the sex and certain genetic conditions of three-day-old embryos at the eight-cell stage of development. Advocates of IVF argue that preimplantation diagnosis avoids the "necessity of later abortions and expands the option of gender choice. The idea that only some lives are worthy to be lived (eugenics) is in direct conflict with the biblical principle that all human life is a gift from God.

IVF increases the likelihood of multiple conception, and thus many physicians now recommend "selective reduction" (i.e., selective abortion) as a legitimate solution to this technologically induced problem.[11] By inserting a needle through the mother's abdomen into her developing child's heart and injecting it with poison, doctors target healthy embryos for destruction—after causing the multiple pregnancy to begin with. Claiming this procedure enhances the survival of the remaining unborn children does not change the fact that the technique is designed to deliberately destroy human life in the womb.

IVF poses unknown risks to women and children.[12] It is not yet known what long-term effects may come from the high doses of hormones women receive while undergoing IVF. Furthermore, it is unknown what effect these hormones will have upon their offspring. In addition, developing ova and embryos receive multiple exposures of ultrasound, which has yet to be declared universally safe in humans by the American Institute of Ultrasound in Medicine. Embryos are created "by hand" under artificial light, in manmade media, and incubated in a nonhuman environment. Whether this will negatively affect the health of those so created is currently unknown.

Like AID, IVF technologies are increasingly using anonymous donors to obtain results.[13] In the high-tech realm of laboratory reproduction, the wonder of conception is desexualized, disembodied, and divorced from the design of natural procreation. Consequently, the words *mother* and *father* take on entirely new and different meanings. Definitions of parenthood dissolve and are refashioned through experimental study and barely tested scientific methods. Assorted couplings, tangled destinies, and genetically disenfranchised offspring are the result.

"Anonymous donors become breeders," explains John T. Noonan, a professor of law at the University of California, Berkeley. "Its acceptance brings us to the worlds of Huxley and Orwell in which the final trick is played on the champions of procreation as a private choice. . . ."[14]

Points to Consider: Extramarital Insemination (AID)

Extramarital insemination commercializes, disembodies, and dehumanizes the father's role in procreation. There are a number of sperm banks around the country who make it their business to provide for the collection and sale of human semen. Lori B. Andrews, an attorney specializing in reproductive technology issues, reports that "donors" are often paid to masturbate in soundproof booths—with pornographic material readily available—for a set fee.[15]

Semen is kept in frozen storage and anonymously advertised in computer sheets listing such things as the sperm vendor's height, weight, hair and eye color, frame size, ethnic background, occupation, and favorite hobbies.[16] Vials of frozen semen are shipped to physicians who perform artificial insemination in their private offices or clinics. In recent years "do-it-yourself" at-home AID has become an attractive alternative to women desiring to bear a child outside of marriage.[17]

Extramarital insemination fractures family bonds.[18] Since the sperm is disembodied from its anonymous source, any child conceived by this procedure is automatically cut off from his or her father. Essentially only the maternal side of one's genetic tree remains; the other half of a person's heritage is completely severed. This can lead to later problems. An engaged couple in Israel discovered shortly before their wedding that they had the same father and could not marry. Both had been the product of artificial insemination by donor.

Lest one compare this too closely with adoption, consider the primary difference. Adoption is the rescue of a child from abortion or abandonment who has already been conceived. AID is a prearranged third-party pregnancy that consciously creates a child to satisfy the wishes of the mother and nurturing father. Adopting a child who already exists is an act of self-giving and compassion, whereas the prearranged splicing of genetic bonds to obtain reproductive fulfillment is child-tampering.

It is a well-known fact that adopted children often desire to meet their birth parents in order to better answer the question "Who am I?" What will happen when the children created by the new techniques are told that they were conceived with computer-selected gametes in a dish or rinsed out of an anonymous donor mother's womb after she was artificially inseminated at the doctor's office? *No one knows the answer to this question; we have no studies to tell us what genetic disenfranchisement will mean to these youth.* Sperm, ova, and embryos become commodities in the medical marketplace. What is this going to mean to the child who was "bought" from anonymous donors?

Extramarital insemination often results in deception about one's origins. Very few children conceived by heterosexual married couples using AID are told the truth about who their dad really is. Consequently, the child is brought up believing that the nurturing father is also the biological father. One eighteen-year-old woman was told at her mother's graveside that she was the product of AID—by the man she had always assumed was her father until he disclosed the facts of her conception.[19]

Extramarital insemination splits the couple in two from the moment of conception. Only one spouse—the mother—has a biological connection to their child. During the pregnancy, she carries another man's baby in her womb. Even if her husband claims it doesn't matter, he will constantly be reminded of his own inability to conceive a child with his wife as her equal partner in procreation. Just because the act is mechanical rather than physical, isn't extramarital insemination actually a form of procreative adultery?

"In the average situation, two parents with equal genetic investment in the child are unified by their mutual relationship to their child," explains Ms. Sidney Callahan, Professor of Social Psychology at Mercy College in New York. "They are irreversibly connected and made kin through the biological child they have procreated."[20] She adds:

> With third-party or gestational donors, however, the exclusive marital unity and equal biological bond is divided. One parent will be related biologically to the child; the other parent will not. True, the bypassed parent may have given consent, but consent, even if truly informed and uncoerced, can hardly equalize the imbalance. While there is certainly no real question of adultery in such a bypassing situation, nevertheless, the intruding third-party donor, as in adultery, will inevitably be a psychological reality in the couple's life. Even if there is no jealousy or envy, the reproductive inadequacy of one partner has been reified, and superseded by an outsider's potency, genetic heritage, and superior reproductive capacity. Fertility and reproduction have been given an overriding priority in the couple's life.

THORNY TOPICS AND SCIENTIFIC SCENARIOS

Beyond the questions surrounding how society defines "life worthy of life," other thorny topics crop up with ARTs. In what ways do family bonds change when five "parents" (sperm donor, egg donor, birth mother, and nurturing parents) are involved in making and raising a baby? What happens when people are told they were conceived with computer-selected gametes or rinsed out of a surrogate mother's womb? How will ARTs' availability shape our grandchildren's views of marriage, sexuality, and procreation? Where do you draw the line in designing your baby—sex, intellect, body shape, eye color? What are the moral limits as we face the possibilities involving future developments in reproductive medicine? We have yet to collectively answer these questions. There are no long term studies, no prior generation's experiences to predict ARTs' outcomes.

Looking Toward the Future: At the Frontiers of Life

What future developments may bring us new questions to answer and new ethical decisions to make?

Fetal farming. Unwanted fetuses and extra embryos may one day supply stem cells and organs for medical treatment in much the same way that fetal brain tissue is being used to treat Parkinson's disease today. According to *Time* magazine, ethicists are now debating the morality of transplanting ovaries from aborted fetuses into aging women. *USA Today* reports that "the prospect of scientists creating babies from the eggs of aborted fetuses—children whose 'mothers' were never born" may be accomplished within three years in humans. (British scientists have already perfected the technique in animals.)

R. G. Edwards suggests: "To grow fetuses to later stages of growth when they take a recognizable human shape and then extract their organs would be an utterly repugnant concept," he says in *A Matter of Life*, "but to obtain cell colonies from minute embryos useful in medicine for the alleviation of certain human disorders—is that not a legitimate target to aim at?" UCLA cryogenics expert Paul Segall advocates a head-to-toe approach using a body clone. Once the clone grew to an appropriate size by intravenous feeding and hormone injections and was placed in frozen storage, it could later serve as the equivalent of a brain-dead organ donor with the same genetic makeup as the person from whom it was derived, thereby avoiding the possibility of transplant rejections.

Artificial wombs. Italian researchers have kept a surgically removed uterus functioning for fifty hours. They believe that breakthroughs in organ preservation techniques will eventually allow machine-assisted uteris and implanted embryos to remain viable for much longer. With artificial placentation systems employing ECMO *(extracorporeal membrane oxygenation)* currently in use, it's only a matter of time before babies might be medically grown from "sperm to term," making biological motherhood technically obsolete.

Cloning, embryo "splitting," and selective breeding. Tests on cows' fertilized eggs proved that sixteen-cell embryos can be divided into four equal groups, cultured for a few days, and then redivided to yield sixteen identical clusters—each of which will grow into a genetically identical cow. The first laboratory duplication of human embryos by American researchers Jerry Hall and Robert Stillman in 1993, in which seventeen embryos were split into forty-eight, provoked intense ethical debate, but so far, no governmental restrictions. "It's up to the ethicists and the medical community, with input from the general public, to decide what kind of guidelines will lead us in the future," Hall said on the Larry King show.

Primate surrogacy and male pregnancy. Someday scientists may be able to medically manipulate men to carry babies via hormones or implant human embryos in primate surrogates for gestation. A British scientist, Dr. R. V. Short, has proposed the creation of chimeras—a genetically combined ape-human species—to create a subclass to perform hazardous labor. Sounds like science fiction, but some researchers are dead serious about pushing the boundaries of reproductive technology to the outer reaches of man's imagination.

Many look at the reproductive frontier and urge caution. "Although the proof of a baby—unlike that of a pudding—does not rest on its consumability, and in the case of man not even on its being born, efforts toward proving what is good for vegetables is also good for human beings are being continued in many places," the co-discoverer of DNA, Dr. Erwin Chargaff, asserts. "The life of man is, however, an unrepeatable experiment: no controls, no placebos."

Perhaps Professor Lewis says it best: "The Christian tradition—the Christian's notion of what God's purposes are—would lend itself to caution in pursuing these technologies. It calls us to radically redefine what it means to flourish."

For infertile couples trying to find their way through the wilderness of today's ARTs, it may also mean finding a path to parenthood that bypasses the rocky road of high-risk, low-yield techniques and treatments.

A CHRIST-CENTERED APPROACH TO INFERTILITY

There are no easy answers to the pain and anguish infertility causes for a couple. *It can be a life crisis more devastating than any other*, producing a wide range of emotions over a period of time—from anger to despair, to a sense of hopelessness and overwhelming fatigue. The following suggestions may help to ease the pain a little, as well as enable you to move through this time with greater understanding and discernment.

If you are having difficulty becoming pregnant, take time to assess your lifestyle and learn how to observe signs of fertility before resorting to medical therapy—if there are no unusual symptoms of reproductive disease or disability. Stress, diet, weight, age, exercise, and a woman's current health status all contribute to her ability to carry a baby. In addition, remember that many women have at least one or two anovulatory cycles per year (cycles in which menstruation occurs but not ovulation) and that the average length of time it takes to conceive is eight months. For further information on how to chart cycles and detect signs of ovulation, read chapters 6 and 7.

Because infertility diagnosis and treatment often involve expensive procedures without guarantees of success, it is essential to proceed carefully when selecting a health-care provider or making decisions about infertility therapy. An excellent resource covering consumer issues in infertility treatment is *Infertility: Medical and Social Choices*, available from the U.S. Government Printing Office.[21]

The selection of a physician is one of the most important health-care decisions an infertile couple seeking medical treatment will ever make, so it is essential to shop carefully. One cannot emphasize strongly enough how important this is. Read Part Three to become better informed about health-care consumerism.

Don't rely solely on friends for recommendations; get references from at least four or five different consumer-oriented services and life-affirming groups such as your local crisis pregnancy center. At least one or two names will probably be mentioned by several people you talk to.

Join or start a Christ-centered support group for infertile couples. Only those who are experiencing a similar situation can truly understand what you are going through. Secular organizations can only go so far in ministering to hurting hearts, yet many churches have been slow to respond to the anguish of infertile couples. Providing appropriate avenues to express this pain and grief with other believers within the body of Christ is vital.

Explore the alternative of adoption. If a child needs a home, adoption is a redemptive act that mirrors God's willingness to accept us as Christ's coheirs in His kingdom. It is not just an alternative method of having children, but a way of responding to a very real need—the need of a baby or little child who might have been aborted or abandoned to know what it means to be unconditionally loved and accepted.

Prayerfully consider adopting a child of a different ethnic background or physical/mental capability than yourselves. While it has become increasingly difficult since the legalization of abortion to adopt a "perfect" or genetically similar child, special-needs children in the United States account for about 60 percent of those waiting to be adopted. Only about one-third of the approximately 36,000 available special-needs kids will be taken in any given year. The federal government has responded to this crisis by taking legislative measures to make the adoption of special-needs children more attractive. In 1980 Congress passed an extensive reform of adoption laws that included offering a stipend—$200 to $300 per month—to qualified adoptive parents.

"With the great scarcity of babies for adoption now, adoptive parents are looking for children of different racial color, children of ethnic backgrounds far different from their own, and, yes, even handicapped children, some of whose handicaps are staggering as one contemplates the special care and love that will be necessary to see the adoptive process through to the end," says former Surgeon General Dr. C. Everett Koop. "It is an example of Christian love, of Christian fortitude, and of the kind of social action by Christians that we talk about more than we see."

Above all, be encouraged! *God hears your prayers and knows your heart. The desire to become parents honors God. If you are willing to trust Him to control and direct this important area of your life, His grace will sustain you in remarkable and unpredictable ways.*

You don't have to turn to extreme techniques and expensive technologies to bear beautiful fruit for the Lord through ministry to your family and to the world. The Author of life hears the cry of all who diligently seek Him.[22] Count on this: God's love never fails.

Part III

DOCTOR-PATIENT

COMMUNICATION

Is There a Crisis in Women's Health Care Today?

Several years ago my husband arrived home eager to locate a newspaper article he had heard about at work. It was one of those hot and humid early evenings Georgia is famous for—sticky, sweaty, soaking-wet summer heat.

After dinner we hunted together through our recycling pile until we found the correct copy. We leafed through several sections. Unable to locate the article, Dave grew increasingly more frustrated. He frowned and then sighed loudly. Finally we simply gave up looking and started back toward our nice, cool, air-conditioned kitchen.

Dave set the final section of the paper he had brought with him down on the table. Suddenly he noticed the article he had been trying to find: It was exactly in the middle of the front page. "How could I have missed it?" he said, laughing in disbelief as he pointed to a large black-and-white picture beneath a boldface headline.

Later that evening, it hit me: Life can be a lot like that. It's often easy to "miss the obvious" when it's right in front of our eyes. Sometimes it's because we are looking in the wrong places due to false assumptions we have made. Or our frame of mind makes it difficult to see things clearly or objectively.

For example, do you remember when *Life* magazine carried a beautifully photographed, awe-inspiring picture of a child developing in the womb on its cover, accompanied by the phrase, "How Life Begins"? The article inside was incredibly detailed; the moment of fertilization, early embryonic stages, and fetal awareness were all highlighted in close-ups that defied simple scientific explanations. But because of the social and moral climate we live in, many readers may have "missed the obvious"—the fact that the tiny developing persons shown in the photo essay represented fragile human lives worth respecting, protecting, and nurturing from the earliest moments of their existence.

ENLARGING OUR VISION

The beauty and mystery of human sexuality inspire and challenge us. Our attitudes, beliefs, needs, values, and assumptions can significantly enhance or stubbornly prevent our ability to see obvious truth that's worth noticing.

Consider this story. A twenty-four-year-old woman—the daughter of a close friend—made an appointment with her gynecologist for a premarital exam several months before her wedding. During the office visit, the doctor told her that oral contraceptives are the ideal form of birth control for most patients, especially newly married women. After a quick discussion that lasted less than three minutes, he wrote out a prescription for a popular brand of the drug under discussion. The young woman left the office, fully satisfied with her physician's subtly biased, too-brief explanation. Then she stopped at a local discount pharmacy on her way home to pick up the plastic packet containing the first month's supply of the pills.

At first glance, this story seems fine, certainly nothing out of the ordinary. But when we take a closer look, a number of key questions come up: What are the young woman's ideas and values about sexuality, conception, and the early stages of human life? Does she clearly understand how this drug works to prevent pregnancy? Do the pills control birth by blocking conception, as the doctor implied, or are they designed to prevent birth in other ways as well?

If my friend's daughter believes that each person's life begins at conception and continues until death occurs—a life that possesses eternal value and is watched over by God, as David's poignant psalm describes—then she has missed the obvious in much the same way my husband did while overlooking his article on the newspaper's front page. Assumptions powerfully shape our vision, and sometimes it's only much later that we realize "the facts" are not as we had originally pictured them.

SEEING THE BIG PICTURE

By taking a closer look at the connections between women's health care, human sexuality, current birth control methods, and abortion, we gain wisdom regarding how our attitudes and assumptions affect our responsibility to act upon what we believe. Our knowledge and actions, in turn, will guide our personal health-care decisions to more consistently reflect our core beliefs about what it means to be created in God's image and bear His likeness.

Whether we like it or not, the trend in reproductive medicine is toward the surgical, technological, and chemical control of fertility, pregnancy, and prenatal life. Since the Pill, *Roe v. Wade*, and the birth of Louise Brown, women's reproductive health management has been revolutionized.

One in every three pregnancies is ended by surgical abortion in the United States each year. New methods of birth control—RU486, Depo-Provera, and progestin skin implants (Norplant)—may act not only to prevent the union of the sperm and egg, but may also enable a woman's body to end a life after it begins.

Prenatal diagnosis contributes worldwide each year to the killing of thousands of babies deemed unworthy of life—children in the womb who are afflicted by genetic or developmental conditions such as Down's syndrome, cystic fibrosis, and spina bifida. Assisted reproductive technologies (ARTs) have created an unprecedented era of embryo experimentation, DNA testing, surrogate parenting, cloning, postmenopausal mothering, and human cryopreservation, raising a multitude of thorny moral, ethical, social, and legal issues. Many of these complex questions remain unanswered.

In addition to these concerns, there are others. Between 1970 and 1986, the cesarean rate in the United States skyrocketed from 5 to nearly 25 percent—a fivefold increase. Is this what our Creator intends for us? Should nearly one million women each year require major surgery in order to have a baby safely?

According to recent statistics, one in three American women will have hysterectomies before they turn sixty years of age, with only 10 percent of these surgeries performed due to a cancer diagnosis. Is the uterus designed so poorly that amputating it is often the best solution to "female problems"?

Given the current ethical and moral controversies in reproductive health care, we can no longer pick a doctor's name out of the yellow pages and simply accept his or her medical advice. We are living at a time when our choices concerning our physicians, hospitals, and medical treatment options are often vitally connected to our commitment to following Christ, our understanding of sexuality, and our respect for the value of human life.

The status of women's health care in the United States is a mixed blessing. There is much to praise and celebrate about the vast array of medical services, information, and treatments available to us. Yet there is room for improvement. Given the latest statistics, we have cause for concern, as well as for admiration, whenever we make decisions regarding our reproductive health. With our active participation, it is my prayer that twenty-first-century reproductive medicine will reflect our educated health-care choices.

FIGURES AND FACTS

In the next few pages I've put together a quick-study section containing a concise summary of the figures and facts you need to know about today's crisis in women's health care. Use it as a reference guide whenever you need some extra motivation to ask the hard questions at your doctor's office. Three of the five most common surgical procedures performed in the United States today involve the uterus—surgical abortion, cesarean section, and hysterectomy. It's about time for a change, don't you think?

Elective Abortion

In each of the twenty-five years since *Roe v. Wade*, elective abortion has been the most common surgical procedure in the United States. (See Figure 52.) More than 1.25 million abortions are performed each year. Four out of ten women of reproductive age have had at least one surgical abortion; and if current rates are sustained, an estimated 43 percent of American women will have an abortion in their lifetime.[1] In some states, there are three or more abortions for every live birth in certain segments of the population.[2]

Abortions in the United States After *Roe v. Wade*
Figure 52

YEAR	NUMBER OF ABORTIONS	ABORTION RATE*
1973	744,610	19.3%
1975	1,034,170	24.9
1980	1,553,890	30.0
1985	1,588,550	29.7
1990	1,608,600	28.0

YEAR	NUMBER OF ABORTIONS	ABORTION RATE*
1992	*1,528,930*	*27.5%*
1993	*1,330,414*	*22.0*
1994	*1,267,415*	*21.0*

* Percentage of pregnancies ending in abortion.

SOURCES: Alan Guttmacher Institute and the Centers for Disease Control. Based on the most recent statistics available.[3]

Cesarean Section

In 1995, 785,000 cesarean sections were performed, making this operation the second most common surgical procedure in the United States. Twelve million American women have had at least one cesarean section. Four million of these were unnecessary, and millions more have had automatic and largely unnecessary repeat C-sections with all subsequent births.[4] The national cesarean rate went up 400 percent in sixteen years between 1970 and 1986.[5]

Hysterectomy

According to the National Center for Health Statistics (NCHS), about twenty-five million American women have had a hysterectomy. In 1995, approximately 583,000 hysterectomies were performed, at a cost of almost $5 billion.[6] Given the current hysterectomy rate, nearly 600,000 women will have their wombs surgically removed this year; one in three will have the operation by age 60.[7]

There is a tremendous variation in regional hysterectomy rates. Compared with women living in the Northeast, women in the South are 78 percent more likely to have a hysterectomy; in the Midwest, 41 percent more likely; and in the West, 20 percent more likely.[8]

In addition, the rate of hysterectomy in Great Britain is half that of the U.S.—with no significant health gains for American women.[9] By the age of 44, women in the United States have a rate of hysterectomy (21 percent) five times higher than that for women in six European countries, where the rate is 4 percent.[10]

Related Facts: Your Quick-Reference Outline
for Fast Reading and Review

A. Uterine fibroids account for 30 percent of hysterectomies performed in the U.S.[11]

   1. FACT: Fibroids are normally not a dangerous condition, often do not require treatment of any kind, and shrink after menopause. (See chapter 17.)
   2. FACT: Between 1982 and 1984, 551,752 hysterectomies were performed to remove these benign growths.[12]

B. Repeat cesarean sections accounted for one-third of all cesareans performed in the U.S., and contributed to 48 percent of the rise in the cesarean rate between 1980 and 1985.[13]

   1. FACT: Following an in-depth survey of U.S. hospital records, the *American Journal of Public Health* stated that "except for the uterine scar from the previous cesarean, VBAC (vaginal birth after cesarean) mothers appear to have about the same history and frequency of complications as mothers with other vaginal deliveries."[14]
   2. FACT: Approximately 250,000 cesareans could have been safely avoided in 1995 if a nationwide policy of encouraging VBAC had been consistently implemented.[15]

C. In their support of elective surgical abortion, both the American Medical Association and the American College of Obstetricians and Gynecologists have successfully legitimized abortion as a method of birth control.

   1. FACT: At least 60 percent of women having abortions did not make any attempt to use contraceptives at the time they became pregnant, according to Dr. Luella Klein, M.D., president of the American College of Obstetricians and Gynecologists.[16]
   2. FACT: When almost 2,000 women having abortions were interviewed by the Alan Guttmacher Institute, 76 percent said the procedure was being performed because "pregnancy would interfere with work or school."[17]

Is there a conflict of interest?

A. Current figures regarding the high numbers of operations being done on the uterus combined with evidence of unnecessary surgery raises questions about some health-care practitioners' professional training and financial motives.

B. The more expensive, more extensive, and more extreme the technology used is, the greater the benefit to the practitioner. But is this also true for the woman being treated?

C. Where treatments are physician-referred and physician-monitored at the client's expense, it is the client and not the physician who pays the physical, emotional, and economic price of the treatment.

Estimating Unnecessary Surgical Deaths

What is the death rate associated with unnecessary surgery? A formula developed by Dr. Robert G. Schneider, a board-certified internist with a subspecialty in cardiology, may be used to estimate the number of deaths that theoretically can be caused by unnecessary surgery.[19]

Total number of annual operations in the U.S. = 20-25 million.

Overall mortality rate for all major surgery = 1.33 percent.

Unnecessary surgery estimates = 15-25 percent for some operations; 40-80 percent and more for tonsillectomies, hysterectomies, and cesarean sections.

The formula works as follows:

15-25 percent unnecessary operations X 20-25 million total operations = 3 to 6.25 million unnecessary operations.

1.33 percent mortality rate X number of unnecessary operations = 40,000 to 83,000 unnecessary deaths per year.

Note: Since this equation was formulated in 1982, the number of unnecessary operations (and deaths) has increased.

Some doctors will say that Dr. Schneider's equation is misleading, since death rates associated with common reproductive surgeries are lower than for other types of surgery. Here's a way to reply to their concern: If even one woman dies as a result of an unnecessary cesarean section or hysterectomy, that's too many.

Other important questions

A. Why is there so much unnecessary surgery in the field of reproductive medicine?

    1. Possible answers provided by the medical profession

      a.   To avoid a malpractice lawsuit.

      b.   Because women request it.

      c.   Because "after the last planned pregnancy, the uterus becomes a useless, bleeding, symptom-producing, potentially cancer-bearing organ and therefore should be removed."[18]

      d.   To improve women's quality of life.

2.   Possible answers provided by health-care consumer groups

      a.   Money.

      b.   Power.

      c.   Gender bias.

      d.   Professional bias.

      e.   Inadequate peer restraint.

      f.   Doctors' medical training.

      g. Lack of patient education and informed consent.

3.   My own opinion

      a.   Both doctors and health-care consumers are responsible for the current crisis in reproductive medicine.

      b.   Insurance companies should monitor unnecessary surgery, set more stringent standards concerning criteria for cesarean section and hysterectomy, and reimburse clients for effective alternative treatments.

      c.   Since most unnecessary surgeries are elective surgeries, it is the patient's responsibility to give her informed consent wisely.

B.   Should women "trust" their doctors?

C.   Can women avoid unnecessary reproductive treatments, tests, and surgeries? How?

    I would not be writing this book if I did not think women can take an active part in the prevention of unnecessary surgery in our country. The following chapters will encourage you to participate—on a very personal level—in becoming better informed about how to communicate with your health-care provider. As you consider the skills that every woman needs to navigate the complicated terrain of today's trends in reproductive medicine, it's my hope that you will gain the knowledge and confidence you need to approach your doctor with gentle dignity.

Communicating with Your Doctor About Her Most Important Client—You

This book wouldn't be worth a dime if it didn't include let's-get-right-down-to-it practical tips on doctor-patient communication. When it comes to talking with our doctors, most of us are wimps! That's right—we're wimps. Now that I've said it, I'll explain why.

Even the best bargain hunters among us become wimpy when it comes to discussing health-care purchases with our doctors. First of all, most physicians speak in terms that ordinary non-Latin speaking people have difficulty understanding. I suspect that this is in no small measure due to the medical establishment's ongoing—and perfectly understandable—concern for its professional and legal status. But if we can't understand what our doctors are saying, how can we ask them questions that make sense? We end up feeling just plain stupid.

Here's a prime example. Betsy, who is nine months pregnant and ready to give birth any day, goes in for a routine prenatal exam and asks, "How are things going, doctor?" Upon examining her filled-to-capacity belly, her doctor replies, "Honey, you're doing just fine. The fetus is in a vertex position in the pelvis, lying in the womb against the cervix, which is dilated to one centimeter."

Now for the everyday English translation: "Betsy, everything's normal. (I know that part wasn't in Latin, but I decided to translate it anyway.) The child you're about to bring forth is lying head down in its nest against the nest's neck, which is opened up to about half an inch wide."

See what I mean? I love learning the English equivalents to Latin terms because it *demystifies* the language of medical-ese. These are two of my favorites so far: *dura mater* ("tough mother"), which is the dense covering surrounding the spinal cord; and the *pudendal* ("shame") nerve, which is the structure that provides feeling to the genitals. Can you picture a doctor administering spinal or pudendal anesthesia and saying, "Drats! I can't seem to get the needle through this *tough mother*" or "The baby's almost here, Cindy, but first I'm going to numb your *shame* nerve down here"? We'd think the doc was a quack!

Wouldn't it be hilarious if doctors started speaking that way? Since that isn't likely to happen, we need to discover ways to reach a compromise somewhere between these two extremes—Latin and plain English—if we're to communicate clearly with one another.

THE REASON WE NEED TO TRANSLATE OUR DOCTOR'S JARGON

It only stands to reason that average, nonmedical people (i.e., plain folks like you and me) are awed by doctors' ability to describe the functions of the human body in technical terms. Their communication seems to come from a lofty height far above common ways of speaking. This is the second reason why it's hard for clients to talk to doctors—they sometimes seem almost godlike.

I realize that this is an unreasonable as well as blasphemous and idolatrous assumption. Yet what else can possibly explain the veneration and submission people show toward the medical profession? Can you picture any of us treating our bankers, lawyers, teachers, and insurance brokers this way? Why *do* we treat doctors so differently from other professionals?

Perhaps doctors represent the parent so many of us wish we could have had but didn't—all-knowing, invincible, wise, powerful, authority figures. In attributing these qualities to doctors, we obviously make many false assumptions. You and I both know that doctors are not godlike, and they're not necessarily good parent figures either. So what are they then? Let's just say that doctors are highly skilled students who professionally interpret and treat what's going on in the human body in exchange for money. (Not masters, mind you—the best doctors become, and forever remain, students.) Needless to say, this puts the medical profession in quite a different light.

There are a number of things we can do to overcome our awe/fear of doctors to obtain the health care we need. The first step is to find out the level we are currently communicating on and then identify the style of communication we need to use.

There's a useful tool you can use to discover and improve the quality of your communication with your doctor. It's a questionnaire developed by nurses (thank the Lord for nurses!) at the University of Colorado. (See Figure 53.) The questionnaire was designed to heighten our awareness of how timid or bold, soft-spoken or loudmouthed, obstinate or communicative, compliant or assertive we are when talking to our physicians. Feel free to jot down any comments, notes, or questions you have as you go.

Assertive Health-Care Questionnaire
Figure 53

Below are a series of statements made by health-care consumers. In the box to the left put a number—from 1 to 5—that best describes you. (1 is most unlike you in your situation, and 5 is most like you in your situation.)

_____ When I go to a health-care provider, I want him or her to tell me what to do.

_____ If I feel unsure about what the health-care provider has said even after an explanation, I will usually seek another opinion from another provider.

_____ I have questions when I see the health-care provider, and I see to it that I get answers.

_____ I adhere to the health-care provider's orders more often than not.

_____ My rights as a patient are most important to me. I stand up for my rights in dealing with most health-care providers, hospitals, and insurance companies.

_____ Health-care providers are busy people. We really shouldn't take up their time. I'll find answers to my questions somewhere else.

_____ My health-care provider almost always has something new to teach me about my health, and I always have some new information to share with my health-care provider about my health.

_____ I can't remember the last time a health-care provider had time to really explain something to me about my state of health.

_____ When I disagree with a health-care provider or want another opinion, I always tell him/her directly.

_____ Frankly it's not my place to tell the health-care provider what to do. If I don't agree with his or her recommendation, I'd rather not say this to the health-care provider directly. I'll handle it on my own.

_____ It's a mess when I want another medical opinion. I never know how to handle the situation with my own health-care provider.

_____ I usually will do what the health-care provider recommends, but I also add my own ideas—and I've told my doctor I usually do this.

_____ I have questions when I see the health-care provider, but frequently they don't get asked, or they go unanswered.

_____ I'd like to share decision-making with a health-care provider, but I usually don't try it.

_____ I am well aware of the fees for services from my health-care provider. If I don't know, I always ask before consenting to the service.

_____ I am uncomfortable disagreeing with a health-care provider.

_____ I like to share decision-making with my health-care provider and do so.

_____ There's too much risk in disagreeing with a health-care provider.

_____ My health-care provider and I have a relationship in which he or she always asks if I agree with the recommendations or if I would like to change them in some ways. Sometimes I suggest a change, which is OK with my health-care provider.

_____ If a health-care provider prescribes something for me, I want to know what it is, why it's needed, and what to watch for.

[Developed at the University of Colorado Health Sciences Center, School Nurse Practitioner Program, Denver.]

Improving Your Skills as a Health-Care Consumer

After you have completed the questionnaire, look over your responses. Which of your replies reflect assertiveness? A reluctance to communicate clearly? Fear of your doctor? Confidence in your ability to say what you need—and why? Overall, do you think you are *assertive* or *passive* when conveying your needs and concerns to your health-care provider? In what ways would you like to change?

You aren't alone if you discovered that you're not especially assertive when talking with your physician. Physicians are powerful figures in our society. (If you doubt this, visit some place with a national health-care system like Great Britain. What a shock!) It takes a considerable amount of determined self-instruction to overcome the cold-sweat, butterflies-in-the-stomach, frozen-smile approach so many of us have used with our doctors all these years. But let me assure you—*it can be done*.

WHAT WOULD YOU DO?

It's time to think through a few situations that can come up during a visit with an ob-gyn. Based on real-life cases, each of these six scenarios offers you the unique opportunity of sitting in with another woman while making health-care decisions. Evaluate each woman's response as if you were in the situation, and choose ways that you might respond.

Each case is divided into five sections:

1. BACKGROUND INFORMATION. The first section contains details of the situation—who is seeking medical help, what actually took place, what the doctor's recommendations were, and what the woman's reaction was.

2. WHAT WOULD YOU DO? Before reading any more, take time out to think about and record how you would respond in this particular situation. What questions could you ask? How might you feel? What does it mean to be gently assertive as a Christian woman? How can you express this through your words and actions?

3. THINGS TO ASK. These are questions I suggest women ask, included here only as an example of how Christian women I know have communicated with their doctors.

4. HOW THE SITUATION WAS RESOLVED. A straightforward, no-nonsense explanation of what happened in each case.

5. FOLLOW-UP. Details how each woman responded in her situation, in

case you were curious. All the classic fundamentals in assertiveness training related to doctor-patient communication are here—finding a second opinion, informed consent, putting things in writing, self-teaching skills—you name it.

Consider returning to this section again after reading the other chapters in Part III and redoing your answers in the "What Would You Do?" sections. I have a hunch that you will do even better the *next* time around (and the next and the next and the next).

Case One: Lynn

Background information. Lynn, age twenty-four, is seven weeks pregnant when she notices some spotting on the toilet tissue after going to the bathroom. In a few hours she is bleeding more heavily. It's late in the evening, so her husband takes her to the closest emergency room rather than her doctor's office. The E.R. physician tells her she is having a miscarriage and needs a D&C right away in order to avoid hemorrhaging. Lynn hesitates. Hasn't she heard something about D&Cs causing an abortion if the baby is alive?

What would you do?

Things to ask. Lynn was right. A D&C, which involves scraping out the lining of the uterus and removing the "products of pregnancy," is a commonly used method of abortion in America. In order to be certain that she is not having an abortion performed on a living child, Lynn should ask: 1) What proof exists that the baby has already been lost? 2) Before I consent to have a D&C, is there any reason why I can't have an ultrasound to determine if the fetal heartbeat has stopped? 3) If the baby has been lost, is a D&C absolutely necessary, or can we wait and see what happens first? 4) What are the major risks and most common complications associated with a D&C? 5) Why would a D&C be beneficial to me at the present time?

How the situation was resolved. Lynn refused to give consent for a D&C until an ultrasound was performed, against her doctor's advice. She had a strong feeling that she was carrying twins and believed that just one of the babies might be dying—a good reason to not go ahead with surgery. To the doctor's surprise—and to everyone else's—the ultrasound revealed that Lynn was in fact carrying two babies instead of one. Even more important, they were both still alive! Lynn carried both babies to term, and they are now twenty years old.

Follow-up. Why wouldn't an E.R. physician offer a woman an ultrasound to check for fetal heartbeats if she was not in imminent danger of losing her own life? How might the availability of abortion have changed some doctors' attitudes about human life during its earliest stages? About miscarriages?

Case Two: Cathy

Background information. Cathy is the forty-three-year-old mother of two children, ages thirteen and eleven. Four months ago she began bleeding heavily during her period—much more than she ever had before. It was so bad that she woke up in the middle of the night and asked her husband to drive her to a nearby hospital emergency room. The doctor assured her that she was not having a miscarriage, nor was she in imminent danger of hemorrhaging, detecting her fears. After making sure that her bleeding was within normal limits, he recommended she come back to the hospital in the morning for an ultrasound to try and find out what was causing the bleeding.

The next morning, an ultrasound showed that Cathy's uterus had several uterine fibroids. The gynecologist on duty recommended she have a hysterectomy as soon as possible to prevent further heavy bleeding. Cathy was stunned and completely surprised by the sudden announcement that she would lose her uterus. Even though she was forty-three, Cathy was considering have more children and was not ready to surrender her potential for childbearing.

What would you do?

Things to ask. Before consenting to any major surgery, it is essential to ask the following questions: 1) Is this surgery absolutely necessary? 2) If it is necessary, why? 3) Are there any alternatives to surgery in treating this condition? 4) What are the possible risks associated with this surgery? 5) How much does the surgery and hospital stay cost? 6) What complications are associated with recovery from this surgery? 7) How long does recovery normally take? 8) What books do you recommend I read about my condition before having surgery?

How the situation was resolved. Cathy called me long distance in a panic. I told her: 1) Uterine fibroids are not an absolute indication for hysterectomy if cancer and uncontrollable bleeding are not present. 2) She should read *Hysterectomy—Before and After*, by Dr. Winnifred Cutler, before consenting to have a hysterectomy. 3) She should get a second opinion. 4) She should let her new doctor know that she views hysterectomy as a last resort because she might be having another child at a future date. 5) She should ask if laser surgery or hormone therapy might be useful alternatives to hysterectomy in her situation.

As soon as Cathy got a copy of *Hysterectomy—Before and After*, she calmed down. Evidently her doctor was either unaware of alternatives to hysterectomy for the treatment of fibroids or wasn't willing (or able) to offer these alternatives. Of course, this made Cathy angry. It also made her angry that many of her friends at church, when they heard about her situation, said things such as, "Oh, Cathy, just go ahead and have your uterus taken out. It's such a bother anyway."

At Cathy's appointment with a new gynecologist for a second opinion, she: 1) wisely brought her husband along to add additional credence to her arguments; 2) began the visit by telling the doctor that she did not want a hysterectomy because she wasn't ready to give up the possibility of having more children; 3) asked what alternatives were available.

Although the doctor was initially surprised and defensive, having her husband there paid off for Cathy. She noticed that the doctor looked at her husband more often than he looked at her during their discussion. Amazingly, Cathy's new gynecologist told her that fibroids disappear after menopause in the natural course of events and that a hysterectomy could most likely be avoided. He recommended that she come in for follow-up visits every six months to monitor the growth of the fibroids in the future.

While visiting with her recently, I congratulated Cathy when I heard the news. "I'm glad you still have your uterus!" I exclaimed. While not all women will empathize with this sentiment, we both shared a secret smile before going our different ways.

Follow-up. Would you have done the same thing in Cathy's situation—or gone ahead with a hysterectomy? What do you think the reasons are behind the high hysterectomy rate in this country? Why are so many women willing to have a hysterectomy rather than seek less invasive alternatives to common reproductive problems?

Case Three: Diane

Background Information. Diane is twenty years old and plans to be married in four months. At her premarital exam, she asked her doctor about various types of contraceptives, including oral contraceptives, the diaphragm, and condoms. Her doctor told her that since she is a nonsmoker, the Pill would be an excellent choice for the first several years of marriage. Then Diane remembered reading something about the Pill possibly interrupting pregnancy if the egg is fertilized "accidentally" and asked her doctor to explain how this might happen. Diane's gyn informed her that this risk is merely "theoretical" due to the Pill's effect on cervical mucus and therefore not worth being concerned about.

What would you do?

Things to ask. Diane should ask her doctor: 1) By what mechanisms of action does this drug work? 2) What are the side effects and risks of oral contraceptives? 3) What are the effectiveness and risks of barrier methods and natural family planning in comparison to oral contraceptives? 4) When does human life begin?

How the situation was resolved. Diane's doctor became quite huffy when she began asking him specific questions about oral contraceptives and the beginning of human life. As a Christian "prolife" physician, he was apparently offended that she was implying that he would prescribe anything that might ever act as an abortifacient. When pressed for details, however, he was unable to answer Diane to her satisfaction. When it came to discussing natural family planning, he cracked several jokes about the "rhythm method" and suggested she be fitted with a diaphragm if she would be uncomfortable taking the Pill.

Diane's use of a diaphragm caused repeated urinary tract infections after her marriage. She called me in desperation soon after her honeymoon and asked if Dave and I could come over to discuss natural family planning with her and her husband. Later we had a good discussion about why natural family planning would be an excellent alternative to barrier methods and the Pill in their case.

Along with her husband, Diane subsequently decided to take a course in natural family planning and was surprised at its effectiveness in enabling them to live with the reality of their fertility as a couple—as well as to avoid those nasty bladder infections!

Follow-up. Why are some Christian physicians reluctant to become certified natural planning practitioners, yet so willing to criticize something they know so little about? Why are they prescribing potential postconception birth control drugs? What can we do to promote life-affirming alternatives to OCs, Norplant, IUDs, and sterilization within our churches?

Case Four: Michelle

Background Information. Michelle, thirty-one, is a single woman who was sexually molested as a young girl. Because she had never had a pelvic exam—she was terrified of the memories of violation, shame, and pain that it might trigger—Michelle made an appointment with her family physician to discuss how she could overcome her fear.

What would you do?

Things to ask. I suggested that Michelle: 1) tell her doctor about her concerns to the degree that she was comfortable doing so; 2) ask why a Pap test and pelvic exam are important for a woman her age; 3) see if she could have an external exam before scheduling a pelvic exam and Pap test at her next appointment; 4) find out about all of the procedures involved; 5) be sure to have a friend or a nurse she is familiar with present to comfort and reassure her during the exam; 6) wait to have the pelvic exam until she had worked through some of her feelings about it and had developed a good rapport with her physician.

How the situation was resolved. Michelle visited her doctor several times before making an appointment for her pelvic, taking several steps to reach her final goal. When the day finally arrived, she felt okay about going ahead with the procedure in order to "get it over with." Nonetheless, she was very nervous (who wouldn't be?) and didn't know if she could actually make it past this major hurdle in her life. Thankfully, she did make it, albeit with a few tears and much anxiety, and never again has to wonder what a pelvic exam is all about.

Follow-up. Why was having a pelvic exam and Pap test beneficial for Michelle? Traumatic? What would you recommend to a woman facing a similar situation? How would you rate her doctor's response?

Case Five: Andrea

Background information. Andrea, age twenty-eight, had been trying to get pregnant for nearly a year. Her family doctor suggested she see an ob-gyn for infertility testing and recommended a colleague in the same building. After a pelvic exam, an evaluation of her medical history, a sonogram (ultrasound exam), and a hysterosalpingogram, Andrea's gynecologist recommended that she begin taking a fertility drug called Clomid to induce ovulation, and he wrote out a prescription. How did Andrea know if she should take the drug?

What would you do?

Things to ask. Andrea needs to ask her gynecologist: 1) Why do you think I'm not ovulating? 2) Why do you think the Clomid will help? 3) What are the risks and benefits of the drug? 4) What do you believe is causing our infertility? 5) Are there any alternative treatments that apply in our situation?

How the situation was resolved. Immediately after her doctor's appointment, Andrea called to ask me what I thought about his recommendation. Apparently her gynecologist had not explained the cause of her infertility to her satisfaction, nor did he deny that she might already be ovulating. Naturally this caused Andrea a great deal of concern. I told her: 1) She should definitely get another opinion about the cause of her inability to conceive. 2) If at all possible, she should find a doctor who could determine if she is ovulating before trying to induce ovulation with Clomid. 3) She should be prepared for further tests and expenses to track down why she wasn't getting pregnant. 4) She should become familiar with alternatives to Clomid before deciding whether to take it.

Andrea subsequently made an appointment with another infertility specialist sixty miles away. He recommended that she chart her menstrual cycles for a couple of months before trying drug therapy. Once he evaluated her charts, checked her hormone levels, and did additional ultrasound studies of her reproductive organs, he decided to perform a laparoscopy several months later (see chapter 16). During the surgery, Andrea's new doctor discovered she had extensive endometriosis, as well as endometrial hyperplasia (a potentially pre-cancerous change in the lining of her uterus).

Had Andrea gone along with her earlier doctor's recommendation, the primary cause of her infertility would have continued to be left untreated. As it was, her new gynecologist performed laser surgery to remove the endometriosis and scar tissue in her pelvic cavity and then placed her on progesterone therapy. Andrea is now the mother of an eight-year-old boy, conceived shortly after her final surgery.

Follow-up. Was there anything Andrea might have done differently with her first doctor, or was a second opinion necessary in her case? Should she have let her first doctor know why she didn't follow his recommendation? If so, how should she have told him? Do you think fertility drugs are being overprescribed today? What can women do to avoid taking drugs that might not do them any good, or worse yet, might do them more harm than good?

Case Six: Jennifer

Background information. Jennifer is thirty-five years old and recently started experiencing terrible mood swings prior to starting her period. After becoming familiar with the signs and symptoms of PMS and trying a variety of self-help remedies, she decided to make an appointment with a well-known physician famous for her expertise in treating PMS.

Due to extensive background reading, Jennifer realized at her appointment that this physician was recommending a risky experimental therapy not currently accepted by the medical community. Suspecting that she might be collecting statistics in this area, Jennifer wondered if she will inadvertently become a research subject if she continues seeing this particular physician. Disappointed and confused, Jennifer left her doctor's office.

What would you do?

Things to ask. When Jennifer called me, I suggested that she had two options. The first was to try a new doctor, but my friend told me that she likes her gyn too much to give her up so quickly. The woman was a terrific advocate for life-affirming medicine, and Jennifer had already recommended her to lots of women. She opted for choice number two instead— to confront the PMS specialist directly with her questions about using patients as research subjects without their informed consent. Gulp! Gasp! Could she really do it?

How the situation was resolved. Jennifer couldn't figure a way to get back into the office without paying for a visit, so she wrote a letter that included several concerns. In it Jennifer asked: 1) what guidelines the physician was using to set her protocols (i.e., rules and policies) for conducting research with clients; 2) to be informed of any experimental treatments she might be recommending to Jennifer; 3) if she would provide Jennifer with separate, detailed informed consent forms to sign before prescribing or performing specific PMS treatments. Jennifer presented these questions within a positive, upbeat framework, emphasizing her respect and appreciation for the physician's work within the Christian community. She did this to keep the door open for future medical care if she decided to continue in this doctor's care.

Follow-up. Should all physicians be required—either ethically, professionally, or legally—to provide informed consent forms to clients before rendering treatment? (The closest thing I can think of to compare this to are consent forms now in use for tetanus, DPT, polio, and MMR immunizations. If you haven't seen this standard form, ask to see one at your local public health department.) Is it ethical for physicians to do research without their clients' informed consent? How can women best safeguard themselves from medical exploitation and experimentation?

IN SUMMARY

If you think you're ready to improve your communication with your doctor (and, believe me, this isn't an easy step for many—most?—of us), here's a checklist of what you'll be actively involved in:

_____ Determining the changes to make in communicating your needs and concerns to your health-care provider.

_____ Selecting a health-care provider who you feel is responsive to your needs and concerns.

_____ Becoming better informed about issues you discuss with your health-care provider.

_____ Making sure to cover all your questions and concerns to your satisfaction at office visits and consultations with your health-care provider.

_____ Learning about alternative treatments and side effects to recommended treatments, drugs, and procedures.

_____ Comparing the risks with the benefits of all recommendations made by your health-care provider.

_____ Taking an active role in improving your health through lifestyle and dietary habits.

_____ Joining (or starting) a support group and/or a local organization with members who share your needs and concerns.

_____ Understanding your legal rights and responsibilities as a health-care consumer.

_____ Becoming sensitive to your style of communication and making any necessary changes to enable yourself to convey your needs and concerns directly and clearly.

_____ Obtaining a second opinion whenever your health-care provider's recommendations need further professional support or evaluation.

Ask Before You Leap: What It Means to Give Informed Consent for Medical Treatment

H ave you ever faced a medical situation in which you wanted to know more about a treatment or procedure that your health-care provider had recommended to you but were afraid to ask? If so, I have some very good news for you: You don't ever have to be afraid to ask again.

Over the years I have heard many stories, positive and negative, from women about how they have been treated by their health-care specialists. I presented several of these cases to you in the previous chapter. It is my hope that the real-life examples I've shared will encourage you to ask your own questions and, when necessary, to seek second opinions. And don't forget to keep praying.

Wouldn't it be great to see a true revival sweep through the medical profession? But until that day arrives, we must be very choosy about our medical care. I realize this is a bona fide luxury. In many places of the world, there aren't even any doctors to choose from. Not so in America. Large metropolitan areas teem with women's health specialists. All one has to do is pick up a copy of the local yellow pages to confirm this. In more isolated areas, any community of more than 50,000 people is bound to have several reproductive health-care providers. This is comparable to many other aspects of American life. Go into a well-stocked supermarket or department store, and what do you find? A wide variety of different brands of similar items.

I'll never forget the time when my mother, visiting us in Nebraska for Thanksgiving, accompanied me to the store to prepare for the big dinner on Thursday. Suddenly she disappeared. I continued to move my cart up and down the aisles, selecting all manner of treats and goodies for our annual family feast, thinking that she had gone to use the bathroom. But guess where I found her? In the pickle aisle *weeping*.

You see, my mom had been living in Zacatecas, Mexico, for some time, and they just don't have our kinds of pickles in Mexico, let alone the zillion brands available in most grocery stores here.

No American thinks anything about the stacks of shelves of pickles and rows of price stickers until it's time to make a purchase. Then—what happens? I don't know about you, but this is my approach:

I check my coupon file. I will probably buy whatever brand I find a coupon for *unless* I can get a better deal on a store brand or a name brand on special sale. Since most brands of pickles are pretty much the same, I'll buy the cheapest brand, *no matter what,* if it's going to be used in something like tuna fish sandwiches for the kids' lunches.

For a special occasion, I may buy a particular brand of pickle that someone especially likes, even if it costs a little more.

I make it a point not to buy any brands of pickles that we have tried and disliked.

I spend as little time as possible in the pickle aisle while making these choices. And I have never actually wept for joy while making my selection.

I have never lived in a Third World country, although I have visited Mexico a few times and can relate to what my mother experienced at the market. Instead, I have been blessed—and challenged—by American life during my pilgrimage on earth thus far. We have so much here to choose from! It is both a blessing and a burden—a blessing because we have the best "quality of life" in the world, and a burden because choosing between available products and services can get really complicated at times. *This is just as true of medical products and services as it is of pickles.* When it comes to your personal health care, however, there's a lot more at stake than the satisfaction of your palate.

MAKING THE BEST CHOICES

Because we live in a free market society, we have the right and the privilege to select the medical care we think will be best for us. And yet how many of us actually get as picky about our medical care as we do about a brand of pickles? Amazing.

This chapter covers the legal doctrine of *informed consent*—the legal idea behind health-care delivery that allows *you* to decide what medical treatments and procedures to buy. When it comes to purchasing medical services, *the law is on your side*—just as it is when it comes to your right to buy a certain brand of pickles.[1] In other words, it is against the law for doctors to coerce their patients to do anything against the patient's best interest. This includes everything from having blood drawn for testing to having a hysterectomy.

Without informed consent, patients can become victims of medical abuse. With this consent, we can avoid expensive drugs and treatments we think may actually do us more harm than good.

Understandably, many doctors don't really like the idea of informed consent, health-care laws, and lawyers who represent consumer concerns because their freedom to practice medicine becomes more limited. But with the current crisis in reproductive medicine, we need good laws to protect ourselves from unnecessary or harmful tests and treatments. Once we realize how beneficial many health-care laws are, we can use them to our full advantage *without* waging unwinnable mini-wars with the medical profession.

Please, let's not fight with doctors. Instead, let's be a witness to them as the apostle Peter admonishes, with gentleness and respect (1 Peter 3:8-17). Having said this, I think it's just as wrong to surrender the stewardship of our bodies as it is to hate those who harm or offend us. My body belongs to God, not to me—and certainly not to my health-care provider.

RULES TO REMEMBER

To simplify medical decision-making, it helps to consider the legal doctrine of informed consent as a set of rules that enables you to wisely choose the best treatment from among several recommended to you—including nontreatment. Informed consent governs all decision-making related to your health care. Unless the laws change, the following rules *always* apply:

Rule 1: Ethical and Legal Basis

Informed consent is the ethical and legal basis upon which you give your health-care provider permission to treat you. The doctrine of informed consent relies upon several sensible components, according to the Department of Health and Human Services. Put together, these five interrelated parts spell BREAD—benefits, risks, explanations, alternatives, and decision-making. This is an easy way to remember what informed consent means each and every time you need to apply it (Figure 54).

The BREAD List
Figure 54

WHAT IT STANDS FOR	WHAT YOU NEED TO KNOW
Benefits	What will I gain from having this treatment or procedure?
Risks	What are the possible discomforts, adverse reactions, common complications, and major risks (no matter how rare) associated with this treatment or procedure?
Explanations	Was all the information I need to make an informed choice presented to me in terms I can understand? Did my doctor encourage discussion? Were all my questions answered to my satisfaction?
Alternatives	Were alternatives explained to me with enough information about each to allow me to decide between possible courses of treatment—including nontreatment?
Decision-making	Was I generally supported in the decision-making process by my physician without feeling pressured to decide in favor of a certain treatment?

Rule 2: Voluntary and Competent Permission

You must give your permission voluntarily, competently, and with understanding in order for your decision to qualify as "informed consent." You should be able to answer yes to all of the following questions after making your decision:

- Did I feel free to decline or consent to the treatment?
- Was my health-care provider willing to discuss the pros and cons (i.e., risks and benefits) of this treatment prior to asking for my permission to treat me?

- Did my doctor support my decision without unduly pressuring me to decide either way?
- Was the probability of success presented accurately, including my doctor's own success rate with this treatment or procedure?
- Were possible alternatives provided to me, including enough information about each option to permit me to make a fully informed decision about what would be best for me?

Rule 3: Understandable Information

The information your doctor gives you must be complete, accurate, and in terms you are able to understand. This necessarily includes but may not be limited to:

- The treatment's probability of success.
- Details of the potential of death and serious injury (if such a potential exists).
- The most common adverse effects.
- Possible complications.
- The availability of alternative treatments, along with their probable success rates.

The Mayo Clinic Health Letter suggests ten sensible questions to ask your doctor before treatment (Figure 55). It's an effective communication tool to keep handy.

Ten Sensible Questions for Any Treatment
Figure 55

1. *What do my symptoms mean?*
2. *Does this medication have any side effects?*
3. *What is this test for?*
4. *What risks are involved in my treatment?*
5. *Do I have any options other than the treatment you've prescribed?*
6. *How do the benefits of my treatment compare with the risks?*
7. *What kind of emotional reaction can I expect from my illness?*

If you're going to be hospitalized:

8. *How long will I need to stay in the hospital?*
9. *Do I have any limitations on my activity at home after release?*
10. *What should I call you about once I'm home?*

Rule 4: Freely Given Consent

Your consent must be freely given and can be freely withdrawn at any time. In a famous court opinion in 1914, a judge named Cardozo wrote: "Every human being of adult years and sound mind has a right to determine what shall be done with his own body; and a surgeon who performs an operation without his patient's consent commits an assault for which he is liable in damages."[2]

Any treatment performed on your body and not authorized by you may be considered *battery* (illegal touching of another person either directly or with an object). I realize this sounds extreme, but that's what it's called.

If you decide to withdraw your consent for treatment, it isn't a bad idea to obtain the original consent form and destroy it or to complete a new form stating that you do not consent to treatment. Include the date and time of day along with your signature.

Rule 5: No Waiver of Rights

You cannot legally waive your right to sue your doctor or hospital in the event of malpractice while giving your consent to treatment. While none of us ever plans ahead of time to file a malpractice suit, it is sometimes justifiable to do so. Like it or not, when you give your doctor permission to treat you, you cannot agree not to sue him in the future.

Rule 6: No Written Requirement

No form is required to make your consent to treatment valid. In fact, no writing is required to make *most* contracts. (What is a contract? A contract is an agreement made between two or more people to do something.) In days gone by, a person's status (such as master-slave) exclusively determined his or her rights. Today citizens enter into *contractual relationships* instead: employer-employee, debtor-creditor, buyer-seller, and doctor-patient, for instance. What a relief!

In the doctor-patient relationship, your rights are *never* subordinate to the doctor's rights due to his "status." Legally your doctor is recognized as owing you a special or "fiduciary" duty to be responsible for your welfare if you ask her to treat you—and she agrees. In real-life terms, the principles of contract and fiduciary duty are especially exemplified by the requirement of obtaining your informed consent *before* treatment.

Your consent may be implied by your actions as well as by taking the form of a written document. For example, if you ask and then allow your doctor to treat you—by giving you a shot or sewing up a cut, let's say—that in and of itself can mean that you have given your consent. Another good example of medical treatment being provided without obtaining written consent first is when such consent becomes impossible. This might happen in a life-and-death situation when a patient is unconscious and there is no next-of-kin available. Society gives doctors this privilege under extreme conditions only.

Putting things in writing provides a record about what was agreed to—for both you and your health-care provider's protection. The purpose of executing a written agreement is to preserve the terms of your consent in case a disagreement arises between you and the provider in the future. While it's not a bad idea in many situations, it's important to remember that *you can withdraw your consent for treatment at any time*. This is especially helpful to remember if you change your mind *after* signing a consent form. In court, consent forms have been considered invalid when patients have refused treatment after signing them

Rule 7: Full Disclosure

The more elective a procedure is, the more important full disclosure becomes in obtaining your consent. As stated above, true emergency situations do not allow enough time for lengthy discussion of recommended treatments and alternatives.

In other cases, there may be no other alternatives other than nontreatment, and a specific treatment may be the only option available to you. In these cases, the informed consent process won't be very detailed or take very long. However, any treatment or procedure that is not an emergency and not absolutely indicated gives you a great advantage: time.

The more time you have to study and learn about your condition, the better informed you will be before making a final decision. In particular, don't rush into any of these situations without preparing ahead—choosing a method of family planning; having a hysterectomy for any reason other than cancer, uncontrollable bleeding, or life-threatening infection; consenting to infertility treatment; taking hormones to control menstrual irregularities or manage menopause; giving birth; and having an elective cesarean section or any other elective major surgery.

Rule 8: Restrictions Noted

Your doctor has the right to have any restrictions you impose upon her noted in your record, including the fact that the risks of such conditions were fully explained to you—and that you understood your doctor's explanation (Figure 56). This is to release your health-care provider from being liable for your non-consent. In the event of a lawsuit, a court of law or hospital arbitration board would want to know why she treated you the way she did.

Doctors may not like it when their clients don't comply with the treatments they recommend, but as long as you sign a medical release form, your doctor cannot perform a treatment you don't want to have.

Your Right to Refuse Medical Treatment
Figure 56

In 1958 the American Hospital Association approved the *Statement on Jehovah's Witnesses and Blood Transfusion*. Due to subsequent court decisions, the AHA Board of Trustees approved recommendations to cover the broader subject of refusal of treatment in the *Statement on the Right of the Patient to Refuse Treatment* (available from the AHA as leaflet #S81).

The statement suggests that "in the case of persons who, for religious or other reasons, refuse to consent to medical or surgical treatment," health-care organizations and providers:

- ask adult patients of sound mind to provide a written refusal to absolve the hospital, physician(s), and other affected personnel from liability.
- explain the medical consequences of the patient's refusal.
- try to obtain consent for an alternative treatment.
- report the patient's refusal promptly to the hospital and give an opinion about the possible medical consequences of the patient's refusal.

The statement also notes that various states have placed legal restrictions on the right of the patient, or someone on her behalf, to refuse medical or surgical treatment. Consequently, state laws differ on this issue.

Rule 9: Request Any Records

You may request to see your medical records at any time and to have a copy made for your own use for a reasonable fee (Figure 57). The purposes of the medical record are to serve as a basis for planning and continuity of care; to provide a means of communication among members of the health-care team; to document the course of a patient's illness and treatment; to serve as a basis for review of the quality of care; to protect the legal interests of the patient, doctor, and hospital; to provide a data base for research and education.[3]

Obtaining a Copy of Your Medical Records
Figure 57

The Joint Commission on the Accreditation of Health-Care Organization's standards for release of patients' medical records[4] require that its members:

1. Develop policies and procedures that specify the conditions under which medical records may be released and govern the disclosure of information contained in the records.

2. Allow a patient or her representative, with written consent, to request release of such information provided the consent is given on a form that includes the:

- Name of the person, agency, or organization to which the information is to be released.
- Specific information to be disclosed.
- Purpose of the disclosure.
- Date the consent was signed.
- Signature of the person witnessing the consent.
- A notice that the consent is valid only for a specified period of time.

The main reason a patient might ask to see her record is to gain a better understanding of her medical condition. Other reasons include checking the accuracy of one's personal and family histories, to become better informed when asked to give consent for treatment, to familiarize herself with the role her physician has taken in her care, and to become better acquainted with the state of her health in order to prevent a recurrence of her condition in the future.

Most medical records can be deciphered if you use a good medical dictionary (*Stedman's* or *Taber's* are available in libraries and most bookstores), know the meanings of the abbreviations being used (look them up in the back of this book), and can read your doctor's handwriting (perhaps the most challenging task of all!). For a detailed analysis of your record, consult an experienced, cooperative medical practitioner.

While your medical record remains the property of your doctor or hospital, you also have a "property right" in the information because it's about you. Therefore, you should not be denied reasonable access to the information.

Rule 10: No "Abandonment"

Your doctor may not discontinue caring for you as a patient if you decline consent for treatment; that is, she cannot "drop" your case without giving you proper prior notice. (It's legally termed *abandonment* if she does.) On the other hand, your doctor will probably be found to be justified in refusing to perform any treatment she considers inconsistent with good medical judgment.

If you should ever reach an impasse in either of these situations, your doctor can leave your case *only* as long as she gives you plenty of notice ahead of time or finds another doctor willing to take your case.

WHAT ABOUT THOSE "BLANKET" CONSENT FORMS?

A "blanket" consent form, while still required by most doctors and hospitals, is frequently considered legally inadequate as a replacement for informed consent related to specific treatments. A "blanket" consent form may read something like this: "I hereby give my permission to (*name of doctor or hospital*) to perform any necessary treatments upon myself as is deemed advisable." Note that a blanket consent form such as this would fall far short of meeting the doctrine of informed consent as defined by the BREAD list (see Figure 54).

You should know that *the less specific the form is, the less likely it is to be legally binding.* Blanket consent forms do not replace the need for specific forms to be signed if you withdraw your consent for treatment, are making a decision about a non-routine procedure, or decide to add any unusual conditions to your treatment.

Don't forget: For consent to be considered truly informed, it should fit the BREAD model. Here's a handy little pyramid to remind you (Figure 58).

The Informed-Consent Pyramid
Figure 58

AS A PATIENT,

YOU HAVE THE RIGHT:

TO OBTAIN MEDICAL HELP,

TO DISAGREE WITH YOUR DOCTOR,

TO BE CLEAR ABOUT WHAT YOU NEED,

TO HAVE ALL YOUR QUESTIONS ANSWERED,

TO SEEK A SECOND OPINION WHENEVER DESIRED,

TO DELAY MAKING A DECISION UNTIL YOU ARE READY,

TO UNDERSTAND WHAT COMES NEXT IN YOUR TREATMENT,

TO SHARE IN THE DECISION-MAKING WITH YOUR DOCTOR,

TO ASK FOR A PRIVATE CONSULTATION BEFORE AND/OR AFTER TREATMENT,

TO BE RESPECTED AS AN EQUAL PARTNER IN THE DECISION-MAKING PROCESS.

14

Toward More Dignified Office Visits— Getting the Most for Your Time and Money

There's one experience in life that a woman never forgets. Any guesses as to what it is? Her first pelvic exam. There are a number of good reasons for this, which are summed up quite well by the following incident.

It happened in the spring of 1980. I had just learned I was expecting our fourth child. After telling my six-and-a-half-year-old daughter Katy the exciting news, she looked at me and asked seriously, "Mom, I have just one question for you. Do you *have* to take your underpants off to have a baby?"

You see, Katy already knew where babies come *from*. She had seen her younger brother David born three years earlier in 1977. Now for the first time the reality seemed to be hitting home. What was I going to tell her—that I could give birth while wearing my best Carter's briefs?

I knew Katy was verbalizing something that concerns all modest women when it comes to giving birth, making love, and—having a pelvic exam. Like it or not, every one of these activities requires taking off one's undergarments. There isn't any way to get around it, although we've sometimes sincerely wished there was (and I do mean *sincerely*.)

Trying once again to be "instant in season," I decided to explain it this way to my insightful daughter: "Katy, the way God designed us to have babies is to give birth from the same place where babies are made. It's a very private place—a special part of your body called your vagina. Only girls have this place, remember?

"When it's time for a baby to be born, the baby leaves the womb through the vagina. If a woman has her underpants on, the baby wouldn't be able to get out, would she? Of course not! So if the mom takes her underpants off, it makes it easier for the baby to be born.

"You were born this way, the same way Joanna and David were, and the same way I was birthed from Grandma's womb. I'm not embarrassed about having to do this because that's the way God made childbirth to be. Still I think He also made the vagina to be a woman's most private place. That's why we need to wear underpants."

After thinking about this for a moment, Katy started talking about something else, completely satisfied with this answer. If only it were this easy to explain other facts of life that I still struggle to accept or understand!

THE PLACE OF MODESTY IN MEDICAL TREATMENT

Did you know that Mayan women in the Yucatan would almost rather die than have a pelvic exam? (Genital exposure is still totally taboo in most tribes and cultures, for good reason.) Did you know that many women in England have traditionally had pelvic exams while lying on their side, offering them much more privacy? That the first woman in history to give birth while lying on her back with her perineum exposed was supposedly the mistress of Louis "The Sun King" in eighteenth-century France?

Are pelvic exams an unavoidable aspect of modern health care for American women? If so, what can we do to keep our modesty intact?

Female genital exposure in medicine is a relatively new thing. It's unique to our current century as a routine, widely accepted medical practice. Yet how many of us have cringed at the thought of our first (and second and third and . . .) pelvic exam, wondering why and if *that* was absolutely necessary?

I believe it's up to each of us to find physicians who respect the role of modesty in modern medical practice. And I believe just as strongly in the value of Pap tests, bimanual exams to check for pelvic abnormalities, and prenatal checkups. So how do we reconcile this dilemma?

In this chapter, I'll be sharing some ideas and information that will enable women to keep their modesty and sense of dignity intact. Perhaps you've already discovered some of these basic helps on your own. As women, we can come up with some terrific ways to stay modest while being more fully involved in our health care than ever before, as well as providing an example to our physicians.

A pelvic exam need not be a horrible, frightening, or traumatic experience when you know what's involved ahead of time. Although you probably will never actually *like* having a pelvic exam, it's possible to make peace with it. Sort of.

FINDING A PRACTITIONER WHO LISTENS AND WHO VALUES HUMAN LIFE

The first thing is to find a primary health-care provider you can talk to easily and who shares your views on reproductive health. This can be more difficult than it sounds.

For most of us, the idea of shopping around for a health-care provider and then bombarding her with a list of questions is difficult, if not impossible, to imagine. Let's face it: How often do we get a chance to meet a doctor for an initial office visit with all of our clothes on?

We usually talk to a nurse first, who briefs the doctor on what to expect after handing us a disposable paper sheet and telling us to undress from the waist down. By the time our physician shows up, we often have developed cold feet (in more ways than one) and chattering teeth. And under these conditions, as you most likely have already discovered, it isn't usually easy to initiate a comfortable medically oriented dialogue.

Now try picturing an altogether different situation. Your physician greets you in her office rather than the examining room. You discuss your expectations and ask questions about her approach to reproductive medicine. Rather than avoid awkward topics, you directly seek to obtain the information you need.

Surprisingly, many women don't know where their physicians stand on abortion. This is particularly amazing when one considers how strongly we feel about the interrelationship of our sexuality to the value of human life. Think about this for a minute: Have you ever asked your doctor when she believes life begins, under what circumstances she would perform or refer a woman for abortion, what she thinks about OCs, IUDs, and Norplant? Most of us would rather avoid such controversial topics, especially when visiting our doctor's office.

It's important not to assume you know where your health-care provider stands on these vital issues, even if you attend the same church. For example, one Christian ob/gyn I know practiced in the same office with the leading abortionist in our city for many years. A long time went by before they finally parted ways professionally. I can't help but think that it had something to do with all the women I know who voiced their concerns and, in some cases, went elsewhere for treatment.

I also remember the time I found an excellent gynecologist who agreed to perform a laparoscopy on me (my family practice physician—a wonderful, life-affirming Christian—couldn't do the surgery). Later I found out she was on the medical advisory board of an agency that offered abortion services. So I never returned to her office.

I'm angry and frustrated that some of the best physicians in town—the most flexible, down-to-earth, and skilled clinicians—tend to also prescribe OCs, insert IUDs, refer for abortions, and even do abortions. I also understand why this is the way it is. Abortion and abortion-inducing drugs and devices are viewed as an acceptable and necessary part of medical training and practice today. Therefore, some doctors actually believe they are doing women good by providing these life-destructive technologies. Peer (and economic) pressure is particularly strong in medicine, and doctors who refuse to refer for abortion, insert IUDs, or prescribe OCs are few and far between.

Yes, women have the right to choose—and that includes the right to choose life instead of death when we make important decisions related to our reproductive health care. By making clearly informed choices about the services, providers, hospitals, drugs, devices, and technologies we use, we affirm God's grand creation. And we deny death access to our hearts and wombs.

CONDUCTING THE SEARCH

I realize that in all likelihood you already have a primary-care physician. I did before I moved. Even though you may be quite satisfied with your care, I encourage you to ask your doctor where he or she stands on abortion and contraception and to prayerfully consider switching to a new physician if your doctor supports, prescribes, or performs abortive drugs or technologies.

Now that I'm living in a new city, I have many different doctors to choose from, and I'm not familiar with any of them. Since I need to go in for a Pap test next month, where do I start?

I've discovered that the Yellow Pages don't tell me much of anything— just names, addresses, and phone numbers of physicians by specialty. Obviously, I'm not just going to make a random selection. I don't know any other women in our community very well, so I can't ask close friends for recommendations. What *am* I going to do?

Here's my plan:

Step 1: *Look through the Yellow Pages to find out what reproductive health care is available, paying particular attention to listings by specialty and indications of board certification* (Figures 59 and 60). Since I have endometriosis, PMS, and other specific menstrual concerns, I want to find a gynecologist rather than a midwife, general practitioner, or family practice physician.

Types of Health-Care Providers
Figure 59

PRIMARY HEALTH-CARE PROVIDERS BY TYPE
AND TRAINING

General practitioner: medical degree with one year of additional internship training.

Family practitioner: medical degree with three or more years of postgraduate residency training in family medicine.

Internist: medical degree with at least three years of postgraduate residency training in internal medicine.

Obstetrician/gynecologist: medical degree with three or more years of postgraduate residency training in pregnancy, reproductive surgery, and health care for women.

Pediatrician: medical degree with at least three years of postgraduate residency training in child and adolescent medicine (nonsurgical).

ANCILLARY HEALTH-CARE PROFESSIONALS
(DIRECT PROVIDERS WORKING WITH PHYSICIAN BACKUP)
BY TYPE AND TRAINING

Certified nurse-midwife: registered nurse with a Master's degree in nursing and/or a certificate from an accredited nurse-midwifery program.

Physician's assistant: graduate of a four-year accredited university training program for physician's assistants.

Certified (or Registered) nurse practitioner (or clinician): registered nurse who has successfully completed a specialized training program and certification exam in gynecology, pediatrics, psychiatry, or family practice.

What All Those Initials Mean

Figure 60

PHYSICIANS

D.M.Sc.—Doctor of Medical Science

D.O.—Doctor of Osteopathy

M.D.—Medical Doctor

Board Certification by Specialty

F.A.A.F.P.—Fellow of the American Academy of Family Practice

F.A.A.P.—Fellow of the American Academy of Pediatrics

F.A.C.O.G.—Fellow of the American College of Obstetricians and Gynecologists

F.A.C.P.—Fellow of the American College of Pathologists

F.A.C.P.—Fellow of the American College of Psychiatrists

F.A.C.R.—Fellow of the American College of Radiology

F.A.C.S.—Fellow of the American College of Surgeons

NURSES

B.S.N.—Bachelor of Science in Nursing

C.N.M.—Certified Nurse-Midwife

C.N.P.—Certified Nurse Practitioner

F.P.N.P.—Family Practice Nurse Practitioner

L.P.N.—Licensed Practical Nurse

M.S.N.—Master of Science in Nursing

N.P.—Nurse Practitioner

R.N.—Registered Nurse

R.N.A.—Registered Nurse Anesthetist

R.N.C.—Registered Nurse Clinician

ALLIED HEALTH PROFESSIONALS

C.C.E.—Certified Childbirth Educator

C.L.C.—Certified Lactation Consultant

C.L.E.—Certified Lactation Educator

I.B.C.L.C.—International Board Certified Lactation Consultant

I.C.C.E.—ICEA Certified Childbirth Educator

N.F.P.E.—Natural Family Planning Educator

N.F.P.P.—Natural Family Planning Practitioner

A.C.C.E.—Aspo Certified Childbirth Educator

P.A.—Physician's Assistant

R.D.—Registered Dietitian

R.P.T.—Registered Physical Therapist

RELATED FIELDS

M.P.H.—Master of Public Health

M.S.W.—Master of Social Work

Ph.D.—Doctor of Philosophy

Locating a Health-Care Provider

Family advocacy groups. There are active family advocacy organizations in every state, including local member groups of the Christian Action Council and Couple to Couple League. Try contacting several by phone and ask them to recommend several physicians in your area. Crisis pregnancy outreach centers are excellent sources of physician referral as well.

Churches and pastors. Any church body committed to supporting the sanctity of human life will be familiar with local physicians who perform abortions and the places in your area where abortions take place. Find out who and where they are; use other physicians, clinics, and hospitals instead.

If your local church is of little assistance, perhaps you could get involved. For specific information contact the National Prolife Religious Council (NPRC), c/o NAE, 1023 15th Street NW, Washington, DC 2005; (703) 591-6635.

Nurses or friends working in a health-related field. Nurses working with doctors are familiar with the personal and professional reputation of physicians in the community, especially at the hospital or practice where they work. A nurse working in labor and delivery, postpartum, surgery, or gyn knows a great deal about the health-care providers working in her area. She will be able to tell you her opinion of their skills and experience.

Local childbirth or home birth association. Childbirth instructors, lactation consultants, cesarean educators, and home-birth advocates are excellent sources of information on local women's health-care services. They also tend to know specific physicians' cesarean section rates, their attitudes toward clients, their routine practices, and patients' breastfeeding rates. Although you may not get specific details, ask for a recommendation of three physicians who do not perform or refer for abortions and see what happens.

Health-care organizations and consumer groups. Many cities have a section in the back of the phone book called the Blue Pages, filled with every kind of health-care organization and consumer group imaginable. If your community doesn't offer this service, try your local newspaper or write to national organizations listed in the Resources section of this book. Many of these groups will provide a listing of specialists in your area who are members of their organization or have registered with their society.

Federal, state, and county agencies. You'd be amazed at the information public agencies make available to taxpayers for free. (For example, most states require reporting of cesarean section rates by hospital.)[1] Women's commissions have gathered data and released surveys of individual physician's practices.[2] California even has an informed consent law regarding hysterectomies.[3] Many of these developments have been prompted by women's health lobbyists. We can take advantage of these resources and use them for our own benefit.

Hospitals. If you don't know anyone working in an ob/gyn related area, call your favorite prolife hospital, ask for a specific department (L&D, OB or GYN-Surgery) and seek a referral directly from the nurse on duty. In most places, nurses will provide three names when asked. Call once at three different times to hit several shifts—7 A.M. to 3 P.M., 3 P.M. to 11 P.M. and 11 P.M. to 7 A.M. Some names will recur more often than others; those doctors likely have the best reputation at that particular hospital.

State or county medical societies. Medical societies provide membership listings and a list of members by category (female family physicians, etc.)

Step 2: *Conduct an in-depth search to narrow down the possible choices.* If I find that only a handful of ob/gyns in my area claim to have a "prolife practice," I'll make a few more phone calls to several physicians and ask their receptionists a few questions before deciding whom to make an appointment with.

If this sounds like a tremendous hassle, it is, but I firmly believe it's worth it. (I also believe that if more women did this kind of comparative shopping for reproductive health care, doctors would start listening to us more.)

Step 3: *Arrange a pre-exam interview.* Once I am fairly satisfied that I'm not wasting my time and money on a doctor I'll be disappointed with, I'll call to make an appointment for a "pre-exam interview." Expectant parents do this as a matter of course with pediatricians before their baby is born, so why not do this with our ob/gyns as well?

It can be explained this way: "Ms. Smith, I'm new in town, and I've heard that Dr. Jones has an excellent reputation within the Christian community here. I am also actively involved in my church. Nurses at Smith Hospital tell me that Dr. Jones is a well-liked and highly skilled surgeon. Before I actually see him for an exam, I'd like to meet with him and ask a few questions. This way I can better determine if his skills and my medical needs and outlook on women's health care match. Would that be possible? A fifteen-minute consultation would be wonderful."

If the receptionist says yes, we're in business. Private consultations don't come cheap, however, so I'll also ask her to send me information ahead of time on the doctor's fees, billing practices, insurance-reimbursement policies, office hours, and any related things I might need to know.

CONDUCTING THE PRE-EXAM INTERVIEW

Before the interview, prepare a brief list of questions to ask. (Once on that examining table, your mind may tend to go blank.) Jot down a few things about your medical history in case it's needed. Knowing it's best to "never let 'em see you sweat," dress neatly and professionally on the day of the appointment and remind yourself to look and act self-confident even though you may actually be quite nervous.

After the introduction, share a little about yourself, your approach to reproductive health care, and why you requested the interview. Be very clear and straightforward about the kind of health care you're looking for. During your conversation, inform the doctor that you expect:

- To be involved in your health care to the fullest extent possible.
- To share in the decision-making process.
- To have a clear idea of her goals and philosophy.
- To have an honest relationship that works both ways.
- To be given thorough explanations concerning any testing and treatment recommendations, including alternative tests and treatments.

GENERAL REPRODUCTIVE HEALTH MAINTENANCE

Before presenting the pelvic exam process in detail, I think it's useful to review *why* it's important, as well as to describe other tests essential to reproductive health.

Pelvic Exam

How often. Before having intercourse for the first time; if menstruation hasn't started by age sixteen; if you are experiencing severe menstrual cramps, very heavy bleeding, or periods lasting longer than ten days; during a routine Pap test; prior to conception for pre-pregnancy advice and assessment; and if any of the following conditions exist:

- Itching, soreness, redness, swelling, foul odor, blisters, or sores in the vaginal or genital area.
- Unusual vaginal bleeding or discharge.
- After missing a period if you think you are pregnant or have had a positive pregnancy test.
- Difficulty conceiving after six to twelve months of "trying."
- Painful, difficult, or frequent urination.
- To be fitted with a diaphragm or prescribed oral contraceptives.
- Three missed periods in a row (especially if you haven't had intercourse).
- Pelvic pain and/or painful intercourse with or without chills or fever.
- If you have had intercourse with someone who might have a sexually transmitted infection.
- If you have been raped or otherwise injured.

Who does it. Primary-care physician or associated health-care provider.
What's involved. Bimanual pelvic, genital, and speculum examination.

Weight Check

How often. Every time you visit your health-care provider, unless you are under treatment for an eating disorder—in which case, you have probably already been told not to weigh yourself for a while.
Who does it. Nurse.
What's involved. Accurate weighing on a balanced scale.

Urinalysis

How often. During any routine checkup, prenatal visit, or if a urinary tract infection is suspected.
Who does it. You collect the urine. A nurse or medical lab technician tests it.

What's involved. If you're being tested for a possible bladder infection, you'll be asked to provide a "clean catch" urine specimen. This is done by thoroughly cleansing the vulva prior to urination and then urinating a little to rid the urethra of bacteria-laden urine. Then you stop urinating, spread your labia apart, and finish urinating directly into a collection container.

If the urinalysis is being done as a routine urine check during pregnancy or as part of a physical, no special precautions to avoid bacterial contamination are likely to be necessary.

Lifestyle Assessment

How often. Upon health-care provider's advice or at your own request.

Who does it. Health-care providers, wellness centers, health maintenance organizations, hospitals, sports clinics, fitness centers, county extension services, various university programs, and public health departments.

What's involved. Evaluation of your nutritional intake, exercise practices, stress level, safety habits, emotional well-being, and blood cholesterol/blood pressure. For women, lifestyle assessment is especially critical if you are infertile, your periods are irregular or abnormal, you have PMS signs and symptoms, you are pregnant, or you are having menopause difficulties. What you eat, how you exercise, and whether you manage stress appropriately can have a direct impact on your menstrual cycle.

Blood Pressure Check

How often. As necessary, depending on what your blood pressure is.

Who does it. Your doctor or someone connected with any fitness or wellness program you might be enrolled in.

What's involved. Checking the blood pressure with a device called a sphygnomometer, which places external pressure on the blood vessels in your arm. Then a qualified professional listens to your pulse with a stethoscope as the pressure is reduced.

Cholesterol and Lipid Screening

How often. Every four to five years between the ages of twenty and fifty; more frequently if you are at risk for developing high cholesterol (personal or family history of heart disease, diabetes, high blood pressure, or stroke); every year after age fifty.

Who does it. Primary health-care provider.

What's involved. To get an accurate reading on your blood lipids, you should fast for fourteen hours before the test. A sample of blood will be taken from your arm. You may ask that a test be done for fasting blood sugar at the same time. To get the most accurate results possible, be certain that your blood sample is evaluated by an accredited medical laboratory. If the test is abnormal, you may want to be retested again before beginning treatment.

Cancer Screening

Note: The American Cancer Society (ACS) recommends a routine annual exam that includes cancer screening for all women age forty and older. If you are younger than forty, you should follow the ACS guidelines as described below.

Pap Test

How often. Soon after first intercourse or by age twenty, whichever comes first. Another Pap test should be performed a year later. If the results are normal and you are in a low-risk category for cervical cancer, a Pap test every three years thereafter is advisable. (See chapter 18 for a list of related risk factors.)

Pap Test

Figure 61

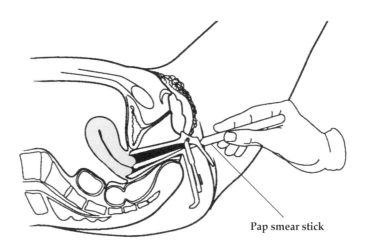

Pap smear stick

Who does it. Primary health-care provider or an associate health professional.

What's involved. A Pap test is performed during a pelvic exam while the speculum is in place. After visualizing the cervix, your health-care provider uses a small, narrow wooden or plastic spatula to gently scrape the surface of your cervix to remove a thin layer of cells (Figure 61). Sometimes, a sample of cells is taken from your vagina and/or cervical canal as well. The cells are spread onto a glass slide, which is then sprayed with or immersed in a fixative solution to preserve them. The slide is sent to a laboratory to be stained and examined microscopically by a pathologist or cytotechnologist. There should be little or no discomfort during this procedure, although you may notice slight spotting or bleeding afterwards.

The Pap test is not intended to provide an absolute diagnosis of cervical, vaginal, or uterine cancer. Its purpose is to detect precancerous or cancerous changes that might be present so that any abnormal findings may be followed up with other tests. It is not 100 percent accurate; nevertheless, it is a reliable test, especially when:

- It's done halfway between menstrual periods.
- You do not have intercourse or place anything inside your vagina for two days before the test, including medication, lubricants, douching solution, barrier contraceptives, or spermicides.
- The test is analyzed by a skilled clinician who specializes in reading Pap tests.

If you are experiencing any symptoms related to uterine, cervical, or vaginal cancer (see chapter 18), do not wait to schedule a Pap test even if you are not at an "optimal time of the month." Do, however, be certain that your Pap test is sent to the most reliable laboratory in your area.

Breast Exam

How often. Breast Self-Exam (BSE) should be done each month, starting at age twenty. Breast exam done by your primary health-care provider at least once every three years between ages twenty and forty (more often if you're in for a Pap test anyway); then every year after age forty.

Who does it. In order to learn how to do a BSE correctly, it is absolutely essential, studies have shown, that women be taught by a knowledgeable health-care provider or educator in person. Then, after you learn the procedure, you can do a BSE every month on your own. Also, a breast exam should be included as part of any routine physical. If you're unsure about your findings—or if you suspect breast cancer—make an appointment with your health-care provider for an exam. Note: Any changes in your breasts should be reported to your primary health-care provider.

What's involved. Systematically checking all mammary gland tissue and its associated structures for evidence of disease, including your breasts, nipples, and lymph nodes under the arms. Breast exams should be done in two positions: lying down and standing up (or sitting) to be accurate. (See Figure 62.)

Most breast cancers are first discovered by women themselves. Since breast cancers found early and treated promptly have excellent chances for cure, learning how to examine your breasts properly can help save your life.

Before a mirror inspect your breasts with arms at your sides. Next raise your arms high overhead. Look for any changes in shape or contour of each breast, a swelling, dimpling of skin, or changes in the skin or nipple.

Lie down. Flatten your right breast by placing a pillow under your right

Breast Self-Exam
Figure 62

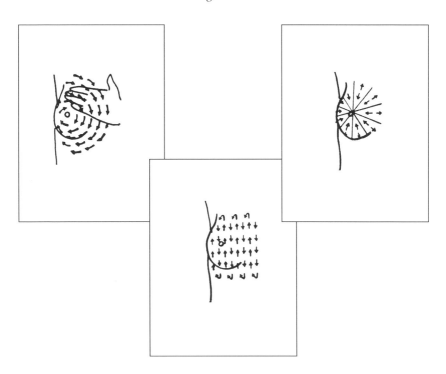

shoulder. Fingers flat, use the sensitive pads of the middle three fingers on your left hand. Feel for lumps or changes using a rubbing motion. Press firmly enough to feel the different breast tissues. Completely feel all of the breast and chest area from your collarbone to the base of a properly fitted bra, and from your breast bone to the underarm. Allow enough time for complete exam.

The diagram shows the three patterns preferred by women and their doctors: the circular clock or oval pattern, the vertical strip, and the wedge. Choose the method easiest for you, and use the same pattern to feel every part of the breast tissue.

After you have completely examined your right breast, then examine your left breast using the same method. Compare what you have felt in one breast with the other.

Finally, squeeze the nipple of each breast gently between the thumb and index finger. Any discharge, clear or bloody, should be reported to your doctor.

If you find a lump or dimple or discharge during BSE, it is important to see your doctor as soon as possible. Don't be frightened. Most breast lumps or changes are not cancer, but only your doctor can make the diagnosis.[5]

Mammography

How often. An initial "baseline" mammogram between the ages of thirty-five and forty, then one every two years between forty and fifty. After fifty a woman should have a mammogram annually. These are the American Cancer Society's current guidelines; other experts question the frequency of mammograms for women under fifty years of age who are not at high risk for developing breast cancer.[6] Mammography is the only test now available that can find many types of breast cancer before a lump is big enough to feel.

Who does it. An X-ray technician. The films are then reviewed by a radiologist—a medical doctor specializing in X-ray analysis.

What's involved. Each breast is placed on an X-ray plate, then compressed. This is temporarily uncomfortable until the breast is released a few minutes later. With the latest X-ray equipment and an experienced radiologist, mammograms appear to be accurate at least 90 percent of the time. False reporting can result in a missed diagnosis or unnecessary biopsy of breast tissue. In addition, the effects associated with the low doses of radiation used in mammography aren't yet clear. Benefits must be weighed against the possible risks, but studies indicate mammograms clearly reduce deaths from breast cancer. When you have a mammogram performed, go to the place with the highest quality equipment and best radiologists available to avoid false reporting of results.

Pelvic Tract Infection Screening—Wet Smear
(also called a "wet prep" or "wet mount")

How often. On an "as-needed" basis when symptoms indicate an infection may be present.

Who does it. Primary health-care provider.

What's involved. Collection of cells present in the vagina and cervix by using cotton swab to get a sample of any vaginal discharge. The sample is then placed on a glass lab slide with several drops of solution. Microscopic evaluation is conducted immediately by your health-care provider and a diagnosis is made while you wait. Note: Chlamydia and gonorrhea are not definitively diagnosed by this procedure. (See below.)

STD Tests

How often. At least once every year if you or your spouse are engaging in intercourse outside of marriage, if you are pregnant and think you could possibly have been exposed to an STD, or if you have any symptoms of these sexually transmitted diseases (see chapter 19 for additional information):

Chlamydia—unusual vaginal discharge, painful urination, chronic pelvic tenderness or discomfort, abnormal bleeding, and/or unexplained fever.

Gonorrhea—symptoms much the same as for chlamydia.

Herpes—painful lesions or blisters on your vulva, genitals, anal area, or buttocks; swelling of lymph nodes in the groin or abdominal area; unexplained fever; and/or swelling of the vulva.

Syphilis—Symptoms vary according to the stage of the disease.

STAGE 1: A characteristic sore called a chancre (a red-rimmed, hardened sore resembling a small boil or a pimple) appears about three weeks after exposure on the vagina, cervix, or anywhere that intimate sexual touching occurred. If the chancre is located deep inside the vagina, it is unlikely a woman will notice it.

STAGE 2: Rash (especially on the palms of the hands and soles of the feet), unexplained fever, sore throat, sore mouth, chronic headache, loss of appetite, nausea, joint pain, lymph node swelling, eye inflammation, and/or enlarged spleen or liver. These symptoms can appear as early as one week and as late as six months after the chancre heals, can last three to six months, and can recur on and off for several years.

STAGE 3: Heart disease, CNS (central nervous system) damage, blindness, insanity, and/or death occur after ten or twenty years if syphilis is left untreated.

Genital Warts (Human Papillomavirus, or HPV)—dry, painless warts on the vulva, cervix, vagina, or rectum. May be diagnosed by Pap test and colposcopy with biopsy (see chapter 16).

AIDS (Acquired Immune Deficiency Syndrome)—Severe fatigue; unexplained weight loss; diarrhea; recurrent, unexplained fever; general malaise, eventually leading to Kaposi's sarcoma, persistent pneumonia, and severe systemic infection.

Why you need this test. To determine if you have a sexually transmitted infection, especially if you have any STD-related symptoms, and/or if you (or your husband) have had intercourse or intimate sexual contact with someone other than each other.

Who does it: These tests can be performed by most health-care providers, including family physicians, gynecologists, internists, general practitioners, nurse-midwives, nurse-practitioners, or physician's assistants.

What's involved: A bimanual pelvic exam; a speculum exam; visual examination of the perineum and cervix; collection of cells from affected areas for microscopic examination and/or culture in the laboratory; and pathogen-specific blood tests.

STAYING COOL AND CALM

Although I am loath to admit it, I am a veteran of dozens of pelvic exams, so I've learned a few things firsthand about how to help myself get through them with minimum discomfort and embarrassment.

Often the examining table is in a flat position. This is more uncomfortable during an exam than a semi-reclining position, which relaxes your abdominal and hip flexor muscles. The semi-reclining position also allows you to have good eye contact and better communication with your health-care provider during the exam. Ask the nurse to reposition the table for you, and be sure to have a pillow for your head.

If your health-care provider is a man, a nurse must be present in the room during the pelvic exam. This is to protect both you and your health-care provider from possible charges of sexual misconduct. The nurse is also there to assist him as necessary and to provide for your comfort during the exam.

When you lie down, the lower half of the table is extended. This is pushed into the examining table before the exam so your health-care provider can sit down comfortably and be able to see better. Before you put your feet into the "stirrups" or over the leg rest, be sure to cover yourself with a sheet.

Female Genital Organs
Figure 63

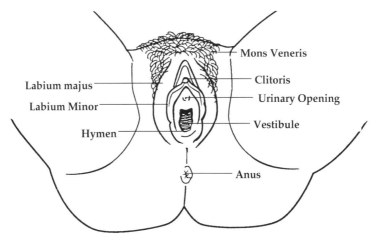

Gynecologic Speculum
Figure 64

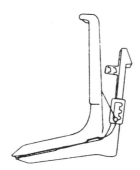

Remind yourself that this exam may be unusual for you, but it is something your health-care provider does on a clinical basis hundreds of times a year. If you like, bring a pair of clean socks to wear; they will keep your feet warm.

A pelvic exam actually involves three separate exams—an external (genital) exam, an internal (speculum) exam, and a bimanual exam. Your health-care provider should tell you what she is doing and why, so that you know what's going to happen next. If you take a few slow, deep breaths, it will help you relax. Thoughtful clinicians put posters on the ceilings and walls of exam rooms to take your mind off what's going on, too.

The external exam involves a visual check of your genitals for any redness, swelling, irritation, or other tissue abnormality (Figure 63). Next your health-care provider will use a stainless steel or plastic device (preferably warmed), called a speculum, to examine your vagina and cervix (Figure 64). The speculum holds the walls of the vagina apart so the vagina and cervix can be examined.

Before your health-care provider places the speculum inside your vagina, be sure your bladder is empty. *Completely relax* the muscles in your pelvic floor—just as you do when voiding. *Concentrate on pressing the muscles down and out* to create an opening, full sensation. This will make the placement of the speculum more comfortable. If you think of it, try to relax your legs—especially your inner thighs—and buttocks as well, as these muscles can contribute to muscle tension in the pelvic floor.

If you've never had intercourse, insertion of the speculum still shouldn't hurt. The vagina is incredibly elastic, much like an accordion or an expandable coffee filter. It's the muscles around it—which you control—that make it "tight." Relax the muscles and, viola, you also relax the vagina.

Some health-care providers place the speculum on a woman's inner thigh before using it and inquire if it's too cold or too hot. This also gives you an advance warning that the internal exam is next, so that it isn't a surprise. Your clinician may also insert a gloved finger into your vagina to enable it to open more easily.

The speculum is inserted with its blades in the closed position, and then, once it is in place, it is rotated until the handle is downwards. The blades are then opened, and the instrument is locked in place to an appropriate width. *If the insertion of the speculum is painful at all, ask your health-care provider to stop.* Sometimes all that's required for a greater degree of comfort is a different-sized speculum or an adjustment in its position. Your clinician doesn't want to cause you any pain or embarrassment and will do whatever possible to make this part of the exam go easier for you.

While the speculum is in your vagina, your health-care provider will collect any necessary lab specimens. (See section above: Pap test, wet smear, and STD tests.) A speculum is also needed for other special tests and procedures as well, such as colposcopy and cervicography.

The speculum is removed as soon as the exam is completed, which normally is over in less time than it took you to read this description. Since a sterile lubricant is used on the speculum to make insertion go more smoothly, you

Bimanual Pelvic Exam
Figure 65

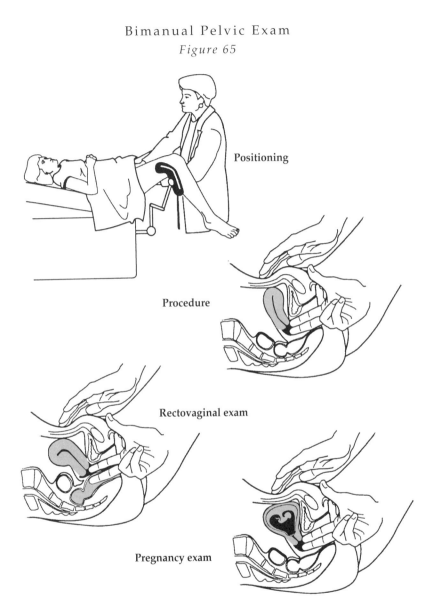

Positioning

Procedure

Rectovaginal exam

Pregnancy exam

will notice some residue afterwards. This can be easily removed with some tissue before you get dressed after your clinician leaves the room. You may also want to use a panty liner to absorb any additional discharge.

Following the speculum exam, your health-care provider will perform a bimanual exam (Figure 65). This involves inserting two gloved fin-

Uterine Placement and Variations
Figure 66

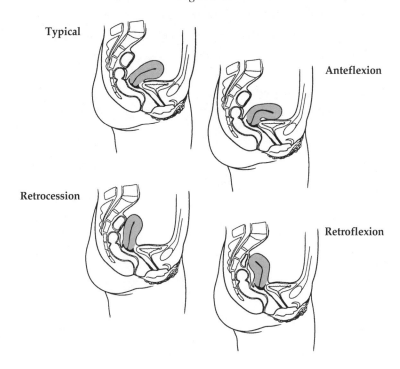

Typical

Anteflexion

Retrocession

Retroflexion

gers of one hand into the vagina while placing the other hand on your abdomen. By manually pressing upward against the cervix and downward on your abdomen at the same time, your clinician can determine the size, shape, texture, and position of your uterus (Figure 66). Your ovaries and fallopian tubes will be checked as well. Your clinician should be able to detect any unusual pain, tenderness, swelling, or growths that might be present.

Some health-care providers follow the first part of a bimanual exam with a rectal exam. One gloved finger is inserted into the rectum while the adjacent finger remains in the vagina. This can find abnormalities in the recto-vaginal wall (the membrane between the vagina and rectum), can check your uterus to see if it's tipped backward, and can detect any unusual growths, pain, or tenderness deeper inside the pelvic cavity.

As a quick review, here are the most essential points to remember about how to survive a pelvic exam:

- Empty your bladder completely—ahead of time.
- Bring socks.
- Don't feel bad about being embarrassed—*everybody* is.
- If it hurts, ask your clinician to stop and try something else.
- Breathe deeply with your mouth *open* (it helps to relax the pelvic floor).
- Don't forget panty liners.
- Keep your sense of humor—and your modesty—at all times.

$\mathcal{P}art\ IV$

REPRODUCTIVE

DISEASES AND TREATMENTS

$\mathscr{E}$ndometriosis:
A Mysterious—and Disabling—
Reproductive Disease

E ndometriosis. What is it? Where does it come from? How do women get this troubling disease? Can they do anything to prevent it?

Endometriosis (*endo*—inside; *metri*—uterus; *osis*—abnormal condition of) is the relocation and growth of small portions of tissue similar to the normal uterine lining away from their normal location. These clumps of endometrial tissue, or *endometrial deposits*, can be located on the fallopian tubes, ovaries, rectum, intestines, bladder, pelvic ligaments, and other places where they definitely *don't* belong.[1]

In extremely rare cases, the cells travel and attach to sites far distant from the pelvic cavity—the lungs, thighs, stomach, spinal cord, brain, chest, or arms, for example—but they are normally located much closer to the uterus within the pelvic cavity.

WHAT ENDOMETRIOSIS DOES ISN'T VERY PRETTY

As with other reproductive disorders, endometriosis is a problem many of us are creatively learning to live with once we receive a definitive diagnosis. But even though endometriosis is not life-threatening for the vast majority of women, it does present a significant reproductive threat. It is an invasive, destructive disease that can be devastating to a woman's ability to bear children.[2] That's why we need to take this disease seriously. It's a prime cause of reproductive disability in women over twenty-five.

When examined under a microscope, endometrial deposits look very much like the cells that line the uterus. They even respond to monthly changes in hormones during the menstrual cycle, just as they would if they *were* inside the uterus. Odd, isn't it?

Every month, displaced colonies of endometrial tissue build up, break down, and bleed in exactly the same way they would if they were still inside the womb (Figure 67). Throughout the menstrual cycle, endometriosis responds to hormones and results in microscopic internal bleeding.

Common Endometriosis Sites
Figure 67

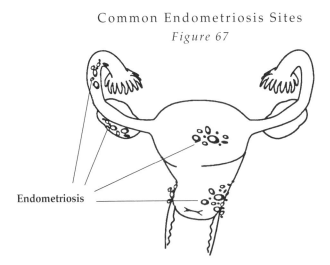

Endometriosis

So where does this little bit of blood go if it's released inside the pelvic cavity instead of within the uterus each month? *Nowhere.* As a result scar tissue and pelvic adhesions form; surrounding structures become inflamed; there is a gradual breakdown of blood and tissue within the pelvic cavity, and the immune system responds accordingly. It's not a very pretty picture, to say the least.

WHAT CAUSES ENDOMETRIOSIS?

No one knows what causes endometriosis yet, but several theories and risk factors are currently under investigation.[3] The first is called the Transportation Theory. The oldest and most popular theory, this idea suggests that endometrial tissue somehow travels outside the uterus into the pelvic cavity where it attaches and grows. There are several different ways this could happen. The blood and lymph fluid could carry them—hence the presence of endometrial deposits in foreign places outside the pelvic cavity. A second possibility is that surgery may cause endometrial cells to be moved to other abdominal locations. Third, endometriosis might be the result of backup, or retrograde, bleeding—the backward flow of menstrual blood up the fallopian tubes and out into the pelvic cavity.

Retrograde bleeding seems to be a plausible explanation in many ways. While it may not be the primary factor in the development of endometriosis, it could very well be a contributing cause, especially when the cervix is blocked or closed from trauma or surgery, the uterus is severely tipped (retroverted or retroflexed), the ends of the fallopian tubes (fimbria) are stuck together, or uterine fibroids blocking the menstrual flow are present. Some researchers have also wondered if orgasm during menstruation and devices that block the menstrual flow (super-size tampons, cervical caps, and diaphragms, for example) might also provoke a backward flow of menstrual blood.

Are shorter, heavier, more painful periods possibly a factor here as well? Perhaps. The truth is, no one really knows—but if the uterus cramps up when bleeding is heaviest, it certainly could result in menstrual "backup."

There is evidence against this theory, however. Most important, we now know that all women (in other words, a full 100 percent) experience backup bleeding. Physicians often view this phenomenon during pelvic surgery. But since not all women have endometriosis, how can backup bleeding be the *primary* cause of endometriosis?

A second theory may help to provide the answer. Called the Transformation Theory, it proposes that cells present at the time of birth mutate into endometrial cells outside the uterus during adulthood (referred to as *metaplasia*). This is best understood by picturing certain cells inside the pelvic cavity as carrying the potential to become one of several different kinds of cells. That is, they are undifferentiated. These cells have the ability to form many different types of tissue, including endometrial tissue.

There may also be a genetic link to endometriosis, predisposing some women to this condition while sparing others. Preliminary studies seem to indicate that heredity does indeed play a role. Endometriosis rates for mothers and sisters were about two to three times higher than rates for comparison groups in one report.[4] The hereditary pattern followed the maternal line (grandmother to mother) rather than the paternal line (grandfather to father) in at least 80 percent of the cases studied. Additional research has revealed that sisters have a six times greater risk of developing endometriosis than their husband's sisters, and another recent study showed that women carried eight times the increased risk if their siblings had the disease. Though these studies strongly suggest a genetic basis for the disease, the mode of inheritance isn't yet known.

New studies have also turned up another possible piece of the puzzle. There may be differences in how immune cells respond to endometrial implants in women who develop endometriosis, linking the condition with immune system dysfunction. Some researchers have further suggested that the immune system and the hormonal system may then influence one another to create an imbalance that eventually results in endometriosis.

Interesting facts, right? But all the statistics in the world don't make a difference if it happens to *you*. If the individual diagnosis is endometriosis, the incidence equals 100 percent. Still it helps to know the overall picture, so read on.

WHO GETS ENDOMETRIOSIS?

It is quite likely that a number of factors are responsible for causing endometriosis, not just one. Regardless of what the exact causes are, we currently have no way of predicting which women will end up with endometriosis or of preventing its development in those who might be susceptible.

Endometriosis afflicts an estimated five million American women today, or between 6 to 7 percent of all females. Of those who have endometriosis, 75 percent are between the ages of twenty-five and forty-five, but it's also found in teens and women after menopause.

On average, women who have endometriosis are likely to:

- Start menstruation at an earlier age.
- Experience more frequent, heavier, longer, and more painful periods.
- Have shorter cycles than other women (24 to 27 days compared to the average length of 28 to 34 days).

Perhaps most worrisome of all is the fact that *endometriosis is responsible for 30 percent of female infertility nationwide.* It has been estimated that between 30 and 40 percent of women who have endometriosis experience difficulty conceiving.[5]

SIGNS AND SYMPTOMS

Unfortunately, the diagnosis of endometriosis is not an easy one to make because it can mimic several other conditions, including dysmenorrhea, colitis, pelvic inflammatory disease, urinary tract problems, irritable bowel syndrome, and ulcers.

Accurate diagnosis requires careful evaluation by a gynecologist based on a thorough discussion of your symptoms related to your menstrual cycle. Your physician may want to confirm her diagnosis with outpatient diagnostic surgery, called *laparoscopy*, because endometriosis cannot be definitively confirmed by any other method.

Your doctor will be looking for the following signs and symptoms:

Painful Periods (Secondary Dysmenorrhea)

Endometriosis may be suspected if menstrual pain begins two to seven days before your period, is strongest at the time of your heaviest flow, continues throughout your period and afterwards, occurs according to a more constant and less "wavelike" pain pattern, can be felt in other areas besides the uterus (rectum, sides of abdomen, navel), and is associated with heavier flow and blood clots.

Painful Intercourse (Dyspareunia)

Although other conditions can cause painful intercourse, sharp pain during deep penile penetration—especially during the premenstrual phase of your cycle—is often indicative of endometriosis. The penis moves the vaginal wall and cervix during intercourse, putting pressure on ligaments supporting the womb (uterosacral ligaments) (Figure 68). These ligaments are often where endometrial deposits are located.

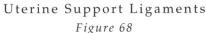

Uterine Support Ligaments
Figure 68

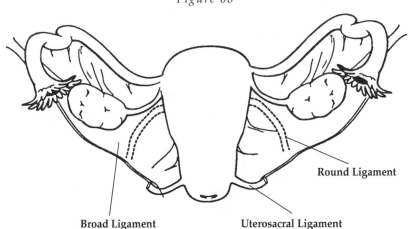

Round Ligament

Broad Ligament   Uterosacral Ligament

Infertility

As endometriosis progresses, it can damage the ovaries and fallopian tubes and cause irregular periods, hormonal imbalances, and changes in the chemical composition of cervical mucus—all factors that directly affect a woman's ability to conceive. Less frequent intercourse due to pelvic pain during lovemaking is also quite common, further decreasing the likelihood of conception. In addition, internal scarring of the fallopian tubes may prevent the passage of fertilized eggs.

The earlier endometriosis is diagnosed and treated, the better the likelihood of preserving your fertility.[6] Also at least one clinician has observed that the likelihood of conception appears to be greater if a woman attempts pregnancy at an earlier age.[7]

Chronic Pelvic Pain and/or Lower Backache

The degree and severity of pain associated with endometriosis depends most on the location of the deposits, not on their size. Even small deposits on the rectum can make bowel movements extremely painful, whereas deposits on the ligaments supporting the uterus may cause excruciating pain during intercourse at certain times of the month. Distinguishing between endometriosis and other conditions that might cause pelvic pain is essential, so keep in mind that pelvic pain from endometriosis is usually worse before, during, and just after menstruation and/or ovulation.

A summary of the signs associated with endometriosis are listed for your reference below (Figure 69). If many of these signs are present, it is very likely that you have endometriosis. If just one or two of these symptoms are present, you still may have endometriosis and should find out what's causing your symptoms.

Signs Associated with Endometriosis
Figure 69

Painful periods (strong menstrual cramps)

Painful urination and/or bowel movements during periods

Pain with intercourse

Difficulty getting pregnant

Gastrointestinal upsets—diarrhea, constipation, nausea

Premenstrual spotting

Urinary urgency

Rectal bleeding

Fatigue

Bloody cough

Sense of rectal fullness during periods

The symptoms of endometriosis are often not in proportion with the extent of this condition. That is, women with the most pelvic or rectal pain may have far fewer endometrial deposits than those with less pain. Even an extensive pelvic exam may reveal nothing abnormal in a woman with an advanced case of endometriosis.

Since the extent of this disease is not related to the degree of its signs and symptoms, a clear, definitive diagnosis of endometriosis must be seriously considered before embarking on a therapeutic program involving any of these symptoms.

GETTING THE RIGHT KIND OF MEDICAL TREATMENT

Endometriosis requires medical treatment—that is, *appropriate* medical treatment—to alleviate its active symptoms and effect on fertility. Unfortunately, endometriosis needlessly remains a major cause of hysterectomy in this country. The surgical removal of the uterus is a radical "cure" that normally is not necessary. In fact, the uterus can be removed and endometrial deposits be missed during surgery, or, worse yet, even "spread" during the operation. And each month, the remaining endometrial deposits will continue to bleed and do internal damage in response to hormonal stimulation.

However, in most cases of endometriosis, there are better ways of treating this condition than taking out the womb. Hysterectomy should be the very last option. In other words, try alternatives first if this is your diagnosis, unless cancer is also present.

Whether you need treatment for endometriosis or can get by with monitoring the condition over time will depend on several factors, including the severity of your symptoms, the degree of reproductive impairment you are experiencing (infertility, painful intercourse, etc.), and your desire for future pregnancy.

Treatments for Endometriosis

Before any treatment is begun, it is essential that your doctor make an accurate diagnosis of endometriosis. Diagnostic laparoscopy—the inspection of the pelvic cavity through a small lighted tube—is currently the only reliable way to confirm that the disease is present. (See chapter 16 for a detailed description of this procedure.) Your doctor may record your laparoscopy on videotape to confirm the diagnosis and help you to understand what is going on inside your body.

In some cases, visual inspection during laparoscopy is not enough to confirm the presence of the disease. Since endometrial deposits vary in color, ebb and flow with the menstrual cycle, and change over time, it is possible to miss them.

If your surgical and/or lab report comes back positive following a laparoscopy, here are a few things you'll want to know:

- How extensive or severe is the endometriosis?

- What surgery was performed during my laparoscopy, if any?

- Are further treatments needed?

- How will this condition and the recommended treatments affect my fertility?

- Should pregnancy be postponed or attempted as soon as possible?

In the absence of cancer, hysterectomy should not be considered until you have been offered less invasive treatments. Remember: the surgical removal of the uterus is *not* the first step in the treatment of endometriosis—it is a last resort only applicable in the most severe cases.

Currently, the best methods of treating endometriosis are laser surgery during laparoscopy or laparotomy, drug suppression of ovarian hormone production, and nutritional supplementation.

Surgical Versus Hormonal Treatment

The surgical removal of endometriosis has significant advantages over attempts to control the condition through hormone suppression treatment. This is particularly true if you can find a gynecologist who is highly skilled in the use of laser surgery. However, you may need—or wish—to try hormone suppression first. The following chart compares the pros and cons to better enable you to make an informed choice between these two options (Figure 70).

Laser Surgery vs. Hormone Suppression Treatment
Figure 70

LASER SURGERY

PROS

Surgery is necessary for a definitive diagnosis of endometriosis. Often endometrial deposits can be removed during a diagnostic laparoscopy.

The removal of endometrial deposits by laser is more likely to give relief from endometriosis for a longer period of time and to prevent recurrence of the disease.

The risks of laser surgery are rare and mostly treatable, whereas the adverse effects associated with hormone treatment are much more common, continue for the duration of treatment (six to nine months), and are disruptive to daily life.

CONS

Your symptoms may be enough for you and your physician to justify hormone treatment first.

Hormone treatment may provide sufficient relief until pregnancy can be established, delaying or preventing the need for surgery until a later date.

The risks of surgery—anesthesia-related complications, infection, hemorrhage, and accidental damage to accessory organs—must be weighed against the side effects of hormones.

HORMONE SUPPRESSION TREATMENT

PROS

Surgery by itself is not always enough to control the spread of endometriosis. New deposits can appear, and some sites may have been missed.

A history of adverse reactions to surgery and/or anesthesia may make hormonal therapy the first treatment of choice.

CONS

There is almost always a recurrence of endometriosis following hormone treatment.

Contraindications to hormone treatment may exist, including: undiagnosed vaginal bleeding, breastfeeding; possibility of pregnancy

HORMONE SUPPRESSION TREATMENT

PROS	CONS
Personal preference for medication over surgery and anesthesia may make hormonal treatment more appealing.	Significant side effects associated with hormones used to treat endometriosis (see Figure 71) may make surgery more desirable.

Laser Surgery. In most cases, endometriosis is diagnosed and treated best during a laparoscopy. But occasionally, a laparotomy may be the only option for diagnosing and/or treating the disease. If the endometriosis is extensive or cannot be adequately removed through a small incision, it may be necessary to reschedule surgery so that a laparotomy can be performed at a later time. (See chapter 16 for a discussion of this procedure.)

Laser surgery uses heat-intense light to cut and remove undesirable or diseased tissue from the body.[8] It has revolutionized surgical treatment for the removal of endometrial deposits. The benefits of laser surgery are many, so be sure ahead of time that your gynecologist is well-trained and willing to perform this procedure during your laparoscopy if necessary. Using a laser beam instead of a scalpel allows for bloodless surgery (the searing heat produced by intense light closes tiny blood vessels at the same time it cuts away affected tissue), the ability to pinpoint and reach poorly accessible areas, and the precise cutting and destruction of endometrial deposits.

Occasionally it is necessary to immediately follow the laparoscopy with a laparotomy to allow for the surgical removal of specific pelvic organs affected by a serious or life-threatening condition, such as cancer. At other times, a laparoscopy may not be possible due to preexisting health problems—obesity or extensive scarring within the abdominal cavity, for example.

Keep in mind that endometriosis is often best located, diagnosed, and surgically treated when it is most active. Therefore, the timing of your laparoscopy should be scheduled just before or during menstruation. At other times of the month, the endometrial deposits may barely be visible and are easier for your doctor to miss. You may also want to request that if a laparoscopy is performed that includes a tissue biopsy (surgical removal of suspicious sections of tissue), the pathology report will be submitted and evaluated while you are still in surgery.

Hormone Suppression Treatment. An alternative or adjunct treatment to laser surgery for the treatment of endometriosis is aimed at stopping or suppressing ovulation for as long a period as possible. Depending on the severity of the disease, your health-care provider may recommend drug therapy with a medication from one of the following drug groups:

- oral contraceptives
- progestational agents (Norplant, Depo-Provera)
- testosterone derivatives (Danocrine, Cyclomen)
- GnRH agonists (Synarel, Suprefact, Lupron, Zoladex)

In mild cases of endometriosis, health-care providers are likely to recommend the use of OCs or progestational drugs to suppress ovulation. (If you choose this route and neither you nor your husband is sterile, you may wish to avoid the potential risk of inducing abortion by using a barrier-method contraceptive.) If your condition is more serious, however, your doctor will likely recommend a drug that will stop ovulation altogether.

The most widely used medicines for stopping ovulation are testosterone derivatives and GnRH agonists.[9] Danazol (Danocrine, Cyclomen), a synthetic form of the male hormone testosterone, reduces the amount of estrogen in the bloodstream while raising the level of testosterone. Consequently, some of the most bothersome aspects of taking this drug are related to its "masculinizing" effects. These include acne, facial hair growth, water retention, weight gain, and deepening of the voice. Danocrine is taken in tablet form by mouth.

The nasal sprays Synarel (nafarelin acetate) and Suprefact (buserelin acetate), and the injectible drugs Lupron (leuprolide acetate) and Zoladex (goserelin acetate), are GnRH agonists (gonadotropin-releasing hormone blockers). They induce a more marked hypoestrogenemic (*hypo*—low; *estro*—estrogen; *nemic*—blood) state than danazol. While this also has significant drawbacks, the adverse effects associated with the administration of a male hormone are avoided.

The suppression of estrogen with all of these hormonal medications stops menstruation and subsequently reverses the growth of endometriosis. Both danazol and GnRH agonists cause the uterine lining to shrink and the endometrial deposits to be reabsorbed into the body, greatly reducing pelvic discomfort. The length of therapy with danazol or a GnRH agonist varies—

between three months to nine months in duration—depending on a woman's reaction to the drug.

Danazol and GnRH agonists are often effective in temporarily treating the symptoms of endometriosis. Because these drugs simulate menopause by decreasing estrogen levels, symptoms such as depression, hot flashes, and insomnia are not unusual. A comparison of the adverse effects of each class of these two types of drugs is shown below (Figure 71). Note: Treatment with danazol or a GnRH agonist should be begun only during menstruation and/or when pregnancy tests are negative. Pregnancy should not be attempted while using these drugs as they may cause abnormalities in the unborn child.

Danazol and Nafarelin: A Comparison of Possible Adverse Effects

Figure 71

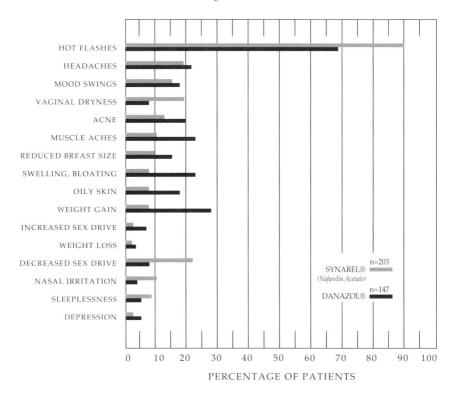

*Adapted from *Physician's Desk Reference*, 45th edition (Oradell, N.J.: Medical Economics Co., Inc., 1991), p. 2207.

In addition to the adverse effects listed, the use of a GnRH agonist for a six-month period or longer has been proven to result in a small loss of bone density (osteoporosis), some of which may not be reversible. For women with major risk factors for osteoporosis (chronic alcohol or tobacco use, strong family history of osteoporosis, or the ongoing use of anticonvulsants or corticosteroids), GnRH agonists pose additional risks. For this reason, the risks and benefits of such treatment must be carefully weighed. In any case, repeated courses of treatment with a GnRH agonist are not advisable.

Variations of Endometriosis

Externally located endometrial cells are normally not cancerous in any way. While normally benign, endometriosis can become malignant. In some situations, the growth of endometriosis on the ureters (tubes that carry urine from the kidneys to the bladder) can result in the obstruction of urine and eventually kidney failure. Both of these complications of endometriosis are potentially life-threatening disorders. They require immediate medical evaluation and attention by a well-qualified gynecologist. However, cancer and kidney failure are very rare complications.

When endometrial cells inside the womb invade the deeper muscle of the uterus itself, the condition is called *adenomyosis*, not endometriosis. Severe menstrual cramps and/or an enlarged uterus may be the result. An alternative name for adenomyosis is "internal endometriosis." Like endometrial deposits outside the uterus, adenomyosis involves tissue that responds to the hormones of the menstrual cycle.

In the healthy womb, there is a natural barrier between the endometrium and the deeper layers of the uterus. This protective border normally defends against the invasion of endometrial tissue. For reasons that are still unknown, this dividing line breaks down in some women. Adenomyosis is the result.

Diagnosing Adenomyosis

Just as with endometriosis, there is a range in the severity of symptoms associated with adenomyosis. Up to 40 percent of women who have adenomyosis have no symptoms whatsoever, while approximately 20 percent experience heavy bleeding and painful cramping during their periods.[10] It is a very difficult condition to diagnose because its symptoms are either silent or seemingly related to other disorders.

In the past, adenomyosis has only been discovered and diagnosed "after the fact," that is, by a pathologist in the lab following hysterectomy. It is unusual to obtain a correct diagnosis for this condition before surgery. The following steps may help you save your uterus if you have adenomyosis.

First, try to discover the cause of chronic pelvic pain, heavy bleeding, and menstrual cramps. Take your menstrual profile and diary to your physician and evaluate your cycles. Ask for a diagnostic ultrasound evaluation and hormone check before surgery or beginning medication. *Magnetic Resonance Imaging,* or MRI, may eventually be employed to great advantage in distinguishing adenomyosis from other reproductive diseases.

Second, if, during a diagnostic laparoscopy, no endometriosis, uterine fibroids, or cancer is found, ask your doctor to take small biopsy samples of the uterus. Laparoscopy can be successfully employed after preliminary diagnostic steps have been taken. Using a needle, your gynecologist can extract a narrow column of tissue from any suspicious areas without damaging your womb. These tissue samples can be sent to a pathologist to be examined while you are still on the operating table. The lab report may indicate whether endometrial tissue has invaded the uterine muscle. On rare occasions, adenomyosis may be present in uterine fibroids, turn into a tumor, or actually grow right through the uterus. If adenomyosis emerges on the outside wall of the uterus, it would appear as endometriosis during a laparoscopy and must be evaluated carefully by your physician and pathologist.

Third, request that your physician remove affected tissue by laser if possible, which is far preferable to a hysterectomy. As one wise physician once said, "Why burn the whole house down in order to catch the mouse?"

Fourth, consider hormone therapy as an alternative to surgery. Like its sister disease, endometriosis, adenomyosis often responds favorably to hormone treatment and nutrition supplements. Danazol or a GnRH agonist may be prescribed to shrink endometrial tissue both inside and outside the uterus. The same comparison of pros and cons should be considered here as for endometriosis (see Figure 70).

Like endometriosis, adenomyosis is not cancer, has not been shown to cause cancer, and is not believed to predispose a woman to developing cancer. In extremely rare cases, it is associated with malignancy, but please put the emphasis here on the words *extremely rare.*

LIVING WITH ENDOMETRIOSIS IS NO LAUGHING MATTER

I doubt if it is possible to have a lighthearted *laissez-faire* attitude about endometriosis. I have it, and I certainly don't. With effective treatments available, I am not considering having a hysterectomy unless another complicating factor arises—continuous, intractable pain, uncontrollable bleeding, or cancer. I'm convinced my uterus offers biological benefits beyond its childbearing role and want to avoid losing it unnecessarily.

If your childbearing years are largely ahead of you, I recommend finding a competent gynecologist to diagnose, evaluate, and treat your endometriosis quickly—the earlier the better.

16

Old and New Diagnostic Techniques— Laparoscopy, Hysteroscopy, D&C, and Laparotomy

Every year about twenty million Americans undergo some type of surgery. Only 20 percent of these operations are emergencies in which neither the patient nor the doctor has a choice about whether or not to operate. The remaining 80 percent are elective surgeries—operations in which the patient, based upon a doctor's recommendation, chooses to have the surgery. Therefore, in the vast majority of cases, there is time to consider alternative therapy and decide how, when, where, and by whom the operation will be done.

Most surgeries do not involve life-threatening conditions, including those discussed in this chapter. They are performed to improve a person's quality of life. As the most operated-on society in the world, Americans have the highest ratio of surgeons per capita and accessibility to the most sophisticated health-care system (hospitals, drug companies, medical suppliers, outpatient clinics, insurance companies) in the world.

As with everything else in life, there are both positive and negative sides to this equation—and consumers are often in the middle. We make the decisions, we have the surgeries, and we pay the bills—either directly or indirectly. This rather complicated fact of life requires us to be smarter than patients have ever had to be before.

In coming years, it is going to get even more complicated as new technologies appear, more options become available, prices continue to escalate, and cost-cutting measures (such as health-care rationing) are forced upon the public. Thus there's no time to waste in acquainting ourselves with ways to negotiate the ins and outs of modern medical care and diagnostic surgery.

All operations are serious and potentially life-threatening—even the most commonplace—as well as being expensive. Surgery should never be taken lightly. Yet when one is absolutely certain that the benefits of a given surgery outweigh the risks after considering all available alternatives, it's possible to be more calm and collected than you might think, especially if you understand what exactly is going to be done and why.

Laparoscopy and Hysteroscopy
Figure 72

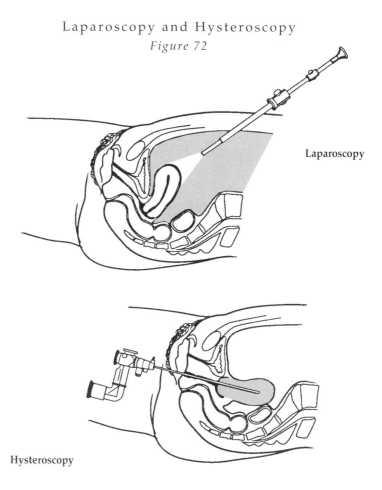

Laparoscopy

Hysteroscopy

Until relatively recently there was little that could be done short of performing major surgery to explore inside the pelvic cavity. Today specially trained surgeons use the technique of laparoscopy (*laparo*—midpelvis; *scopy*—to examine with a lighted instrument) or hysteroscopy (*hystero*—uterus) to see what's going on inside the abdomen or uterus (see Figure 72).

Although laparoscopy and hysteroscopy require the use of anesthesia, these procedures are much less invasive than laparotomy (*laparo*—midpelvis; *tomy*—to perform surgery on), which necessitates at least a five-inch incision through the layers of the abdomen and a four- to six-week recovery period.

Are laparoscopy and hysteroscopy as easy and convenient as some doctors say they are? Not necessarily. As with any other surgery, proceed with caution.

LAPAROSCOPY

Although laparoscopy is performed on an outpatient basis and is not considered major surgery, it *is* surgery. Consequently, it's not without risks. About one woman out of every 120 will experience a significant complication.[1] Approximately one death occurs in every 20,000 laparoscopies performed for diagnostic reasons, whereas the rate of death associated with laparotomy is about one in 1,000—exactly the same as for a hysterectomy.[2]

The risks of complications are lowest for young, healthy women whose gynecologists perform more than 100 laparoscopies annually. Medical factors that increase the risks of laparoscopy are diabetes; obesity; respiratory problems such as asthma, emphysema, and bronchitis; and previous pelvic surgery or pelvic infection.[3] While serious complications and deaths are very rare, you should be familiar with the relative risks of laparoscopy before consenting to the procedure (Figure 73).

Laparoscopy: Possible Risks, Complications, and Contraindications
Figure 73

POSSIBLE RISKS/COMPLICATIONS

Risks of anesthesia, including cardiac arrest, stroke, allergic response to anesthesia or medications used, or respiratory distress.

Accidental surgical damage to the stomach, intestine, bladder, or abdominal blood vessels, with possible resulting infection.

Abnormal blood clot formation in leg or pelvic veins (thrombophlebitis) or a dislodged blood clot in the lungs (embolism).

Formation of scar tissue and adhesions within the pelvic cavity, making additional surgery necessary.

Problems with gas inflation, causing gas to enter the wrong structures—for example, the stomach or bowel.

Upper respiratory problems, including pneumonia or bronchitis.

Irregular heart rhythm patterns due to abdominal stretching or disruption of blood gas levels.

Infection of the urinary tract, the wound, or pelvic organs.

Pelvic infection resulting in permanent damage to the uterus or fallopian tubes.

Peritonitis (infection or inflammation of the lining of the abdominal cavity).

Internal bleeding resulting from accidental damage to a pelvic organ or blood vessel that may occur during surgery or recovery.

External vaginal bleeding caused by instruments used in the cervix or uterus during surgery.

Unsuccessful laparoscopy, resulting in discontinued surgery or laparotomy.

CONTRAINDICATIONS

Absolute—a laparoscopy should not be performed at all if the following condition is present:

> Known or suspected intestinal obstruction.
> (A laparotomy should be performed instead.)

Relative—a laparoscopy should be delayed or performed only if the benefits of the procedure clearly outweigh the possible risks if any of the following conditions are present:

> Uterine (as opposed to tubal) pregnancy.
>
> Severe heart or lung disease.
>
> Peritonitis (inflammation or infection of the abdominal lining).
>
> Hernia of the abdomen or diaphragm.
>
> Large abdominal mass.
>
> Previous abdominal surgery.
>
> Previous pelvic or abdominal infection.
>
> Body weight substantially below or above normal range.

Reading a list of possible problems and risks associated with surgery understandably causes some concern. To determine your risks, discuss your concerns with your doctor. Then you will have a clearer idea of how these risks in your individual case compare to the benefits of laparoscopy for you. When the benefits outweigh the possible risks, then you will be able to proceed with greater peace of mind.

What a Laparoscopy Involves

Indications. Laparoscopy is now a common diagnostic procedure that provides valuable information previously unavailable to physicians without performing major surgery. The conditions for which a laparoscopy is often indicated include:

- Suspected endometriosis, tubal pregnancy, or pelvic infection.
- Pelvic pain of unknown origin.
- Infertility assessment if 1) an X-ray dye test (hysterosalpingogram) shows possible tubal or uterine abnormalities; 2) endometriosis or tubal damage from pelvic infection is suspected; 3) a woman's age makes early diagnosis of the cause of infertility preferable; 4) tubal repair might be advisable; or 5) four to six months of treatment for infertility problems pass without pregnancy taking place.
- Laser surgery to remove and treat a variety of reproductive disorders, including endometriosis, scar tissue (pelvic adhesions), ovarian cysts and tumors, or an early tubal pregnancy.
- Removal of an IUD lost in the pelvic cavity.

If a laparoscopy is indicated. You will be scheduled at the short-stay surgical center of your choice and asked to report sometime in the morning. You will need to have blood drawn prior to the procedure to check your hematocrit (blood count and iron level) as well as your blood type. Since a laparoscopy is an elective (nonemergency), prescheduled surgery, you should be in generally good health when the procedure is performed. On the night before surgery, you will be asked to have nothing to eat or drink after midnight. This is to minimize the risk of involuntary vomiting while you are under general anesthesia.

Hospital admission. When you check into the hospital, you will go through the admissions office and then be taken to your room. A nurse will give you a gown, check your vital signs (blood pressure, pulse, and temperature), take your medical history, and ask you to sign a consent form (see chapter 13 for everything you need to know about informed consent). Before surgery, you may be given a Fleet enema to empty your lower bowel and an injection to dry the secretions in your upper respiratory tract. This makes intubation during anesthesia easier. The upper border of your pubic hair and your abdomen will then be shaved with a disposable razor to allow for a "clean" incision to be made.

Anesthesia. Once you are in the operating room, you will be greeted by your anesthesiologist (a physician who has been specially trained to administer all types of anesthesia) or nurse-anesthetist (a registered nurse who has received additional training to be able to administer general anesthesia). This person will have talked to you beforehand about the type of anesthesia he or she will be using, what you can expect to feel, how it will affect you, and the risks of the anesthesia.

An IV (intravenous tube) will be placed in the back of your hand to administer a drug to cause you to lose consciousness. If you are prone to nausea and/or vomiting, let your anesthesiologist know ahead of time so that a drug can be put in your IV to counteract this tendency. As soon as the medication enters your bloodstream and reaches your brain, you will "go under," and your gynecologist will proceed with the surgery.

What Happens During Surgery

A tube or needle is inserted into the lower abdomen through a small incision just above the pubic hairline to inflate the pelvic cavity with a gas. This distends the area and separates the pelvic organs from the abdominal wall in order to allow your gynecologist to see better. Then the surgeon makes a one-inch incision just below the navel.

In the uppermost incision, a small, lighted stainless steel tube (laparoscope) allows the physician to view all of the reproductive organs—the uterus, ovaries, oviducts, rectum, bladder, and other surrounding structures. These are all clearly visible unless dense scar tissue blocks the view or makes movement of the laparoscope impossible. By moving the laparoscope within the abdomen, your physician can inspect each part of the pelvic cavity carefully.

During the surgery, your doctor may use a laser beam or electrocautery (*electro*—electric current; *cautery*—burning) to remove strands of scar tissue or endometrial deposits if they are not too numerous. Tissue samples may be taken (and preferably analyzed on the spot by a pathologist, if needed), as well as certain surgery performed.

If necessary, dye may be used to check for tubal blockage. The dye is injected through the cervix and allowed to move up through the uterus into the fallopian tubes and out into the pelvic cavity while your physician watches through the laparoscope. Once all appropriate procedures are completed, the inflation gas will be allowed to escape from your abdomen and the instruments removed. Your incisions will then be closed with a few dissolving stitches and covered with Band-Aids (hence the nickname "Band-Aid surgery").

Recovering from Laparoscopy

Following your laparoscopy, you will be taken from the surgical area to a nearby recovery room where you will awake from the anesthesia. This can be quite an odd experience. Your senses of hearing and sensation will normally be the first to return, so you can listen and feel what's going on before you can actually see or talk about it.

Also it's important to remember that if general anesthesia is used, it will cause a complete loss of memory for the time you were unconscious. From the moment you "go under" to when you "come to," there is no sense of the passage of time. It is not the same as sleeping. During sleep, there is both a consciousness of time passing and of body weight and placement. Dreams occur often during sleep but are not experienced during general anesthesia.

Waking up from anesthesia and going home. Upon awaking, you will immediately feel discomfort from the incision and be groggy and possibly dizzy or nauseated. After spending fifteen to forty-five minutes in the recovery room for observation, you will be taken on your cart back to your room, where you will stay until leaving for home. Within two to six hours following surgery, you should feel quite alert and be able to walk without difficulty, although you will be sore. Someone will need to take you home from the hospital since you should not drive for the first twenty-four hours.

Postoperative pain and discomfort. Pain and discomfort after a laparoscopy should not be severe. Pain medication will be prescribed for you to take at home and should effectively manage your discomfort. In addition, some muscle soreness (from muscle relaxants used during surgery), a mild sore throat (from the windpipe tube used for anesthesia), slight vaginal bleeding or spotting (lasting up to two or three days), and shoulder pain (caused by the gas used to inflate your abdomen, which collects under the diaphragm, putting pressure on nerves that affect the shoulders) are common. The gas is usually reabsorbed within twenty-four to thirty-six hours, at which time any abdominal bloating should also subside. Contact your physician immediately if you experience any warning signs (Figure 74).

Warning Signs Following Surgery
Figure 74

Fever: body temperature greater than 100.4 degrees F.

Persistent pain: if lasting longer than twelve hours.

Severe pain or cramps: if not relieved by prescribed medication.

Vaginal bleeding: bright red or heavy bleeding from your vagina that is not a normal menstrual period.

Vaginal discharge: if abnormal or foul-smelling.

Fainting or dizziness: if lasting more than a few seconds.

Breathing difficulties: chest pain, coughing, shortness of breath, difficulty breathing, or coughing blood.

Red or tender skin: if at the incision site.

Bleeding or oozing: from the incision.

Persistent bladder discomfort: burning with urination, blood in your urine, or inability to urinate.

Constipation: more than three days without a normal bowel movement.

If you experience any of the warning signs listed above, contact your physician immediately or go to a hospital emergency room.

At-home care. Watch for danger signs for the entire first week after surgery. Normally the incisions will heal quickly and will itch during the healing process. Keep your incisions covered with Band-Aids—as well as clean and dry—while they are healing. Bathing and showering immediately following a laparoscopy is usually permitted, but double-check with your physician first. If nondissolving sutures were used, they will need to be removed at your doctor's office about a week after your laparoscopy.

As the incisions heal, you will probably notice thickening of the underlying tissue—a firm, tight, knobby area just under the skin. If painless, it means a perfectly normal "reknitting" together of connective tissue is taking place. After several months, this will most likely disappear, and your incisions become lighter in color as the scars form and then almost disappear.

It is normal to feel an increased need for sleep after having general anesthesia. Easily digested foods and snacks, with plenty of liquids you enjoy, will be your best bet the first few days. Get all the rest you can to hasten the healing process.

Follow-up visit. A follow-up visit will be scheduled about two weeks after surgery. The cost is normally included in your bill for the operation. At this time, your doctor will check to see how the incisions are healing, remove any fragments of suture remaining, and discuss recommendations for further treatment, if indicated.

HYSTEROSCOPY: WHAT IT IS AND WHY YOU MIGHT NEED IT

While laparoscopy permits your doctor to view inside your pelvic cavity, hysteroscopy allows her to see inside your cervical canal and uterus using a *hysteroscope* instead of a laparoscope. No incision is necessary. Hysteroscopy can also be performed under general anesthesia in conjunction with a laparoscopy, as part of an infertility evaluation, for example. In some cases, it is possible for a hysteroscopy to be done in your doctor's office under local anesthesia. If the necessary equipment is not available or extensive manipulation of the uterus must be performed, a short-term surgical center is the place to be.

Indications. Hysteroscopy is an excellent way to inspect the cervical canal and uterine cavity to pinpoint or confirm a diagnosis. Over time, it is becoming more widely available as a useful procedure in the evaluation and treatment of such problems as[4]:

- Uterine polyps.
- Uterine fibroids lying just beneath the surface of the uterine lining.
- Abnormal uterine bleeding of unknown cause.
- Uterine cavity abnormalities, including scar tissue blockage, suspected uterine septum (thin sheet of tissue dividing the uterus that can cause infertility and pregnancy problems), diagnosis of the shape of the uterus—especially if you have had repeated miscarriages or an abnormal hysterosalpingogram (X-ray dye study).
- Retrieval of an IUD embedded in the wall of the uterus.
- Evaluation of precancerous cervical abnormalities extending into the cervical canal.

Serious complications are rare. Hysteroscopy is considered minor surgery because instruments do not enter your abdominal cavity and no incisions are made (Figure 75). Instead a telescopelike instrument, called a hysteroscope, is inserted through the vagina and cervix, allowing your gynecologist to view the inside of your uterus.

Hysteroscopy: Possible Risks, Complications, and Contraindications
Figure 75

POSSIBLE RISKS/COMPLICATIONS

Anesthesia complications (paracervical block), including severe allergic reactions or overdose. (For risks related to general anesthesia, see Figure 73.)

Infection via introduction of harmful bacteria into the uterus or spread of a preexisting infection

Damage to the cervix, uterus, or surrounding structures, including perforation of the cervix or uterus, cervical tears, and injury to the bladder, bowel, or blood vessels. The risk of perforation is about one in five hundred, with women at higher risk if they have a very narrow or tight cervical canal.[5]

CONTRAINDICATIONS

Absolute—a hysteroscopy should not be performed at all if any of the following conditions are present:

> Pregnancy
>
> Cervical cancer
>
> Pelvic infection

Relative—a hysteroscopy should be delayed or performed only if the benefits of the procedure clearly outweigh the possible risks if any of the following conditions are present:

> Current menstrual flow
>
> Cervical infection or cervicitis (possibility of bacterial infection)
>
> Possible gonorrhea or chlamydia infection, or recent possible exposure to gonorrhea or chlamydia
>
> Narrow, tight cervical canal (cervical stenosis)
>
> Recent full-term pregnancy, miscarriage, or abortion

A Step-by-Step Guide to What to Expect

If you are going to have a hysteroscopy along with a laparoscopy or as an out-patient in a short-term surgical center, the same information applies as covered in the section above. If you are going to have the procedure done under local anesthesia and/or in your doctor's office, you will be positioned on an exam table with your feet in stirrups as you would be for a normal pelvic exam. Regardless of where the procedure is done, you will want to make absolutely certain you are not pregnant—to avoid inducing an abortion. In addition, you should be checked to make sure that there is no infection in your uterus or fallopian tubes. (Hysteroscopy can cause infection to spread into the pelvic cavity.)

Administration of anesthesia. First, your doctor will perform a bimanual vaginal exam to assess the size and position of your uterus. Next, a speculum will be placed inside your vagina to permit visual access to your cervix. Your vagina and cervix will then be washed with an antiseptic solution before your doctor gives you the local anesthetic. Called a *paracervical block,* injections are made on each side of the cervix to temporarily numb the opening of the uterus. Crampy discomfort is not uncommon during the administration of the anesthetic.

You will still be able to feel sensation in your vagina and abdomen—movements as your physician uses the hysteroscope and/or cramping if the procedure causes the uterus to contract. Patterned breathing will enable you to relax more than if you block your breath or tense up. (Try "IN-two-three; OUT-two-three" at a slow or moderate pace, but be careful. Overbreathing can cause you to hyperventilate.) Concentrate on relaxing your shoulders, abdomen, buttocks, face, hands, and perineum to the maximum extent possible.

If a narrow hysteroscope is used, it probably won't be necessary for your doctor to dilate your cervix. Otherwise your cervix will be dilated as for a D&C (see the last section in this chapter). When ready, your doctor will insert the hysteroscope through your cervical canal and then proceed to carefully examine and inspect each part of your cervix and uterine cavity.

If you require more extensive treatment during your hysteroscopy, the procedure will be done on an outpatient basis at the hospital. Your doctor will need to use a larger hysteroscope, requiring that he expand your uterine cavity slightly with carbon dioxide gas or a liquid solution. The gas or solution is flushed into the uterus gently, holding the walls of the uterus apart to allow your physician to have better visual and manual access with the hysteroscope. This irrigation process continues until your physician is finished. As soon as his examination and any treatments are done, the hysteroscope is removed.

Immediate recovery period. If local anesthesia is used, most women can resume normal activities shortly after a hysteroscopy is performed. If general anesthesia is used, it is possible to return home within several hours and feel back to normal within one or two days.

Post-treatment pain and discomfort. Any fluid or gas that escapes into the pelvic cavity through the fallopian tubes may cause shoulder and abdominal pain or discomfort. The pain subsides within a day or two as the gas or fluid is reabsorbed by the body. No evidence exists that this causes any harmful or persistent adverse effects. Your doctor should prescribe or recommend a pain reliever.

At-home care. It is normal to experience light bleeding or spotting for several days after this procedure—or none at all. You will need to watch for warning signs for the first week after the procedure. In addition to the first seven signs listed in Figure 74, if you experience heavy bleeding for more than six to twelve hours, or if you must use five sanitary pads or more in an hour, contact your physician or go to an emergency room immediately.

As a safety precaution, as with a D&C, you will need to let your cervix heal before using tampons, douching, or resuming intercourse. Such activities might introduce unwelcome bacteria into your reproductive system and result in infection.

DILATION AND CURETTAGE (D&C)

Dilation and curettage, commonly called a D&C, is simply the medical term for "opening and scraping." What is being opened is the cervix, followed by scraping of the uterine lining with a sharp, spoon-shaped instrument called a *curette*, from the French word for cleansing. Approximately one out of every two hundred women in the United States undergoes this procedure every year, making it one of the most frequently performed surgical procedures.[6] Except in an emergency, the primary reason to have a D&C is for your doctor to carefully and thoroughly explore the inside of your uterus and treat specific uterine conditions, which is not possible in an office setting.

A D&C or one of its related procedures allows your doctor to scrape away a part of the uterine lining—the endometrium—for diagnosis (Figure 76). Examining the size, shape, and arrangement of cells obtained during a D&C enables a pathologist to determine whether cancer is present. Precancerous changes in the uterine lining may be detected as well. Furthermore, hormonal irregularities and polyps (small protruding growths attached by a stem) can show up during the pathologist's microscopic examination of specially prepared slides.

Dilation and Curettage
Figure 76

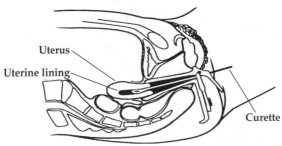

Uterus

Uterine lining

Curette

Prior to *Roe v. Wade*, most of us didn't think of a D&C as a method of abortion, although it was frequently used in this way. Today D&C—used along with vacuum aspiration of the uterus—is the most common method of surgical abortion in the United States. In spite of this, a D&C can be a life-enhancing rather than a life-destroying procedure when performed for an appropriate reason (see Figure 77). This procedure is normally done to evaluate or treat abnormal uterine bleeding. Since abnormal uterine bleeding can be an early sign of uterine cancer or may indicate precancerous changes in the lining of the uterus, it's important to try to find out why the bleeding is taking place.

Reasons to Have a D&C
Figure 77

- To treat heavy bleeding or hemorrhage as an emergency measure.
- To remove fragments of placental tissue remaining after childbirth.
- To evacuate the uterus after a baby has been lost during the early stages of pregnancy if heavy bleeding precludes a safe, natural miscarriage.
- To remove uterine polyps (a condition that causes tissue to thicken in one area instead of throughout the entire uterus).
- To fully assess the extent of uterine cancer after it has already been diagnosed.
- To identify and evaluate endometrial hyperplasia (an overgrowth of the uterine lining).
- To identify and evaluate hormone response of the uterine lining.
- To identify and evaluate any existing cancer.
- To distinguish between endocervical and endometrial cancer.

A Common Diagnostic Alternative to D&C

A type of diagnostic scraping of the uterine lining that is simpler and less invasive than a complete D&C is available. Called *endometrial biopsy*, this procedure takes a few shreds of the uterine lining for microscopic evaluation and requires little or no cervical dilation. Though a local block may be used to numb the cervix, it is possible that no anesthesia will be required. A slender plastic tube is inserted into the uterus through the cervical canal. The uterine lining is then scraped using suction (*aspiration curettage*, or *vacuum scraping*).

In the past, D&C was commonly used to diagnose causes for abnormal vaginal bleeding. Today endometrial biopsy is commonly employed as an alternative.

If a D&C Is Indicated: What to Expect

If your medical condition indicates that a D&C is the preferred diagnostic choice, you will want to review the hospital admission and surgical preparation information listed under the section on laparoscopy. Also be sure that you discuss the benefits and risks associated with a D&C with your gynecologist prior to the procedure (Figure 78).

D&C: Possible Risks, Complications, and Contraindications
Figure 78

POSSIBLE RISKS AND COMPLICATIONS

Complications of anesthesia (see Figure 73)

Infection

Hemorrhage

Damage to the uterus or adjacent organs—blood vessels, bladder, or bowel

Scar tissue formation inside the uterus (Asherman's syndrome—can result in infertility and the absence of menstruation.)

CONTRAINDICATIONS

Absolute—a D&C should not be performed at all if the following condition is present:

A viable pregnancy

CAUTION: A D&C WILL INDUCE ABORTION. IF YOU ARE PREGNANT, DO NOT HAVE A D&C UNLESS IT IS NECESSARY TO SAVE YOUR LIFE.

Relative—a D&C should be delayed or performed only if the benefits of the procedure clearly outweigh the possible risks if any of the following conditions are present:

Uterine, tubal, or cervical infection

Heart, kidney, or respiratory problems, placing one in a
high-risk category for anesthesia

Any blood clotting disorder that could result in excessive bleeding

---

The procedure itself. General anesthesia (loss of consciousness) or a regional anesthetic block (loss of sensation from the diaphragm to the toes) will be administered to you to eliminate the pelvic pain caused by intense cramping that cannot be totally blocked by local anesthesia. After your inner thighs, vulva, and vagina are completely cleansed with a soapy solution, you will be draped with sterile towels and then be given a thorough pelvic examination. A speculum is then placed inside the vagina, allowing your gynecologist to see your cervix. While holding the cervix steady with a clamp called a *tenaculum*, your doctor then assesses the angle of your cervix and the depth of your uterus. Tissue specimens may be obtained from the cervical canal at this time.

The surgeon will follow these procedures by dilating the cervical canal with tapered metal rods in graduated sizes so the cervix is slowly opened. After the cervix is sufficiently dilated, your doctor will carefully collect tissue samples from the uterine lining for microscopic evaluation by a pathologist (Figure 76). Polyps may also be removed at this time. *Caution: Aggressive scraping of the uterine lining may result in permanent scarring and impaired fertility.* Be clear with your doctor about this concern prior to surgery and have a "complete" D&C only if it is absolutely necessary.

When necessary, the uterine cavity is "evacuated" to assist the process of a miscarriage or delivery of the afterbirth if fragments of the placenta remain attached following childbirth. This is done in order to prevent or treat heavy bleeding (*hemorrhage*).

Recovering from D&C. Once anesthesia has been given, the entire procedure takes about ten to fifteen minutes. As with a laparoscopy or a laparotomy, you will be kept in a recovery room until you awaken. Then you will return to your hospital room until you're ready to be discharged and go home.

Light bleeding or spotting for a few days following a D&C is normal. Elevated body temperature, severe cramps, persistent abdominal pain, heavy vaginal bleeding (lasting more than twelve hours or requiring more than five pads in one hour), a feeling of faintness or dizziness for more than a few seconds, or an abnormal or foul-smelling vaginal discharge are not. (See Figure 74 for a complete list of warning signs following surgery.) *Contact your gynecologist or go immediately to a hospital emergency room if you experience any of these symptoms after your surgery.*

Any lab reports related to your D&C should be completed within one week of your surgery, though if cancer is suspected, some surgeons ask for an evaluation to be made while you are still under anesthesia. Most hospitals are not equipped for this, however. For this reason, when you give your consent for an in-hospital D&C, look for the wording "and a possible hysterectomy" on your form. If you want to wait before having a hysterectomy (in order to have your lab report confirmed by an outside source and/or to seek a second opinion), do not sign the form until it has been reworded to your satisfaction.

Note: The interpretation of pathology specimens on slides varies with the expertise of the clinician performing the evaluation. For this reason, some gynecologists *routinely* request an outside opinion on their patients' slides.

It is advisable to avoid intercourse, tampons, and douching (i.e., don't put anything in your vagina) until the uterus has healed in order to prevent infection-causing bacteria from being introduced into the uterus. The cervical canal should return to its normal size in about two weeks, at which time you should see your gynecologist for a follow-up appointment to check for signs of uterine infection and to make sure your cervix is healing properly.

LAPAROTOMY

Compared to laparoscopy, hysteroscopy, and D&C, a laparotomy (or "exploratory surgery") is major surgery and should be approached cautiously (Figure 79). It requires an incision five to six inches long, including incisions through several layers of abdominal tissue and several major muscle groups. As a result, postoperative pain and discomfort are significantly greater, both in length and severity. Laparotomy involves a greater amount of anesthesia, an inpatient hospital stay, and longer recovery. Also internal scarring (*pelvic adhesions*) is much more common following a laparotomy. This scarring can produce later discomfort as well as impair a woman's fertility in the future.

Laparotomy: Possible Risks, Complications, and Contraindications
Figure 79

POSSIBLE RISKS AND COMPLICATIONS

Anesthesia-related complications (see Figure 73)

Infection in the wound, uterus, tubes, or pelvic cavity

Hemorrhage, possibly necessitating blood transfusion

Accidental damage to the uterus, bladder, bowel, ureters, or blood vessels

Urinary tract problems—infection, inability to urinate, burning with urination

Burn injury to the bladder or bowel if cautery is used to remove endometriosis

Abnormal blood clot formation (thrombophlebitis) in leg or pelvic veins, with potential for pulmonary embolism (clot could break loose and travel to the lung, resulting in serve respiratory distress, stroke, or death)

CONTRAINDICATIONS

Absolute—there are no absolute contraindications to this procedure when laparotomy is used as an essential or life-saving procedure.

Relative—a laparotomy should be delayed or performed only if the benefits of the procedure clearly outweigh the possible risks if any of the following conditions are present:

Uterine pregnancy

Severe heart or lung disease

Diabetes, heart, kidney, or respiratory problems, placing one
in a high-risk category for anesthesia

Any blood clotting disorder that could result in excessive bleeding

Indications. The advantage of a laparotomy over a laparoscopy is that it allows the gynecologist to confirm a diagnosis and treat the problem all in one step. Sometimes this is warranted. If your doctor thinks internal hemorrhage, overwhelming infection, or invasive cancer are present, laparotomy may be the best option. It is *not*, however, a usual "first step" in the treatment of endometriosis or many other disorders unless serious contraindications to laparoscopy exist.

Laparotomy is indicated:

- To examine and treat an enlarged ovary.
- To correct a structural abnormality of the uterus.
- To remove benign uterine fibroids.
- To remove extensive endometriosis.
- To repair damage to the fallopian tubes.
- To diagnose and treat internal hemorrhage or severe infection.

Note: Laparotomy may be your best—or only—option when laparoscopy would be too limited a procedure to treat the problem correctly or is contraindicated by your medical condition.

What to Expect

Hospital admission and anesthesia. The preliminary steps leading up to a laparotomy are similar to those for a laparoscopy, but you will be admitted to the inpatient surgical section of the hospital instead of the short-stay center. In addition to the preoperative performed prior to a laparoscopy, you will also need to have a tube inserted into your bladder, called a *catheter*, for a longer period of time—both during and after surgery.

An incision is made into your abdominal cavity just above the pubic hair line. If extensive surgery is anticipated, a vertical incision may be required instead. The incision opening involves several layers: the skin, muscles, and connective tissue, and the peritoneum, the thin membrane that lines your pelvic cavity. Your intestine, gall bladder, liver, kidneys, and other abdominal organs will be checked for abnormalities after the incision is made. Instruments will then be used to hold the incision open and move your intestines out of the way to allow for access to your ovaries, fallopian tubes, and uterus.

Depending on the reason for your surgery, any procedures that you have previously discussed with your physician and consented to will be performed at this time. Unexpected findings may require additional steps beyond what you had anticipated, but a thorough discussion beforehand will have prepared you for this possibility.

The internal incisions will be closed with dissolving sutures, whereas the incision on your skin may be closed by temporary stitches or metal clips (removed after several days), or by absorbable stitches.

Recovery period and postoperative pain management. You will be in the recovery room for about an hour and then moved back to your hospital room. For the first couple of days, patients report experiencing a significant degree of pain following laparotomy. Pain shots will be given periodically to reduce discomfort until you are able to swallow and absorb pills. Since you cannot eat or drink for a few days, IV fluids will be given instead. This is because bowel activity stops temporarily after any major abdominal surgery.

The hospital stay. The usual hospital stay following laparotomy is five to seven days. The length of time will depend on how much surgery was involved, what you were being treated for, and how your recovery is progressing. If you experience any of the warning signs listed for laparoscopy (see Figure 74), you need immediate medical attention.

For the first four days after surgery, your incision will need to be kept clean and dry. After this, no special precautions concerning bathing or showering are necessary. It is normal for the incision to form a firm, tender cord just beneath the skin as it heals, which will eventually decrease in size over the next six to twelve months. Surgical incisions appear pink initially, then fade in color; numbness in the area is also not uncommon. Sensation should return within the next few months. Most postoperative problems women encounter are in the first few days following surgery before returning home, so be sure to talk to your nurse or doctor about any questions or concerns.

At-home care. Recovering at home is preferable to the hospital—once you are up to it—because it is more familiar to you and usually much quieter. Also there are fewer germs in your home environment, so there is less chance of acquiring a hospital-induced infection. You also have greater choice over what you eat and when you eat. And last but certainly not least, home recovery is obviously much less expensive.

For the first week or two, you will need lots of rest and someone to perform all household tasks, including child care, cooking, shopping, and the laundry. If you have young children at home, consider staying with a friend or relative for the first five to seven days after being released or having someone come to stay with you to watch the children while you stay in bed. A return to full household duties or outside work should not be planned until six weeks after surgery.

$\mathcal{W}$hen Is
Hysterectomy Needed?

H ysterectomy, the surgical removal of the uterus, which may also include removal of the fallopian tubes, the cervix, and/or the ovaries, can be an extremely valuable operation when a woman's condition indicates that it is necessary or unavoidable.

If the problem you have is serious and alternative treatments are ineffective, the possible risks of hysterectomy should be carefully considered against the possible benefits. Since newer treatments are being developed all the time, it is especially important to obtain up-to-date information. (See "Resources.") In addition, not all treatments are currently available in all places. If this is true in your case, you may need to travel outside your community to locate a skilled gynecologist.

Nearly 600,000 hysterectomies are done in the United States annually.[1] The procedure is the second most frequently performed major surgical procedure among reproductive-aged women. An estimated 8.6 million women had a hysterectomy between 1980 and 1993.[2] Hysterectomy for a cancer or precancer diagnosis accounts for only 9 to 10 percent of the total number of operations performed; uterine fibroids, pelvic relaxation, endometriosis, and adenomyosis—conditions considered to be relative indications for hysterectomy—account for almost 80 percent.[3] With innovative advances in laser and laparoscopic surgery, I believe this will change as women become increasingly aware of their options to hysterectomy.

ABSOLUTE INDICATIONS FOR HYSTERECTOMY

In the following situations, a hysterectomy may save your life:

- You have invasive uterine, cervical, vaginal, tubal, or ovarian cancer.
- You have severe, uncontrollable bleeding.
- You have a severe, uncontrollable infection (pelvic inflammatory disease, or PID).
- You have a life-threatening blockage of the bladder or intestines and the primary problem cannot be treated without also removing your uterus.
- You are having a cesarean section or giving birth and experience severe, uncontrollable hemorrhage.

In all other medical situations, hysterectomy is an elective procedure. If you are not facing one of these life-threatening problems, you have time to consider the pros and cons of hysterectomy—as well as to find out about possible alternatives—before deciding to have this operation.[4]

In addition to the critical, life-threatening problems that are absolute indications that a hysterectomy should be performed, there are a number of relative indications for hysterectomy. In the following cases, hysterectomy is not performed to save a woman's life, but to alleviate significant discomfort and treat serious or disabling symptoms:

RELATIVE INDICATIONS FOR HYSTERECTOMY
(INCLUDES PERCENTAGE OF ALL HYSTERECTOMIES PERFORMED)

- 30 percent—Uterine fibroids (also called *myomas, myofibromas, fibromyomas,* or *leiomyomas*).
- 19 percent—Endometriosis.
- 16-29 percent—Pelvic relaxation involving bladder or bowel dysfunction, and uterine prolapse (the uterus "dropping down" into the vagina).
- 10-19 percent—Chronic pelvic pain (CPP).
- 6 percent—Endometrial hyperplasia (overgrowth of the uterine lining).

- Excessive vaginal bleeding.
- Recurrent pelvic infections or chronic infection.

UTERINE FIBROIDS: #1 REASON FOR HYSTERECTOMY

As many as one in four women will be diagnosed with uterine fibroids during their reproductive years—most between the ages of thirty and fifty. (See Figure 80.) Research suggests that 40 to 75 percent of all women develop fibroids during their lifetime. Many of those affected will never know they have the condition because the majority of women experience no symptoms or complications.

Facts About Fibroids
Figure 80

Fibroids occur in women of all ages:
Fifty percent of women over age fifty and at least twenty percent of women over age thirty have them.[5]

Fibroids are almost always benign:
Approximately 99.8 percent of all fibroids are benign. In two cases out of 1,000, a fibroid is found to be malignant.[6] Fibroids may be removed to check for cancer without removing the uterus.

Fibroids vary in size and symptoms produced:
They can range in size from 1 cm. ("pea-size") to more than 15 cm. ("cantaloupe-size"); occur singly or, most often, in groups; and can cause heavy menstrual periods, cramps, spotting, frequent urination, abdominal pressure, and infertility. However, most women with uterine fibroids have no symptoms at all.

Fibroids may be hereditary:
Three times as many black women suffer from fibroids as do white women. There may also be an increased risk if a woman's mother has a history of fibroids.

Fibroids should be left alone unless they are very large, cause distressing symptoms, or are growing rapidly:
Bleeding, excessive discomfort, or interference with normal uterine, bladder, or kidney function all warrant appropriate medical treatment.

Fibroids are not an absolute indication for hysterectomy:
Hysterectomy should be considered only when symptoms warrant removal of the uterus, especially for women of childbearing age. Less radical treatment—laser surgery, myomectomy, drug therapy, even nontreatment—should almost always be considered as possible alternatives to hysterectomy.

No one yet knows why uterine fibroids develop, though some researchers believe that they grow in response to estrogen. The fact that fibroids are stimulated to grow during pregnancy (when estrogen levels are very high) and shrink after menopause (when estrogen levels drop) lends credence to this theory.

A complex hormonal mechanism may be responsible for this phenomenon—the existence of *estrogen receptors* inside fibroid tissue. What these receptors may do is "lock up" the ability of cells to grow in a healthy way when they "pick up" estrogen molecules.[7] In other words, the absorption of estrogen by uterine muscle cells may be what causes fibroids.

Uterine fibroids have a characteristic "whorling-band" pattern to identify them. These abnormal masses of tissue can be soft, firm, hardened, or liquid-filled; they may be "encapsulated," (inside a membrane as a separate structure from the uterine wall) or "invasive" (embedded within the uterine wall by means of a network of microscopic rootlike fibers). They can grow on all levels of the uterus, but are thought to originate from within muscle tissue within the uterine wall.

Specific names have been assigned to different types of fibroid growths (Figure 81).

Types of Fibroids

Figure 81

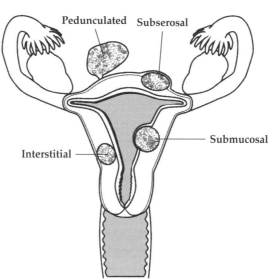

- *Submucosal fibroids* bulge out from beneath the uterine lining into the uterine cavity.

- *Interstitial (or intramural) fibroids* grow deep within the uterine wall.

- *Subserosal* fibroids bulge outwards through the surface of the uterus.

- *Pedunculated fibroids* grow on a "stalk" and are usually of the submucosal or subserosal variety.

Getting the Treatment You Need

Remember: *Fibroids are usually not cancerous or dangerous.* Many medical experts believe that fibroid growths should be left alone unless they interfere with normal reproductive or urinary function. Symptoms requiring medical evaluation include:

- Prolonged, irregular, and/or heavy menstruation.

- Painful or crampy periods.

- Abdominal swelling.

- Pressure or obstruction of pelvic organs (due to fibroid growth) resulting in frequent urination; abdominal, back, and/or pelvic pain; or constipation.

- Problems with pregnancy (infertility, miscarriage, or premature birth).

- Vaginal bleeding after menopause.

The smaller the growths are, the less likely a woman is to experience any symptoms. Diagnosis is often made during a bimanual pelvic examination when the physician finds that the uterus is lumpy, enlarged, or an irregular shape. Further examination by pelvic or vaginal ultrasound enables a gynecologist to obtain a clearer picture of what is going on. An endometrial biopsy, D&C, or hysteroscopy may be recommended in the case of abnormal menstrual bleeding, at which time the physician may detect bumps indicating fibroids.

Sometimes a physician misses the diagnosis. If you suspect you may have a fibroid tumor due to your symptoms, see your doctor again later, ask for an ultrasound scan (sonogram), or obtain a second opinion.

So how do you know when—and how—to deal with fibroids if your doctor confirms that you have them? There is *no rush to proceed with immediate*

surgery unless you are experiencing severe, uncontrollable bleeding or intense pain.
Take time to ask your gynecologist any or all of the following questions:

- What can I expect if we do nothing to treat the fibroid?
- If treatment is recommended at this time, what are the possible alternatives to hysterectomy?
- Are you trained to perform laser surgery or traditional myomectomy? If not, to whom can you refer me?
- What is your opinion of hormone treatment for fibroids?
- How might this affect future pregnancies I might have?
- Is the fibroid located in an area that might endanger my fertility later on?

Examining Your Options

My friend Sally was told that she needed a hysterectomy for fibroids and called to ask if I thought it was really necessary. We discussed her symptoms. Sally didn't want to permanently close the door on childbearing and understandably felt reluctant to have her uterus taken out. She decided to seek a second opinion, emphasizing to her next gynecologist that she might want to have another baby.

Firmly and politely, Sally informed the physician of her preference, saying that she did not want to have a hysterectomy unless it was absolutely necessary. Her new doctor quickly got the point. He did not recommend a hysterectomy, but offered her several alternatives. What surprised Sally most of all was how well he explained why she didn't need a hysterectomy at present, in spite of what she had previously been told.

A range of alternatives are available to the majority of women with uterine fibroids:

Monitoring. Also called waiting, this approach offers the option of periodic pelvic exams to evaluate the rate and amount of fibroid tissue growth. If growth accelerates, do not panic. Cancer is a remote possibility and can usually be detected without a hysterectomy. Hysterectomy should not be considered solely because there is a risk of cancer.

"Monitoring" the growth of uterine fibroids is sometimes misleading. The disadvantage of this option is that it can fool women into thinking their doctor has given them a "reprieve." Be aware that some fibroids, if not treated early, become much worse over a relatively brief period of time. This may actually *increase* your likelihood of having a hysterectomy in the long run. Consequently, women frequently find themselves being offered hysterectomy once symptoms have convinced them that it's finally necessary—*after* it's too late to have less radical surgery that spares the uterus.

Another drawback to a passive "let's-wait-and-see" attitude is that pelvic exams and ultrasound scans don't always provide all the data you need to make an informed choice. A bimanual pelvic examination does not normally determine the location of all possible fibroids or their rate of growth. Furthermore, if you are in much pain, your physician cannot apply enough external pressure to check all suspected tumor areas. In addition, if you have excessive fatty deposits overlying the uterus, the thickness of the abdominal wall may preclude a reliable exam.

The drawback to an ultrasound scan is that it can appear that you have a fibroid when actually you don't. That's because other conditions can look like some types of fibroids on ultrasound. Ultrasound also may not reveal the number and location of all the fibroid growths you might have—just as a pelvic exam does not. *Only surgery can determine the true extent of the fibroids,* and even then some fibroids can be missed.

If your fibroids are not very large, not growing rapidly, or not causing uncomfortable symptoms, monitoring your condition may be the right approach for now. But watch diligently. Keep track of any changes in your symptoms and schedule appropriate exams with your gynecologist frequently. Most of all, be prepared to intervene with a D&C, hysteroscopy, laparoscopy, and/or myomectomy (see below) when indicated to avoid a hysterectomy in the future.

If you decide to wait, you may want to use a pain reliever (such as those listed in chapter 2) for menstrual cramps—but *don't ignore any pelvic pain that continues to get worse or suddenly becomes severe.* Fiber supplements for constipation may be helpful as well. In any case, you will benefit from reaching (or maintaining) your ideal weight to lower your blood level of estrogen. Eat nutritious low-fat, complex carbohydrate foods.

Drug treatment. Hormonal treatment of fibroids merits serious consideration for some women.[8] The hormones used are called GnRH agonists (see chapter 16), synthetic hormones that suppress estrogen production and imitate menopause. In addition to effectively shrinking fibroids prior to surgery, GnRH agonists are also used to treat other diseases affected by ovarian hormones, including endometriosis, breast cancer, and polycystic ovarian disease. Note: GnRH agonists (Lupron, Synarel) should always be administered under close medical supervision.

Drug treatment to shrink uterine fibroids prior to surgery facilitates the procedures of myomectomy (see below) or hysterectomy. Tumor shrinkage can improve the likelihood that the surgery will be successful. It also may reduce the risk of excessive blood loss and permit the use of vaginal (versus an abdominal) hysterectomy if removal of the uterus becomes necessary.

Hormonal treatment for fibroids is not long-term. While this treatment is used primarily before fibroid surgery, for women nearing natural menopause surgery may be avoided altogether by using a GnRH agonist. (However, if hormone replacement therapy using estrogen becomes necessary, the fibroids will most likely be stimulated to grow again.) The adverse effects associated with any hormonal treatment must be seriously weighed against possible benefits.

In recent years more physicians are prescribing oral contraceptives as an alternative drug treatment for both uterine fibroids and endometriosis. Research suggests that women who take OCs for these reasons experience less bleeding and reduced pain.

Myomectomy. Myomectomy is the surgical removal of uterine tissue or fibroid growths (Figure 82). It is a uterine-sparing procedure that has traditionally been reserved for women who wished to remain fertile or as a treatment for infertility. It is an exacting, time-consuming operation requiring advanced surgical training and, as such, is not offered by many gynecologists as an alternative to hysterectomy.

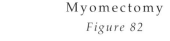

Myomectomy

Figure 82

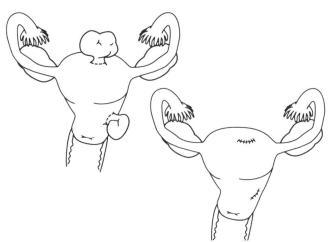

Because the uterus is a highly vascular (supplied with blood) organ, a myomectomy can cause profuse bleeding, requiring a blood transfusion. However, laser surgery and presurgical hormonal treatment significantly decrease this potential problem.

In the past myomectomy could only be performed in conjunction with laparotomy. With advances in fiber-optic technology and laser surgery, some types of fibroids can be excised during laparoscopy or hysteroscopy.[9] As with laparoscopy for any other condition, the advantages are significantly less pain after surgery, a much shorter hospital stay, quicker recovery, and a faster return to a normal activity schedule.

A commonly cited disadvantage to myomectomy is that fibroids may recur. Research reports on the incidence of this recurrence vary widely—from 2 to 3 percent,[10] to 10 percent,[11] to 25 percent,[12] and up to even 40 percent[13]. The availability of what may perhaps be the best surgical alternative to hysterectomy—myomectomy using laser surgery—is limited at present.

Depending on the extent of the incision(s) made on the uterus, a vaginal birth following myomectomy may not be advisable. If the uterine muscle is weakened by the surgery, labor contractions may cause the scars to separate during childbirth. Cesarean section may become medically necessary, so be sure to discuss this possibility with your gynecologist ahead of time. If your desire is to have children in the future, this may be acceptable to you.

Endometriosis may make the timing of your myomectomy critical. To prevent the spread of endometriosis into the muscular portion of the uterine wall as a result of surgery, it has been recommended that surgery be scheduled during the first eight days of the menstrual cycle.[14]

PELVIC RELAXATION AND PELVIC PAIN

In addition to uterine fibroids, endometriosis, and bleeding difficulties, there are two more relative indications for hysterectomy—pelvic relaxation and pelvic pain.

Pelvic Relaxation

Imagine the base of your pelvis as a muscular sheath similar to a hammock. Over the years the weight of your pelvic organs places pressure on the hammock, causing it to sag and stretch. Pregnancy, large fibroids, hormonal disturbances, obesity, and the long-term effects of gravity can all contribute to the stretching and sagging process, eventually leaving the uterus with little support.

In its downward descent, the uterus can fall forward, backward, or straight down. Accompanying pressure on the bladder, rectum, bowels, or vagina may cause further tissue damage, pushing these organs out of their normal position as well. This is not a new problem, needless to say, since women have been having babies ever since Eve.

Degrees of Uterine Prolapse
Figure 83

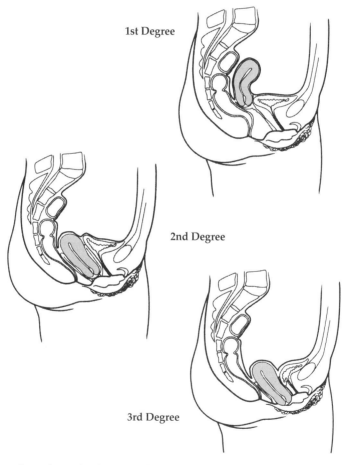

1st Degree

2nd Degree

3rd Degree

Reading about the history of treatment for uterine prolapse, one quickly is convinced that there has never been a perfect solution to this problem. Honey paste, pessaries, uteroabdominal supporters, astringents, cold sitz baths, seawater douches, postural exercises, and even leeching have been tried. Today hysterectomy is the most common medically prescribed solution for this condition.

In the most severe cases, the uterus sags down into the vagina and can even protrude from the body (Figure 83). This is not a pleasant experience, to say the least. For a married woman, lovemaking and her self-image as a sexual person may suffer. Nothing compares to being told by a doctor that your vagina is in bad shape for "a woman of your age." (It's not as if there is an abundance of highly specialized fitness classes to correct the problem, if you know what I mean.)

Short of having a hysterectomy, what can be done? First of all, it's important to remember that prolapse is a normal phenomenon that comes with the process of aging. Second, if the degree of prolapse is not severe enough to cause disabling symptoms, you don't need to worry about it. Third, exercising the pelvic floor muscles correctly at the first sign of prolapse may help to prevent it from getting worse. Fourth, hormone replacement therapy (HRT) for postmenopausal women may contribute to genital muscle strength and slow the rate of prolapse. If you are considering this approach, become informed about the full spectrum of risks and benefits related to HRT first.

Note: Beware of doing pelvic floor (Kegel) exercises without being taught on an individual basis how to do them correctly—it's easier than you might think to do them the wrong way. Biofeedback specialists trained to use a device called a *perineometer* offer a type of fitness class that trains women—in private—how to contract and relax pelvic floor muscles to counteract pelvic relaxation. The perineometer is placed in the vagina to measure the strength of contractions and allow the woman to see how she may voluntarily control specific muscles to increase strength. Check your local Yellow Pages. I'm serious. It just may save your uterus.

If you have any of the following symptoms, you may have a significant degree of uterine prolapse worth doing something about:

- Lower abdominal pressure that increases as the day passes.
- Lower backache.
- Pain during intercourse.
- Frequent urination.
- Difficult bowel movements.

As an alternative to hysterectomy, the uterus can be surgically resuspended in its normal position higher in the pelvis. This is done by cutting the ligaments that suspend the uterus and shortening them. Like myomectomy, it has traditionally been a rarely performed procedure reserved for women who want to have more children. Consequently, if you are considering having this surgery done, you would need to find a surgeon who has plenty of experience doing it.

Surgical repositioning can be used on all degrees of uterine prolapse, avoiding the loss of the uterus and the long-term effects of hysterectomy. The advantages of this approach also include a much shorter hospital stay and recovery period, preservation of fertility and normal menstrual and hormonal function, no shortening of the vagina, and no impediment to normal sexual intercourse.

Results can be mixed. If the prolapse is especially severe, uterine resuspension may be less than 100 percent successful. Also prolapse can recur. However, doctors rarely discuss the possibility of secondary prolapse following a hysterectomy. Because the uterus is placed centrally within the pelvic cavity, its removal may cause inadequately suspended organs (the vagina, bladder, and rectum) to fall. If surgery during hysterectomy doesn't repair these weakened areas, a secondary prolapse may result.

Some women avoid hysterectomy by using a latex ring-shaped device called a vaginal pessary. It is manually inserted into the vagina in much the same way as a diaphragm. Designed to hold the uterus in place, it must be fitted and inserted by a physician and be removed periodically for cleaning. The disadvantages to this device are that the pessary can interfere with lovemaking; it may cause an irritating discharge with an unpleasant odor; and most gynecologists are no longer trained to fit pessaries—they're trained to do hysterectomies instead.[15]

Pelvic Pain

In his book *Women's Health Alert,* Dr. Sidney Wolfe asserts that "the perplexing problem of chronic pelvic pain (CPP) remains a huge gray area because by definition the problem can't be pinpointed to a specific disease. Unfortunately, too often the 'solution' is a hysterectomy where a completely healthy uterus is removed."[16] This is especially disturbing when one considers that 10 to 19 percent of all hysterectomies in the United States are performed for this reason.[17]

If a thorough physical examination and laparoscopy show that no abnormality exists, a hysterectomy should not be performed. Gynecologist and researcher Dr. Robert Reiter, at the University of Iowa, puts it this way: "When you don't see anything there, it doesn't make much sense to take out normal tissue."[18]

In a significant study published in 1990, Dr. Reiter and his colleagues reported following 250 women for CPP after they had been told they needed hysterectomies despite a normal laparoscopy. Fifty of these women had already had hysterectomies and still had chronic pelvic pain.

Amazingly, what Dr. Reiter discovered was that half of the women in the group had identifiable reasons for their pain that had been missed. Even more astounding is the fact that for 80 percent of these 125 women, the cause of their pain was not gynecologic.[19] Instead, the pain was being caused by bladder and abdominal wall problems, irritable bowels, and other conditions not related to the reproductive organs. What this means is that none of these women needed a hysterectomy, and a hysterectomy would not have cured their chronic pelvic pain.

For the remaining 125 women, Dr. Reiter found the pain to be psychological in origin, caused by sexual abuse, stress disorders, and/or depression. Many of the women had been sexually molested or assaulted—a fact that previous physicians had not even discovered.

"What is tragic about this," says Dr. Reiter, "is that the doctor, even with the best intentions, doesn't realize that the last thing in the world a woman needs is to have another assault on her sexual organs, as if the original trauma were not enough." He goes on to say that these women "continue to pay and pay, because, as our research shows, they continue to experience multiple physical symptoms which keep them returning to doctors, searching for physical explanations."[20]

Dr. Wolfe makes this recommendation to any woman suffering from relentless pelvic pain whose physician immediately recommends a hysterectomy: *Shop for a new physician.*[21] Any woman with CPP should be given a full range of diagnostic tests, including a psychological evaluation, and be offered alternatives to hysterectomy. It's essential to find a cause for the pain, including possible emotional or lifestyle causes, and then to treat the cause—not simply remove the uterus.

NON-INDICATIONS FOR HYSTERECTOMY

Just so you know, hysterectomy is not indicated as a treatment for:

- Pelvic pain of unknown origin.
- Small fibroids with no symptoms.
- Mild abnormal uterine bleeding.
- Menstrual cramps.

- Pelvic or abdominal pressure.
- Cervicitis (irritated cervix; heavy discharge).
- Pelvic congestion (menstrual irregularities; low back pain).
- Fertility (sterilization).

TAKE TIME OUT TO RECONSIDER

Why make such a big deal about this? Haven't many women had hysterectomies who were glad to be done with menstruation, birth control, cramps, and other "female problems"? Since the uterus can develop cancer, is it a good idea just to take it out? After having her last child, what woman needs a womb?

Perhaps I'm somewhat old-fashioned, but I think my uterus is just fine as far as body organs go. I'm not going to lose it without a very good reason. Why should I face the risks, the pain, and the expense of this major operation if it's not absolutely necessary? (See Figure 88.)

Hysterectomy: Possible Risks and Complications[22]
Figure 84

DEATH

There are between 1 and 2 out of every 1,000 cases, or 600-1,200 hysterectomy-related deaths in the U.S. each year. Both a woman's age and her reason for having the surgery have a significant impact on this risk.

At least one-quarter—and as many as one-half—of all women undergoing hysterectomy experience one or more of the following complications:

INFECTION

The risk is significantly greater following abdominal hysterectomy compared to vaginal hysterectomy. Overall, 30 percent of all women undergoing abdominal hysterectomy and 15 percent of those having vaginal hysterectomy require treatment for infection. Most infections are minor and can be effectively treated with antibiotics, but severe infection can still occur—a major cause of hysterectomy-related deaths. And 30 to 40 percent of women experience a fever above 100.4° F.

BLEEDING

Approximately 10 percent of women require blood transfusion during surgery. Bleeding can also occur later, commonly between seven and fourteen days after surgery, possibly necessitating hospitalization and blood transfusion.

INJURY TO ADJACENT ORGANS

Accidental injury to the bladder, bowel, or ureters requiring surgical repair, while uncommon, can occur. About 1 woman in 200 will experience injury to the bladder; 1 in 300, injury to the ureters.

REPEAT SURGERY

Nearly 15 percent of women need repeat surgery for complications related to the original operation.

URINARY TRACT COMPLICATIONS

Nearly half of all women experience a kidney or bladder infection following surgery.

BLOOD CLOTS

While uncommon, abnormal blood clots can form after surgery, posing a threat of impaired breathing and cardiac arrest if a portion of the clot travels to the lungs or heart.

BOWEL PROBLEMS

Problems can occur after any major abdominal surgery, including surgical injury, bowel blockage, constipation, and infection. If scar tissue forms, follow-up surgery may be required. In cases of severe injury, a colostomy must be performed.

DEATH OR PARALYSIS FROM ANESTHESIA

See risks of anesthesia in chapter 16 (Fig. 73).

OVARIAN COMPLICATIONS

Researchers have found that up to 40 to 50 percent of women who have hysterectomies before menopause report symptoms of insufficient ovarian hormone production.

IMPROPER VAGINAL HEALING

The incision made during a vaginal hysterectomy tends to heal slowly. As the vaginal incision heals, it can result in thickened tissue along the incision line that can break open slightly during intercourse or cause an excessive watery discharge. Also scar tissue build-up can make the vaginal lining less elastic. If too much vaginal tissue is removed during hysterectomy, the vagina will be shortened—sometimes to the extent that intercourse becomes painful or even impossible.

IMPAIRED SEXUAL FUNCTIONING

Women have reported a wide range of effects on sexual function—from greater sexual enjoyment to a complete shutdown of the ability to engage in intercourse. Shortening of the vagina, scar tissue build-up, changes in hormone patterns, removal of the cervix, lack of uterine contractions following orgasm, and slow healing after surgery are all possible aftereffects that can impair sexual function.

The womb not only conceives and births and involutes (bleeds), it secretes pleasure hormones (beta-endorphins) and contracts vigorously during orgasm.[23] That's not all, either—the uterus secretes a lubricative, prostaglandin-rich substance in response to sexual arousal that further contributes to a woman's enjoyment of her sexuality.[24] And if that weren't enough to convince us that our wombs are sexually (as well as reproductively) valuable, it should also be noted that the cervix acts to "stop" the penis during intercourse and has sensory nerve endings that respond to coital stimulation.[25]

It makes me sad that women sacrifice one of their primary sexual organs so quickly and that many doctors so readily remove the uterus without valid reasons—even thinking they are doing women (and their husbands) a favor by performing the operation.[26] Unfortunately, alternatives to hysterectomy are not always offered to women.

"There is very little an uninformed consumer can do to distinguish between an appropriate hysterectomy and an inappropriate one," says Dr. Steven J. Bernstein, assistant professor of medicine at the University of Michigan School of Medicine and the lead author of a study on hysterectomy reported in the *Journal of the American Medical Association*.[27]

Using the criteria set by a panel of medical experts, reviewers who evaluated 642 women's medical records found that nearly half of the surgeries were not clearly indicated. In addition, they found that 16 percent of the operations were definitely inappropriate, and another 25 percent were performed for questionable reasons. As a result of these findings, Dr. Bernstein suggests that women act on their own behalf by asking whether alternative treatment might be available.

It won't be only the health-care providers and HMOs that will lower the hysterectomy rates in this country—it also will be the women who value their wombs. As long as we continue to view hysterectomy as a desirable solution for common female complaints like cramps, heavy periods, and vaginal gas, what else can we expect? We need to be more resourceful, protective, and knowledgeable about our bodies, than ever before.

If, after considering effective alternatives, you find that having a hysterectomy is your best option, read everything you can about the surgery, what to expect during recovery, and how to promote the healing process. Become familiar with the types of hysterectomies and surgical procedures available today, and thoroughly discuss the benefits and risks associated with each method with your gynecologist prior to the operation (Figure 85). Several excellent books on this subject are recommended in the Resources section at the end of this book. In addition, you can help prepare yourself for surgery

Types of Hysterectomies
Figure 85

SUBTOTAL HYSTERECTOMY

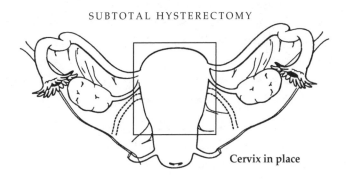

Cervix in place

TOTAL HYSTERECTOMY

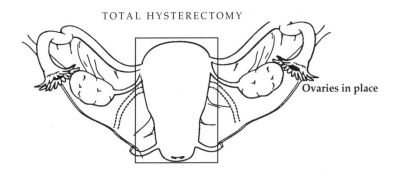

Ovaries in place

TOTAL HYSTERECTOMY
AND BILATERAL SALPINGO-OOPHORECTOMY

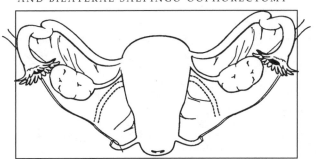

by recognizing and talking about the common feelings associated with hysterectomy:[28]

- A sense of loss of the womb's reproductive role (menstrual cycles, childbearing, and sexual response), causing anger, sadness, anxiety, and/or depression.
- Fears and concerns about surgery, recovery, and afterward.
- An altered sense of femininity or self-worth.
- Anxiety about how hysterectomy will impact sexuality.

By understanding what to expect before, during, and after your surgery, you will feel a greater sense of control throughout the entire process. As much as possible, know the medical indications for hysterectomy, the physiologic and emotional aspects of the surgery, and the related medical treatments (hormone replacement therapy, for example) you will need after surgery. Do not agree to a hysterectomy without being fully informed about why it's being recommended and understanding what's involved during surgery and recovery. Then once you have made the decision that hysterectomy is a valid option for you, do everything you can to enhance your physical and emotional healing.

ASK YOUR DOCTOR ABOUT HYSTERECTOMY[29]

What condition are you trying to treat by performing a hysterectomy?

What are all the methods available to treat this condition?

Why are you recommending one medical approach over all others?

What is the worst thing that can happen if I decide not to follow your recommendation?

What changes can I expect following surgery?

What reading materials can you recommend to enable me to become more informed about hysterectomy and its alternatives?

Will you recommend a specialist for a second opinion? (Many health insurance providers now require a second opinion before surgery.)

How many hysterectomies have you performed? What specialized training is required?

What are the success and failure rates associated with hysterectomy, as well as the possible risks and complications?

Can you recommend any women who have had this procedure who might be willing to talk to me about their experiences?

A Little Worry Now May Save Your Life Later: Prevention and Diagnosis of Women's Cancers

Cancer of the female reproductive tract is something every one of us thinks about. Many of us have friends, grandmothers, mothers, aunts, or sisters who have faced a form of this debilitating disease. Some have survived; others have not. And as the years go by, we hear of more people we know personally who are battling cancer in one of its various forms.

One of the greatest benefits of taking more responsibility for our reproductive health is that our bodies become less a mystery to us. In addition to abstinence and monogamy, our best defense against cancer is this: The more familiar we are with ourselves, the earlier we can detect any changes that may endanger our health.

Think about it: Breast self-exams, monitoring menstrual signs, and noting cervical discharges are all excellent techniques for detecting early signs of cancer of the reproductive organs. Obviously, this doesn't mean we should interpret every unusual symptom as a sign of cancer. It simply means we will worry less by getting help as soon as we discover we need it.

The next section of this chapter presents a no-nonsense approach to covering the symptoms of reproductive cancers, as well as some known risk factors and possible preventive measures.[1] If you are experiencing any of these symptoms, see your gynecologist as soon as possible for a thorough evaluation. If you think you are at risk for developing one of these types of cancer, make an appointment with your health-care provider to determine which cancer-screening technique might be beneficial for you.

SIGNS AND SYMPTOMS OF WOMEN'S CANCERS

Remember, it is possible to have some, all, or none of the symptoms listed here. Also keep in mind that risk factors significantly vary in their cancer-causing capacity. (For example, breastfeeding may slightly reduce a woman's risk of developing breast cancer, while having a sister and a mother with breast cancer significantly increases one's risk.) Research is continually yielding new information about cancer prevention and risk-factor reduction, as well as about cancer treatment. It will be up to you to stay informed.

The symptoms for each type of cancer are followed by further information to aid in your health-care decision-making. Please don't panic if you discover that you're experiencing one of the cancer signs listed below. Instead, you may use the information as a prompt to visit your health-care provider soon for a consultation and checkup.

Cervical Cancer

SYMPTOMS:
- Pain in the vagina, cervix, uterus, tubes, and/or ovaries
- Bleeding after intercourse
- Bleeding after menopause
- Bleeding after douching or pelvic exam
- Spotting between periods
- Thick, increased, unusual, or foul-smelling discharge
- Itching and irritation
- Bladder or urethral pain
- Abnormal Pap test

RISK FACTORS:[2]
- Previous cervical dysplasia (abnormal Pap test)
- First intercourse before ages eighteen to twenty
- Previous herpes, gonorrhea, chlamydia, syphilis, or human papillomavirus (HPV, or genital warts virus) infection
- First pregnancy before age eighteen to twenty
- Multiple sex partners

- Use of birth control pills for four years or longer
- Previous vulvar or vaginal cancer
- Exposure to a male partner who has (or had) penile cancer
- Exposure to a male whose previous partner(s) had cervical dysplasia or cervical cancer
- DES (diethylstilbestrol) exposure during prenatal development
- Cigarette smoking

HOW TO LOWER RISK FACTORS:

- Delay first intercourse until age twenty or older.
- Have sexual intercourse with only your husband. Women who have sex with more than one person—both over a given period in their lives and over their lifetimes—increase their risk of encountering a partner infected with an STD. Their risk rises as the number of partners increases. (For example, compared to the risk for a woman with one lifetime partner, two partners double the risk; six partners increase the risk by 600 percent, and so on).[3]
- Use a barrier method of family planning (a condom or a diaphragm).
- Get a yearly Pap test and pelvic exam.
- Don't smoke.
- Don't use oral contraceptives.
- Take vitamin A, vitamin C, and beta-carotene supplements in recommended dosages.

SCREENING TECHNIQUES:

- Pap test
- Pelvic exam
- Colposcopy or cervicography

DEFINITIVE DIAGNOSIS REQUIREMENTS:

- Biopsy obtained by using endocervical curettage, punch biopsy, electrosurgical loop excision (LEEP), and/or cone biopsy
- Careful evaluation for cervical cancer is justified whenever abnormal bleeding or discharge persists and is unexplained.
- The accurate diagnosis of cervical cancer requires biopsy. Also, careful evaluation for unsuspected cervical cancer is essential before having a hysterectomy. Optimal cervical cancer treatment may include the use of radiation treatment rods placed in the cervical canal and uterus prior to surgery.

There are two types of cervical cancer, noninvasive and invasive. (See chapter 14 for a discussion of Pap tests.)

KEY FACTS ABOUT NONINVASIVE CERVICAL CANCER:

- It takes between three and fifteen years for noninvasive cervical cancer to develop into invasive cancer. Early cervical cancer often doesn't have noticeable symptoms and is often entirely painless.
- About 45,000 new cases of noninvasive cervical cancer are diagnosed in the United States every year. It's very likely that cervical cancer is a sexually transmitted disease. Up to 90 percent of cervical cancers show evidence of HPV infection.[4]
- More than 90 percent of all cervical cancers are *squamous cell carcinomas*, that is, cancer limited to the outermost surface of the cervix. Many researchers currently believe that this type of cancer is actually a sexually transmitted disease.
- Early detection and treatment are essential in preventing the spread of cervical cancer to deeper layers of the uterus.
- Noninvasive cervical cancer is most common in women under forty and is almost 100 percent curable if treated at the time of diagnosis.

KEY FACTS ABOUT INVASIVE CERVICAL CANCER:

- Invasive cervical cancer is found for the first time in about 15,000 women each year. The rate has fallen dramatically in recent years due to better and earlier diagnosis.
- Most of these women are between the ages of forty and sixty, although 25 percent of all cases occur in women over sixty-five. Overall, one or two women out of 100 develop invasive cervical cancer during their lifetime.
- Invasive cervical cancer accounts for an estimated 4,600 deaths annually in the United States.

Ovarian Cancer

SYMPTOMS:

- Dull, persistent pain or vague pressure in the pelvis or abdomen
- Altered bowel or bladder patterns; constant need to use the toilet
- Persistent diarrhea or constipation
- Loss of appetite; unexplained weight loss; feeling full after a light meal
- Enlarged abdomen or enlarged dress size
- Persistent, unexplained digestive system symptoms—indigestion, stomach discomfort, gas distension, bloating; nausea, or vomiting
- Abnormal vaginal bleeding

- Flu-like symptoms, including chest problems, coughing, and difficulty breathing

RISK FACTORS:[5]

- Ovulation for more than forty years
- Family history of ovarian, uterine, or breast cancer, particularly in a mother or sister
- Ovulation induction with fertility drugs
- Previous cancer of the colon or rectum, or hereditary intestinal polyps
- Previous breast cancer or benign breast disease
- No history of pregnancy or having first pregnancy after age thirty
- Ovulation for more than forty years
- Menopause after age fifty-five
- Exposure to herbicides and environmental toxins
- History of irregular or absent menstrual cycles, ovarian cysts, ovarian tumors, polycystic ovarian disease
- Endometriosis
- Obesity
- Hypothyroidism (lowered thyroid function)
- Asbestos exposure
- Use of body talc products, especially in the vaginal area
- Diabetes
- Hypertension (high blood pressure)
- High-fat diet
- Excessive coffee consumption
- Mumps or German measles in childhood or adolescence
- Caucasian, especially Jewish, ethnic background

HOW TO LOWER RISK FACTORS:

- Pregnancy and prolonged breastfeeding may lower risk.
- Avoid asbestos, talcum powder (an asbestos derivative), herbicides, and environmental toxins.
- Maintain healthy weight.
- Eat a low-fat, high-fiber diet high in vitamins C and A.
- Reduce coffee consumption.
- Immunize children for mumps and rubella in infancy.
- Have more frequent pelvic exams and ultrasound scans if you're at high risk.
- Obtain medical attention for any persistent abdominal symptoms, even if mild.

SCREENING TECHNIQUES:

- Pelvic exam
- Pap test
- Pelvic ultrasound
- Ca-125 blood test

DEFINITIVE DIAGNOSIS REQUIREMENTS:

- Evaluation prior to surgery to determine if the cancer has spread—chest X-ray; intravenous pyelogram; stool blood test; CT scan; MRI; routine blood chemistry workup including blood count, kidney and liver function tests, and blood calcium
- Surgical biopsy during laparotomy or, when possible, laparoscopy
- Immediate tissue examination of the entire tumor or a significant portion of it by an in-house specialist

KEY FACTS ABOUT OVARIAN CANCER:

- Ovarian cancer is not common, affecting about one out of every 1,000 women.
- Fewer than 7 percent of women diagnosed with ovarian cancer have any relatives with the disease.
- Although ovarian cancer accounts for only 4 percent of all cancers affecting women, it is responsible for half of all genital cancer deaths.
- Ovarian cancer occurs in ten to twelve out of every 100,000 women in the United States; in many nonindustrialized nations, it occurs at about half that rate or less.
- Symptoms of ovarian cancer during the earliest stages of the disease are often entirely absent or quite mild.
- With ovarian cancer, treatment success depends on the stage and also on the specific type of cancer involved.
- Some experts have observed that for 99.9 percent of human history, women ovulated much less frequently than we do today, due to lengthy periods women used to spend being pregnant or breastfeeding. (One researcher has estimated that our ancestors might have experienced fifty mentrusal cycles in an entire life span, versus the more than 400 cycles women have today.)

Endometrial Cancer

SYMPTOMS:

- Unexplained vaginal bleeding or watery, bloody discharge after menopause

- "Breakthrough" bleeding between periods or increased menstrual flow
- Unusual discharge or spotting
- Enlarged or growing uterus, especially after menopause
- Pain sometimes present in early stages; symptoms listed above are more common

RISK FACTORS:[6]

- Conditions resulting in elevated estrogen levels or prolonged exposure to estrogen without normal progesterone levels, including:
  —history of infrequent or no ovulation
  —history of abnormal hormone patterns
  —estrogen medication exposure
  —postmenopausal treatment with estrogen only (no progestin)
  —previous use of sequential oral contraceptives (now off the market)
  —infertility
  —few or no pregnancies
  —obesity
- Menopause after age fifty-two
- Menarche before age twelve
- Liver disease
- History of abnormal uterine lining
- Family history of uterine cancer
- Previous radiation treatment in the pelvic area
- History of breast, ovary, or bowel cancer
- Tamoxifen treatment for breast cancer
- Polycystic ovarian disease
- Uterine polyps
- Diabetes
- High blood pressure
- Hypothyroidism (low thyroid function)

HOW TO LOWER RISK FACTORS:

- Maintain healthy weight.
- Pregnancy may lower risk.
- Taking combination birth control pills or HRT treatment for at least one year may lower risk.

SCREENING TECHNIQUES:

- Pelvic exam
- Pap test
- Endocervical curettage (ECC)

DEFINITIVE DIAGNOSIS REQUIREMENTS:
- Biopsy of the uterine lining (endometrium) obtained by endometrial biopsy, hysteroscopy, or D&C
- Interpretation of pathology slides by a specialist in pelvic cancers to avoid false-positive reporting

KEY FACTS ABOUT ENDOMETRIAL CANCER:
- If endometrial cancer is present, a hysterectomy may save your life.
- Endometrial cancer is a malignancy of the uterine lining.
- This cancer is most common between the ages of fifty and sixty-four.
- Endometrial cancer is the most common and the least deadly of all female cancers.
- This cancer afflicts approximately 54,000 women annually.
- Estimated survival rate is between 75 and 90 percent.
- Early detection is essential. If detected and treated at an early stage, this type of cancer is highly curable.
- Approximately two or three out of every 100 women develop endometrial cancer, but it is rare before the age of forty.
- Abnormal bleeding is commonly the first sign of endometrial cancer. (About 90 percent of all women with uterine cancer report abnormal bleeding.)
- Endometrial cancer usually appears after menopause. Bleeding after menopause has taken place is the most important sign of endometrial cancer. Any unusual postmenopausal bleeding should be immediately evaluated by a gynecologist.
- Complete evaluation of abnormal bleeding should include a pelvic exam, Pap test, aspiration curettage (endocervical curettage), and endometrial biopsy.

Breast Cancer

SYMPTOMS:
- Persistent lump or thickening in the breast or armpit
- Change in the color, contour, or appearance of the breast or areola
- Nipple retraction or scaliness
- Thickening or swelling of the skin overlying the breast
- Dimpling, puckering, scaling, or a similar change in skin texture
- Abnormal nipple discharge

RISK FACTORS:
- Family history of breast cancer

- Family history of breast-ovarian cancer syndrome
- Personal history of breast or ovarian cancer
- Early menarche (starting menstruation before age twelve)
- Late menopause (ending menstruation after age fifty)
- Alcoholic beverage consumption
- Impaired immune response
- Previous radiation treatment or chemotherapy
- No children, impaired fertility, or first pregnancy after age thirty
- Menstruation for longer than forty years
- Carcinogen exposure, including DES exposure while pregnant
- Uterine cancer
- High dietary fat intake (35 percent or more of daily intake)
- Sedentary lifestyle
- Hormone replacement therapy
- Oral contraceptives (appears to apply only to women at increased risk due to other factors)
- Severe obesity (forty pounds or more over ideal weight)
- Personal history of one or more of the following breast conditions, confirmed by biopsy:
  —moderate hyperplasia
  —papilloma with a fibrovascular core
  —atypical hyerplasia
- Abortion

HOW TO LOWER RISK FACTORS:
- Do monthly breast self-exams.
- Use an alternative to oral contraceptives if you are at high risk for breast cancer.
- Have your children before age thirty.
- Maintain healthy weight.
- Eat a low-fat, high-fiber diet.
- Breastfeed for at least six months.
- Participate in at least four nonconsecutive hours of cardiovascular exercise per week.
- Reduce the use of estrogens after menopause.

SCREENING TECHNIQUES:
- Breast self-exam (BSE) (See Figure 62 in chapter 14.)
- Mammography—the American Cancer Society recommends one baseline mammogram before age forty, mammograms every one to two

years between ages forty and fifty, and every year for women over fifty; other experts suggest a different schedule (see Resources).

- Regular physical exams by a health-care professional
- Ultrasonography

DEFINITIVE DIAGNOSIS REQUIREMENTS:

- Biopsy using needle aspiration or surgical biopsy
- Diagnosis of tissue samples by a qualified pathologist

KEY FACTS ABOUT BREAST CANCER:

- This is the most common type of cancer in adult women.
- More than 180,000 women are diagnosed with breast cancer in the United States annually; approximately 46,000 with the disease die each year.
- The incidence of breast cancer began rising in the 1940s and began to increase sharply around 1980, with breast cancer rates increasing around the world by about 2 percent each year. Most of the increase in the United States has been in women over fifty.
- Up to 30 percent of breast cancer patients have a family history of the disease.
- At the time of birth, American females have a one-in-eight chance of developing breast cancer during their lifetimes.
- Mammography reduces deaths from breast cancer by 30 percent in women between fifty and seventy years of age.

Vaginal Cancer

SYMPTOMS:

- Abnormal vaginal bleeding or bloody discharge
- Bleeding after intercourse or pelvic exam
- Painful and/or frequent urination
- Urge to strain during urination or bowel movements
- Thickening or warty growth on the surface of the vaginal lining

RISK FACTORS:

- Previous cervical or vulvar cancer
- Radiation therapy
- Previous infection with a sexually transmitted disease, especially human papillomavirus (HPV)
- Prenatal DES (diethystilbestrol) exposure
- Use of a pessary (device used to treat uterine prolapse)

HOW TO LOWER RISK FACTORS:

- Have regular pelvic exams and Pap tests.

DEFINITIVE DIAGNOSIS REQUIREMENTS

- Pap test
- Colposcopy
- Biopsy with diagnosis conducted by a qualified pathologist

KEY FACTS ABOUT VAGINAL CANCER:

- Cancer of the vagina is one of the rarest cancers, accounting for about 1 to 2 percent of gynecologic cancers.
- The majority of vaginal cancers occur in women between the ages of fifty and seventy. An even more rare form of vaginal cancer, called clear-cell adenocarcinoma, occurs largely in females under twenty.

Cancer of the Vulva

SYMPTOMS:

- Constant, unexplained itching of the genitals or surrounding skin
- Burning, pain, bleeding, or discharge in the genital area
- Change in a mole or birthmark on or near the vagina
- A lump, ulcer (open sore), wart, or thickening of tissue on or near the labia majora, labia minora, clitoris, perineum, or vaginal entrance
- Changes in the color of the skin (to pink, red, brown, gray, white) in the vulvar area
- Painful urination

RISK FACTORS:

- Infection with human papillomavirus (HPV) or herpes simplex virus
- Immune-system-suppressing drugs and diabetes (may be additional risk factors, but the current evidence is inconclusive)
- History of other gynecologic cancers
- Smoking
- Obesity
- Excessive coffee consumption
- History of vulvar inflammation

HOW TO LOWER RISK FACTORS:

- Have intercourse with only your husband; avoid exposure to STDs.
- Use good personal hygiene habits (wipe front to back after urinating; use unscented toilet tissue; avoid tight panties and clothing; wear panties and hosiery with 100 percent cotton crotch; use mild laundry

detergents, little bleach; avoid scented soaps and personal hygiene products—sprays, wipes, deodorizers, douches, tampons, pads, and panty liners).
- Perform vulvar self-exams once per month, using a mirror to inspect the outer and inner vulva. Check for warning signs: Are both sides alike? Does the skin have a healthy appearance? Are there any lumps, growths, masses? Is the tissue tender or painful?
- Don't smoke.
- Reduce coffee consumption.

SCREENING TECHNIQUES:
- Vulvar self-examination
- Regular pelvic exam

DEFINITIVE DIAGNOSIS REQUIREMENTS:
- Biopsy with diagnosis by a qualified pathologist
- Colposcopy
- Pap test to check for associated genital cancers

KEY FACTS ABOUT VULVAR CANCER:
- Cancer of the vulva is extremely rare, accounting for less than 1 percent of all tumors of the female reproductive tract.
- About 10 percent of women with vulvar cancer have another kind of cancer in another location within the lower reproductive organs.
- Vulvar cancer is three times more common in white women than in black women.
- With early detection, diagnosis, and treatment, vulvar cancer is highly curable.
- The rates for early vulvar cancer have increased among younger women in recent years.
- The best way to prevent vulvar cancers is to avoid voluntary exposure to sexually transmitted diseases.

Cancer of the Fallopian Tubes

SYMPTOMS:
- Abnormal vaginal bleeding
- Spasm-like pelvic pain
- Heavy, watery, or blood-tinged vaginal discharge
- Abdominal distension
- Vague, persistent bladder or rectal discomfort

RISK FACTORS:

- Because a low number of cases of this disease have been reported, there is little data concerning risk factors.
- History of tuberculosis, multiple tubule infections, and chronic pelvic inflammatory disease may be associated with a higher risk.

KEY FACTS ABOUT CANCER OF THE FALLOPIAN TUBES:

- Cancer of the fallopian tubes is extremely rare, representing about one out of 1,000 reproductive tract cancers.
- Diagnosis of fallopian cancer is very difficult because its symptoms are so similar to other gynecologic problems. Thus it is often not discovered until surgery is done to evaluate the symptoms.
- This type of cancer is rare before age fifty and after sixty.
- Like ovarian cancer, cancer of the fallopian tubes involves both tubes in about 15 percent of all cases.
- Surgical treatment is likely to include removing the ovaries and uterus as well as both fallopian tubes.

DIAGNOSTIC TECHNIQUES FOR REPRODUCTIVE TRACT CANCERS

Pelvic Exam

A complete and thorough pelvic exam is often the first step in detecting and diagnosing the presence of gynecologic cancer. However, cancer must be confirmed by obtaining a tissue sample and analyzing the cell structure for abnormalities. A licensed, expert pathologist who specializes in reproductive tract cancers should evaluate a suspicious slide sample in order to avoid false-negative readings (a reading that would indicate cancer or a precursor to cancer when the condition is actually less serious).

Endocervical Curettage, or ECC

An in-office procedure used to obtain tissue samples from the cervix for laboratory analysis if cancer is suspected due to an abnormal Pap test and pelvic exam evaluation.

Cervicography

This procedure is actually a photographic analysis of the cervix that is less expensive than colposcopy (see below). Photographic slides are sent for outside analysis by certified experts, so your physician doesn't need special train-ing, and the camera equipment is less expensive than a colposcope. Having this procedure done along with a Pap test reduces the risk that a significant cervical abnormality may be overlooked.

Colposcopy

Using a diagnostic instrument resembling binoculars mounted on a mechan-ical arm, your doctor can look through a colposcope to view the surface of your cervix and vaginal lining magnified ten to twenty times normal size (Figure 86). A painless procedure, colposcopy involves the insertion of a speculum following a pelvic exam, the patient lying still with feet in stirrups for ten to twenty minutes during the colposcopic examination, the physician swabbing the surface of the cervix with a vinegar-like solution to clear away mucus and make cervical features more visible, and careful examination and identification of any abnormalities for later biopsy. Colposcopy is a painless procedure since the colposcope doesn't touch your body, although the vine-gar solution may sting a little when applied.

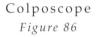

Colposcope
Figure 86

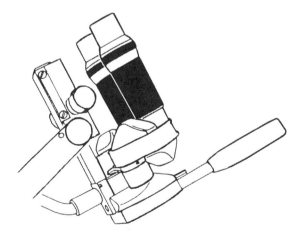

Cone Biopsy

In this procedure, the gynecologist surgically removes a cone-shaped tissue sample from the center of the cervix. It is not used as frequently today as it once was because colposcopy now allows physicians to identify suspicious areas and use punch biopsy (Figure 87). In some cases, cone biopsy may be required to examine a larger tissue sample and/or treat cervical abnormalities. Cone biopsy is considered a major surgical procedure and is performed in a hospital with general or regional anesthesia.

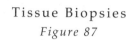

Tissue Biopsies
Figure 87

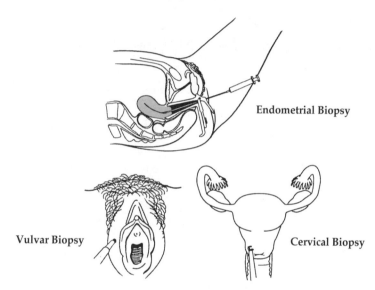

Endometrial Biopsy

Vulvar Biopsy

Cervical Biopsy

D&C

D&C, or dilation and curettage, may be used as a means of assessing precancerous or cancerous changes in the uterine lining.

Electrosurgical Loop Incision (LEEP)

Often done as an alternative to cone biopsy, LEEP uses a thin wire loop containing a low-voltage radio wave to remove abnormal tissue from the cervix for treatment and/or examination.

Endometrial Biopsy

Your physician may obtain tissue samples of the uterine lining for cancer evaluation on an outpatient basis in a short-stay surgical center or in her office by performing an endometrial biopsy (Figure 87).

Hysteroscopy

Hysteroscopy may be used to obtain tissue samples from inside the cervix and uterus and is performed in-office or at a short-stay surgical center.

Laparoscopy

Used to examine inside the pelvic cavity, laparoscopy can also be used as a means of obtaining tissue.

Laparotomy

If previous tests warrant cancer diagnosis and surgical treatment as soon as possible, laparotomy may be advisable.

Pap Test

Pap tests detect changes in the cervix long before cancer develops. If you're at high risk for cervical cancer, you should have a Pap test once or twice every year.

Needle Aspiration Biopsy

After a local anesthetic is applied to the skin, fluid is removed from a breast lump or mass through a hollow needle and examined under a microscope for abnormal cells. This procedure is performed in the doctor's office.

Surgical Biopsy

This simply means the surgical removal of a small sample of tissue for microscopic evaluation by a pathologist, a physician specially trained to identify cell abnormalities. In some cases, the tissue sample can be collected in-office under local anesthesia. Biopsy permits your physician, with the aid of an expert pathologist, to precisely confirm or deny a cancer diagnosis.

Ultrasound (Sonogram, Sonography)

By using sound echoes aimed at soft tissue, clinicians may now gain a fairly clear and immediate picture of structures inside the pelvic cavity. Ultrasound is not X-ray—it's sonar. As sound waves painlessly bounce back and forth, a machine interprets the distance, length, and frequency of the waves on a screen (Figure 88). Photographs may be taken to be read later by your physician if she is not present during the examination.

While there has been no evidence of harmful effects from exposure to diagnostic ultrasound, animal research and studies of cells have shown possible adverse effects with prolonged exposure. Nevertheless, when ultrasound is medically indicated (as opposed to just using it to take a picture of your pelvic cavity or preborn baby), it can enable you and your physician to more accurately know how and when to intervene in your situation.

Ultrasound Exam

Figure 88

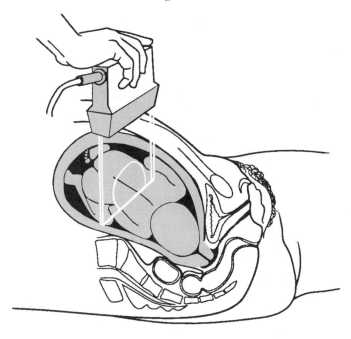

In addition, the following diagnostic measures may be taken in the case of invasive cancer to check for evidence of metastases (spread of the cancer to other parts of the body). If any of these tests are recommended, ask your health-care provider to explain the procedure to you, including risks and benefits.

- Chest X-ray
- Intravenous pyelogram, an X-ray dye study of kidneys, ureters, bladder, and urethra
- Stool blood test
- Routine blood chemistry workup, including blood count, kidney and liver function tests, and blood calcium
- Cystoscopy
- Proctosigmoidoscopy
- Intravenous pyelogram (IVP)
- Lymphangiogram (X-ray study of the pelvic lymph system)
- Urogram (X-ray of the urinary tract)
- Bone scan
- CT scan
- MRI (Magnetic Resonance Imaging)

How to Avoid STDs— and What to Do If You Get One

Wise King Solomon once said, "There is nothing new under the sun." Clearly, people have been "experimenting" with sex ever since Adam and Eve took a taste of that sinfully delicious and, alas, forbidden fruit.

But something *has* changed. Since the Pill, we've had bigger and better and more technology than ever before in history to do our thing *with*. Some might claim this has been a fun and liberating experience. They're wrong. *No one benefits from promiscuity*—not one person. So called casual sex is—at least eventually, if not initially—an emotional, spiritual, intellectual, interpersonal, and physical disaster. Sex outside marriage wreaks havoc with your whole life—your heart, soul, mind, spirit, and body.

We owe it to our daughters and ourselves to avoid using simplistic jargon about "safe sex" and the virtues of virginity with one another. Tough times require tough truths. Our Creator stipulates this for our good: *Sex is for marriage*. Why?

There are lots of reasons. Entire volumes have been penned on this very theme. Seminars are offered internationally on the topic. Videos and sermons abound every season of the year. The Bible teaches that monogamous sexuality is a good thing because it fits our God-made emotional, physical, social, and spiritual makeup.

But are we practicing what we preach? Given the latest statistics on sexually transmitted diseases (STDs), it looks as if lots of people are still rejecting monogamy in favor of multiple sexual liaisons.

We can talk until we're blue in the face about reasons to abstain—as we should—but STDs graphically demonstrate why it's wise to live chastely. In the university classes on human sexuality that I used to teach, I always asked the following questions before my lecture on STDs: How many of you would like to marry someone who has slept with twenty people? Ten? Five? What if a potential marriage partner had syphilis or gonorrhea in the past? Or what if the person has an incurable sexually transmitted infection—herpes, for example?

You know what? *No one* has ever raised a hand. And I believe one of the primary reasons why is that we have a built-in desire within our hearts for exclusive, lifelong sexual intimacy. It's a human quality we're born with, an immutable component of our original design, but not an easy thing to live out. However, if we think we can thwart God's plans for our good by living outside His boundary lines, we're terribly mistaken.

As women, we need to compassionately underscore this critical fact: *Monogamy is our best defense against sexually transmitted sterility and disease.* Women are at higher risk of acquiring an STD than men because our anatomy makes these infections more easily transmissible to us.

Natural law and reproductive biology discriminate against promiscuity in favor of sexual union between one man and one woman for life. The two *do* become one—body fluids and all. There is no other human activity that is more real, more basic, more intimate, more life-giving, more revealing, or more potentially destructive than sex.

Consider what would happen to the current STD epidemic diseases if we all followed God's user's manual for our bodies—the Bible. Here is a vivid example of our Creator's grand design for human sexuality:

> The body is not for sexual immorality but for the Lord, and the Lord for the body. And God both raised up the Lord and will also raise us up by His power. Do you not know that your bodies are members of Christ? Shall I then take the members of Christ and unite them with a man other than my husband? Never!
>
> Do you not know that she who unites herself with a man other than her husband is one with him in body? For it is said: "The two will

become one flesh." But she who unites herself with the Lord is one with him in spirit.

Flee sexual immorality. All other sins a woman commits are outside her body, but she who sins sexually sins against her own body.[1]

Isn't this fantastic? When we consider the physical, emotional, social, and spiritual harm that comes from not listening to—and living by—the Word, why would any of us want to do anything contrary to the Lord's good teachings?

THE HEARTBREAKING TRUTH

I'll never forget a close friend of mine calling me on the phone and tearfully telling me her husband had been unfaithful and consequently had passed on his chlamydia infection to her. She was devastated and filled with anger. Another woman called with a similar story. Her spouse had stayed out all night with a prostitute while she was out of town and ended up with gonorrhea as a result. Both couples subsequently divorced.

Before this happened to my friends, their husbands apparently didn't know there were around six million new cases of chlamydia and gonorrhea in the United States that year, not to mention one million cases of pelvic inflammatory disease (PID), up to a million cases of human papillomavirus (HPV), and around 500,000 cases of genital herpes simplex virus (HSV).

Now they know.

It's not always the man's fault, of course. Often it works the other way around—someone's wife or girlfriend or fiancée is with another man, catches chlamydia, and then passes it on to him. To deny that this happens to Christians as well as to nonbelievers is just plain stupid. *STDs are the most prevalent infectious diseases in the United States today.*

TWENTY SAD FACTS ABOUT
SEXUALLY TRANSMITTED DISEASES

- The World Health Organization estimates that 250 million people—that's one out of twenty worldwide—contract a sexually transmitted disease annually.[2]
- The estimated total number of people newly infected with an STD every year in the United States is twelve million.[3]
- About 27,000 people catch some form of STD *every day* in the United States; one in four Americans between the ages of fif-

- teen and fifty-five today will contract an STD during their lifetime.[4]
- Chlamydia has become the nation's most common STD, accounting for four million new infections each year.[5]
- The highest incidence of STDs occurs among young people ages twenty to twenty-four. Next are those ages fifteen to nineteen, then ages twenty-five to twenty-nine.[6]
- STDs cause about one-third of all reproductive deaths in the United States.[7]
- As of 1979, an average of approximately one death due to pelvic inflammatory disease, or PID, occurred every other day in the United States. There are now one million new cases of PID every year, costing over $4.2 billion annually.[8]
- If cervical cancer is viewed as an STD, then deaths due to this cause alone (approximately 4,600 each year) would far outnumber deaths due to all other reproductive causes combined.[9]
- Women suffer more serious long-term consequences from all STDs except AIDS—including sterility, chronic pelvic pain, pelvic adhesions, tubal pregnancy, infertility, cervical cancer, and PID.[10]
- Due to the "fluid dynamics" of sexual intercourse, women are more likely to acquire a sexually transmitted disease from a single sexual encounter.[11] For example, the risk of acquiring gonorrhea from a single act of intercourse, if one partner is infected, is just 25 percent for men but 50 percent for women.[12]
- In some areas of the United States, between 10 percent and 30 percent of adolescent females are believed to have chlamydia, a disease that can lead to sterility and infertility and infect infants at birth.[13]
- Syphilis cases hit a forty-one-year peak in 1989. Estimated cases: 44,000, compared to 27,000 the year before. Syphilis is passed through sex or birth and can be deadly if left untreated.[14]
- Between 1966 and 1990, first visits to a private physician for treatment of genital herpes virus increased 500 percent.[15] Genital herpes is now detectable in roughly one in five persons twelve years of age or older nationwide.[16] At least 30 percent of single sexually active Americans have been genitally infected with HSV and can give it to their partners.[17] The average male adult has a 50 percent chance of carrying this virus.[18]
- It is currently estimated that between forty-eight and fifty million Americans have been genitally infected with human papillo-

mavirus (HPV), with almost one million men, women, and children becoming newly infected in the United States each year.[19]

- It is now known that over fifty organisms and syndromes are transmitted or occur as a result of sexual activity.[20]

AFTER THE FACT

Once someone has a sexually transmitted disease as a consequence of sexual sin, it's too late to slap that person on the wrist and say, "It's wrong. It's naughty. Don't do it." The time for choosing between right and wrong is—irrevocably—past.

But thank God for the awesome moment when the extent of our brokenness reaches deep into the very center of our hearts, for that is when He is most able to help and heal us. May we never forget that the mercy of God and the power of the blood of Jesus Christ is sufficient to renew us, no matter how great the sin may be. (Read 1 Corinthians 6:9-11 for God's promise about this.)

While spiritual healing proceeds, physical effects may still linger. It's essential to be ministered to in both areas at the same time. *If you suspect that you have a sexually transmitted disease, seek medical attention now.* It's very easy to deny that an STD is present, saying, "This could never happen to me." But Christians are as likely to get an STD as anyone else, especially if they ignore healthy sexual boundaries. It's a fact: The most common STDs in the United States today—chlamydia, gonorrhea, pelvic inflammatory disease, human papillomavirus, and herpes simplex virus—have reached epidemic proportions in recent years. *No one who engages in sex outside marriage is immune.* The following sections will tell you what you (and your mother, sisters, friends, and daughters) need to know about these six sex-related afflictions.

Chlamydia

Also called *mucopurulent cervicitis,* chlamydia is an infectious disease caused by an intracellular bacterium (*Chlamydia trachomatis*). This STD often doesn't produce clear-cut clinical signs. An estimated one in ten adolescent girls and one in twenty women of reproductive age are infected with chlamydia every year. There are an estimated four million new cases annually in the United States, making chlamydia the most common infectious disease reported to state health departments and the Centers for Disease Control.[21]

Up to 75 percent of the women who have been infected with chlamydia have few or no noticeable symptoms, and without testing and treatment the infection may persist as long as fifteen months. Without treatment, 20 to 40 percent of women with the infection may develop pelvic inflammatory disease (PID).[22] Chlamydia is often not detected until PID has developed. (See Figure 89 for specific signs and risks.)

Transmission and incubation period. Chlamydia is transmitted via infected vaginal, oral, urethral, or rectal secretions during sexual contact. Symptoms, when they occur, usually appear one to two weeks after infection.

Possible risks. Results of the disease may be pelvic inflammatory disease, infertility, sterility, pelvic abscesses, and, if the woman is pregnant—miscarriage, stillbirth, and postpartum fever. Chlamydia can be passed from mother to child during birth and can include pneumonia or eye infection.

Diagnosis. The infection is diagnosed during a speculum exam. The clinician looks at the cervix to see if it has red, swollen areas and is secreting a thick, yellowish discharge. If so, a cotton swab is used to collect a specimen for microscopic examination. The discharge is examined immediately under a microscope on a "wet prep." For a definitive diagnosis of chlamydia, however, the specimen must be tested by culture, immunoflourescence, or enzyme immunoassay in a laboratory.[23] The testing is expensive because chlamydia organisms die quickly outside the body.

Treatment. Oral antibiotic therapy using either doxycycline (Doryx, Vibramycin, and others), 100 milligrams twice per day for one week, or azithromycin (Zithromax), a single-dose drug therapy that works as well as doxycycline. Other treatments still being used include erythromycin (PCE, ERY-C, etc.), 500 milligrams four times daily for one week; ofloxacin (Floxin), 300 milligrams twice a day; and, less effectively, sulfisoxazole (Gantrisin), 500 milligrams four times per day for ten days.[24] Sexual contact should be avoided until both partners are free of the infection. An early follow-up exam is necessary if the symptoms persist or recur.

Complementary natural therapies. Use complementary therapies—listed here and in the following sections—in addition to recommended medical treatments. As with other alternative treatment suggestions listed throughout this book, check with your physician about any contraindications that may exist before trying a remedy. To obtain an extra measure of relief during a chlamydia infection, you may want to try:

- Soaking in two or three fifteen- to twenty-minute warm baths every day. Add fifteen drops of one of these essential oils—juniper, peppermint, wintergreen, or rosemary.

- Taking acidophilus capsules to restore a healthy balance of intestinal bacteria eliminated by the antibiotics. Use as directed on the label. Note: Acidophilus works best when taken on an empty stomach. (Many women take acidophilus whenever they are undergoing antibiotic therapy for this reason.)

Also, see Figure 93 for specific suggestions about ways to boost your immune system's infection-fighting ability now and in the future.

Follow-up. There is no need to be retested after antibiotic therapy unless symptoms recur or you are exposed again to the virus. (Make certain that anyone with whom you have had sexual contact is also tested and treated for the infection.) And if you are married, be sure to avoid lovemaking with your spouse until your physician says it's okay to resume sexual relations.

Chlamydia and Gonorrhea Alert: Who's at Risk?
Figure 89

AT RISK:

- any woman currently engaging in intercourse or genital sexual activity

---

THE RISK INCREASES SIGNIFICANTLY IF YOU ARE:

- on birth control pills
- having intercourse/genital contact outside of marriage
- in your teens and early twenties and engaging in premarital or extramarital sex
- married to someone engaging in extramarital sex

WARNING SIGNS:

- unusual vaginal discharge
- cervical irritation
- abdominal pain
- abnormal periods
- fever
- tenderness or swelling in the groin area

- spotting between periods
- bleeding after intercourse
- husband: genital pain or discharge and/or urinary problems

Gonorrhea

Gonorrhea is a bacterial disease (*Neisseria gonorrhoeae*) that causes inflammation of the genital tract. If left untreated, it can cause PID, arthritis, heart disease, and meningitis.

Like chlamydia, gonorrhea can exist in one's body for a long time before being diagnosed during a routine exam that includes a gonorrhea culture (a prenatal exam, for instance). Before 1991 gonorrhea was the most commonly reported STD in the United States, though some experts believe the total number of new cases is somewhere between 800,000 and two million each year.[25] Of these, only 392,848 cases were reported to the CDC in 1995, the last year for which data is currently available.[26]

Transmission and incubation period. Women are many times more susceptible than men to acquiring this STD. The likelihood of a man getting gonorrhea after having sex once with an infected woman is 20 to 25 percent, but for a woman having sex once with an infected man, there is an 80 to 90 percent chance she will catch the disease.

Because the gonococcus organism dies quickly once it is exposed to air, gonorrhea is almost always transmitted by intimate vaginal, anal, or oral sexual contact. These are the most likely sites of infection in women, although gonorrhea can spread to the eyes, causing an infection called gonococcal conjunctivitis, which can cause blindness if left untreated. This is a rare occurrence in the United States today because newborns—who may come into contact with the bacteria during birth—are routinely given antibiotic eye drops to prevent this type of infection. Other places in a woman's body that may be infected with the organism include the blood, heart, joints, skin, brain, and spinal cord.

The incubation period for gonorrhea is currently unknown but appears to be about ten days. Up to 80 percent of women with the disease are without symptoms, making diagnosis difficult unless a woman's partner shares the truth. The signs of gonorrhea are much more obvious in males—painful urination and a thick discharge from the penis—so it's much more likely that the man will be the first to discover the infection. Even so, about one in five infected men have no symptoms at all.

Possible risks. There is a 40 percent risk of scarring, tubal obstruction, and infertility if a gonorrhea infection reaches a woman's fallopian tubes. Women who go untreated for gonorrhea develop PID at this percentage rate and are at risk of PID's consequences—infertility, sterility, pelvic abscesses, and tubal pregnancy. In addition, babies born to infected women are at risk for eye infections, lung disease, rectal infections, and scalp abscesses where internal fetal monitoring was performed.[27]

Diagnosis. Gonorrhea cannot be diagnosed by pelvic exam alone. It requires a highly specialized laboratory culture test that takes about forty-eight hours to complete. Chlamydia is present at the same time as gonorrhea in one-fifth of men and two-fifths of women, so treatment should include drugs to stop both infections.[28]

Treatment. Many strains of gonorrhea are now resistant to antibiotic therapy using penicillin and tetracycline. Cases of penicillin-resistant gonorrhea nearly doubled in one year in the United States (about 9,000 in 1985 compared to 17,000 in 1986).[29] Caused by organisms called PPNH (*penicillin-resistant Neisseria gonorrhea*), these strains of gonorrhea cannot be cured by the same drugs that were used in the past. Penicillin-resistant strains infect 35 to 50 percent of women with gonorrhea.[30]

As a result, newer therapies are commonly used: ceftriaxone (Rocephin) given once as a 125-milligram intramuscular injection; cefixime (Suprax), 400 milligrams taken orally in a single dose; ciprofloxacin (Cipro or Noroxin), 500 milligrams orally in a single dose; ofloxacin (Floxin), 400 milligrams in a single dose; or, for women who are allergic to the previous drugs, spectinomycin (Trobicin) given once in a two-gram intramuscular injection.[31]

Complementary natural therapies. Same as for chlamydia infection.

Follow-up. Same as for chlamydia infection.

Pelvic Inflammatory Disease (PID)

Perhaps one of the most distressing negative health consequences of STDs today, and one of the most avoidable, is PID. It is distressing because PID is now responsible for more than a quarter of a million cases of female sterility each year in the United States. It is avoidable because PID is most often caused by either chlamydia or gonorrhea—diseases transmitted by sexual contact outside marriage. Pelvic inflammatory disease can and does happen to Christian women—and not always as a result of out-of-bounds sexual activity (Figure 90).

Pelvic Inflammatory Disease:
Incidence, Risks, and Symptoms
Figure 90

FACTS[32]

- There are more than one million new cases of PID each year; of these, some 300,000 require hospitalization.

- Between 100,000 and 150,000 American women become infertile as a result of an STD that developed into PID.

- One woman in seven becomes infertile after a single episode of PID.

- Women who have had PID are six to ten times more likely than other women to experience *ectopic pregnancy,* a potentially life-threatening condition in which an early embryo cannot pass into the uterus due to scarring of the fallopian tubes and instead implants itself in a tube or, more rarely, in some other part of the abdomen.

- About half of the more than 88,000 ectopic pregnancies that occur every year are caused by a previous STD infection.

WHAT IS PID?

Infection of any or all of a woman's pelvic organs:
- *endometritis* (infection of the uterine lining)
- *myometritis* (infection of uterine muscle)
- *saplingitis* (infection of the fallopian tubes)
- *oophoritis* (infection of the ovaries)
- *peritonitis* (infection of the peritoneum, the membrane that lines the pelvic cavity).

WHAT CAUSES PID?

- *More than half of all cases of PID* are caused by chlamydia or gonorrhea.

- *Most PID* is caused by more than one pathogen, or microbe.

WHAT ARE THE SYMPTOMS OF PID?

In many cases, the symptoms are silent or subtle. *See your physician as soon as possible if you are experiencing:*
- persistent or mild abdominal discomfort or backache
- slightly increased vaginal discharge
- pain or discomfort during intercourse or movement (walking, coughing, jumping)

As PID progresses, symptoms may become more pronounced. *See your physician immediately or go to an emergency room if you are experiencing any of the following PID warning signs:*

- abnormal pain with urination or bowel movements
- chills, muscle aches, fatigue
- fever greater than 100.4° F.
- cramping or persistent pain in abdomen or back
- vaginal bleeding or spotting
- severe pelvic pain

Note: Few women experience all *warning signs. If you have possibly been exposed to chlamydia or gonorrhea, have an IUD, or have recently had a baby, a miscarriage, an abortion or pelvic surgery,* SUSPECT PID.

HOW IS THE DIAGNOSIS OF PID MADE?

Pelvic exam with STD culture tests for chlamydia and gonorrhea; ultrasound; blood count (to check for elevated number of white cells); and/or surgery (laparoscopy or, in rare cases, laparotomy).

WHAT IS THE TREATMENT FOR PID?

Treatment is done on an outpatient basis *unless* a woman is:

- seriously ill
- pregnant
- has suspected pelvic abscesses, appendicitis, or tubal pregnancy
- does not respond to antibiotic treatment
- attended by a physician unsure of the diagnosis
- unable to be treated on an outpatient basis

Hospital treatment of PID includes complete bed rest and I.V. antibiotic therapy using doxycycline and cefotoxin for a minimum of four days and at least two days after fever has stopped. This is followed by oral antibiotic therapy for ten to fourteen days.

At-home treatment of PID includes complete bed rest, pelvic rest (no activity that jars or bounces the pelvis), avoidance of sex until infection is cured, antibiotics administered orally and/or by intramuscular injection:[33]

- cefotoxin (Mefoxin) intramuscular injection *plus* probenecid tablets (Benemid), taken together, or,
- ceftriaxone (Rocephin) by intramuscular injection *plus* doxycycline, (Vibramycin, Doryx, and others) taken orally for fourteen days, or
- ofloxacin tablets (Floxin) plus clindamycin (Cleocin HCl) orally for fourteen days or metronidazole (Flagyl) orally for fourteen days.

Follow-up treatment for PID includes reevaluation by a physician forty-eight to seventy-two hours after initial treatment for PID. Further tests, hospitalization, and surgery may be recommended.

Permanent damage is likely if PID reaches the fallopian tubes, which are particularly vulnerable to infection (Figure 92). Fluid and pus may cause inflammation, swelling, and scarring, sometimes sealing the end of the tube shut. Infertility can result even when the tubes do not become blocked; however, damage to the tubal lining is enough to cause changes in their shape and function.

Severe infection that is not resolved by appropriate therapy may necessitate removal of the uterus (hysterectomy), fallopian tubes (saplingectomy), and/or ovaries (oophorectomy) to save a woman's life.

Infertility Risk and PID
Figure 91

NUMBER OF PID EPISODES	PERCENTAGE OF WOMEN WHO BECOME INFERTILE
1	11
2	23
3	54

SOURCE: L. Westrom, "Incidence, Prevalence and Trends of Acute Pelvic Inflammatory Disease and Its Consequences in Industrial Countries," *American Journal of Obstetrics and Gynecology* 138:880-892, 1980.

Effects of PID on Fallopian Tubes
Figure 92

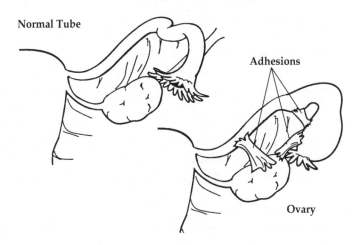

If you have PID, *anyone with whom you have had intercourse must also be treated at the same time* with one large dose of antibiotics followed by treatment with follow-up medication taken orally for seven to fourteen days. *This is necessary whether he has any symptoms or not.*

If you have acquired a pelvic infection resulting from pregnancy, miscarriage, or abortion, it requires different treatment. An ultrasound is done to check for any remaining tissue from your pregnancy. A D&C will be recommended if there is any evidence of tissue or if you do not respond to antibiotic therapy. You will also probably be given a drug to contract your uterus to minimize bleeding. *If you have PID as a result of an IUD*, the IUD should be removed if the infection is severe or does not respond to treatment. (Consider removing it anyway. See chapter 9 for reasons why.)

Human Papillomavirus (HPV)

Human papillomavirus, or HPV, is a highly common, incurable virus that is increasingly being transmitted during intimate sexual contact.[34] Because HPV is a nonreportable STD, epidemiologists are not able to obtain accurate figures on the total number of Americans affected with genital strains of HPV. Since 1987 the number of patients treated annually for HPV has increased 1,000 percent. According to recent studies, 7 to 19 percent of college women seeking gynecological services are found to be infected with a strain of the virus.[35]

Though HPV is now more common than genital herpes, many women remain completely in the dark about this emerging epidemic.

HPV can cause warts anywhere on the body, and these often recur after treatment. When these benign growths infect the genital and anal area, they are called *genital warts*. Genital warts (also referred to as *venereal warts* or *condylomata acuminata*) are usually spread via sexual contact with an infected partner. Condoms do not offer women protection from HPV and genital warts because the scrotum, as well as the penis, can harbor the virus. HPV and genital warts may also be transmitted by touching the genitals with wart-infected hands or, in rare cases, from an infected mother to her baby during birth.

HPV is more easily detected in the form of genital warts than in its "subclinical" form. STD experts believe that HPV occurs in subclinical form in about 70 percent of infected people and causes warts in about 30 percent of infected people.[36] Colposcopy and biopsy are required for the proper diagnosis of subclinical HPV.

At present the primary health concern is HPV's connection to women's cancers. For reasons that are not yet fully understood, women with the virus are at increased risk for both cervical and vulvar cancers. HPV comprises over sixty viral strains; approximately twenty-five can infect the genital area. These different strains of HPV have been assigned numbers, with different numbers producing different kinds of problems. Of these, at least five—types 16, 18, 31, 33, and 35—carry a higher potential for malignancy in subclinical HPV infections.[37] The HPV strains that cause genital warts do not lead to cancer.

Risk factors. A woman's likelihood of getting HPV is greater if she:

- has sexual relations with a man who is not a virgin.
- has a suppressed immune system due to oral contraceptive use, pregnancy, or a condition that has lowered her immunity (leukemia, HIV, or Hodgkin's disease, for example).
- has another STD (chlamydia, HSV, etc.).
- is between twenty and twenty-four years of age.
- smokes tobacco.

Symptoms. In most cases women with HPV do not have any signs or symptoms of infection until an abnormality is picked up by a Pap test. Genital warts are more obvious. They can be located anywhere on the vulva, in or near the vagina or anus, on the cervix (visible during a pelvic exam), on the groin or thighs, or in the mouth. The warts are usually flesh-colored, but they can be pink, red, or gray. Most often they do not hurt, though genital warts in some cases may bleed, burn, itch, or cause considerable discomfort. The warts may appear singularly or in clumps, may be raised or flat, and may start out as small swellings that grow into large cauliflowerlike clusters up to three inches in diameter.

Transmission and incubation. HPV is spread by skin-to-skin contact, most commonly though vaginal, anal, or oral sex. The incubation period for the virus may last as long as six weeks, but for two-thirds of the women who actually develop genital warts instead of subclinically harboring the virus, it can take up to nine months for the warts to appear.

Experts believe the HPV virus enters the body through small breaks in the skin surface, often caused by friction during sex or tampon use, or from another type of infection. Once inside the skin, the virus goes into the skin's deeper layers and stays there for months or even years. After this occurs, the virus may never return to the surface. As a result, a woman may be married for years before being diagnosed with HPV during a routine Pap test.

If you are diagnosed with the virus, try not to jump to any conclusions. Instead, keep in mind that you or your husband could have contracted the infection at any time—including *before* your marriage if either of you had sexual relations with anyone other than your spouse. HPV may raise many questions about your relationship, but if either (or both) of you have had sex with anyone else, you simply cannot say with any certainty when you were exposed to the virus because it could have been weeks, months, years, or decades ago. If you were a true virgin (i.e., had never had *any* type of sexual contact with another man, including kissing, genital touching, or oral sex), then you know it's probable that your husband gave you the virus. But he may have been infected quite a long time ago. On the other hand, you may simply be having a clinical manifestation of an HPV infection you picked up ages ago with someone you engaged in sexual behavior with.

Diagnosis. If you suspect you may have genital warts, seek treatment promptly. There is no blood test or quick lab culture for HPV. In most cases of HPV infection, the virus shows up as an abnormal Pap test and is followed up several weeks later with a colposcopy (see chapter 18). When stained with a vinegar-like solution (acetic acid), areas of the vagina and cervix where HPV is present turn white. The doctor may then take several small samples of tissue via punch biopsy to be later analyzed by a pathologist. Diagnosis of genital warts may simply require a physician's examination of the affected area, though in some cases, a biopsy may be needed to rule out vulvar cancer, which can resemble HPV.

Treatment. Treatments for HPV vary with the size, location, and symptoms of the infection. As with all medical treatments, it's essential to understand the risks and benefits of any recommended drug or procedure. Noncervical warts go away without any treatment 20 to 30 percent of the time. If discomfort persists or interferes with daily activities, external genital warts (not those in the vagina or on the cervix) can be treated with a drug called podofilox (Condylox). The drug is self-applied at home with a cotton swab twice per day for three days, followed by four days without treatment. The cycle can then be repeated up to four times. A burning sensation and localized irritation at the application site are common with this treatment. (Note: *Do not use this drug during pregnancy.*)

Small external genital warts may also be treated with a chemical solution, either podophyllin (Pododerm, Podocon-25) or trichloracetic acid, applied to the affected area by a physician during a pelvic exam. Podophyllin causes localized mild to moderate pain and must be rinsed off one to four hours after application. It may be reapplied once every week for up to six weeks. (Note: *This treatment is not to be used during pregnancy due to its potential for causing birth defects.*) Trichloracetic acid also causes burning discomfort at the site where it is applied and may be repeated weekly for six weeks.

If the warts persist, a physician may recommend electrocautery, cryosurgery, or laser vaporization. With electrocautery, the doctor applies a local anesthetic and then uses an electrical current to burn off the growths. Cryosurgery treatment uses liquid nitrogen to destroy genital warts or abnormal cervical cells. This technique requires no anesthesia, is performed in the gynecologist's office, takes just ten to twenty minutes, and is less risky than electrocautery and laser vaporization. Because laser treatment requires regional or general anesthesia and is associated with a painful recovery period, it is used only when other methods have failed.

Complementary therapies and natural treatments. (See Figure 93.) You may also wish to facilitate healing by:

- Keeping the affected area dry—wear loose-fitting garments and 100 percent cotton underwear; after bathing use a portable hair dryer on a cool setting to dry the area.
- Avoiding irritating, rubbing, or scratching the infected area.
- Applying several drops of tea tree oil to a sterile cotton gauze square and dab on the affected area twice a day.

Follow-up. During treatment it's important to abstain from sexual relations to avoid the possibility of reinfection and to protect the affected area from friction. Later vaginal skin abrasions may be avoided by applying a sterile lubricant prior to lovemaking if vaginal dryness exists, as well as using sanitary pads instead of tampons on days when the menstrual flow is light.

After being treated for HPV and genital warts, a woman should be rechecked by her physician in about six months. In a significant number of cases, additional treatment is needed. Doctors recommend a Pap test be performed every six months for a few years following HPV diagnosis as a precaution to rule out cancerous changes of the cervix.

Herpes Simplex Virus (HSV)

If you suspect you have been infected with genital herpes, *don't panic.* Here's why:

- Blood studies suggest that up to 95 percent of adults living in urban areas have antibodies to the herpes simplex virus—in other words, they have already "caught the bug" at some point during their lifetime.[38]
- It is now believed that 25 to 30 percent of genital herpes is caused by HSV-1 (the "above the waist" strain of the herpes simplex virus that causes cold sores on the mouth, lips, and face), *not* by HSV-2, which has traditionally been associated with below-the-waist herpes infections. *Both strains can infect anywhere in the body.*[39]
- HSV can develop in any woman who has skin contact with the lips, mouth, cheeks, genitals, or anal area of an infected person through kissing, touching, or sexual intercourse. Yet many people remain unaware that HSV-1 may be easily transmitted to the genitals.
- Recent studies show that most people with a genital herpes infection—as many as 75 to 80 percent—don't realize they have acquired the virus because they have no obvious HSV symptoms, making transmission during an infection more likely.[40]

"If there's one thing most people share in the United States, it's the herpes simplex virus (HSV)," states a recent article in the *Harvard Women's Health Watch.*[41] And it's true. Increasingly, HSV has become an infection monogamous men and women are getting from and giving to one another through intimate kissing and touching within marriage.

Consider the following all-too-common scenario: A monogamous woman who has been married for twelve years is diagnosed with genital herpes during a regular pelvic exam. But when the culture comes back positive, her doctor fails to explain one crucial fact: The test did not distinguish between HSV-1 and HSV-2. And because the herpes infection is located on the woman's genitals, she automatically assumes her husband has been unfaithful.

With many tears, the woman tells her husband about the diagnosis, expecting his full confession about an adulterous liaison. The husband is stymied. He *knows* he hasn't been with another woman. Consequently, the accused spouse becomes the angry accuser, heatedly suggesting to his wife that *she* must be the one who has been unfaithful. Without sound medical advice and information, neither partner can fully believe the other because they don't know the herpes infection was passed husband-to-wife when he had a cold sore.

See the problem? HSV has become so prevalent that it isn't possible to figure out whether an outbreak of the virus on the genitals is the type 1 or type 2 form without specific testing. Without a blood test to determine what kind of antibodies a person carries in the bloodstream, there is simply no way to know. So the first step after getting a positive diagnosis of genital herpes is for both partners to believe one another—or to hold off on the accusations until they have their blood checked. Then if both partners show antibodies to HSV-1, it's much more likely that the infection was transmitted within the marriage. On the other hand, if the blood test results show *seropositivity* (*sero*=blood; positive) for HSV-2, it's time to have a serious talk. (There is also a type-specific culture that can be done at the time of the initial test, but it's expensive and takes longer to get the results.)

This doesn't mean, of course, that most cases of genital herpes today are the result of self-infection (passing the virus to one's self from one part of the body to another area) or monogamous sexual contact. According to a recent study published in the *New England Journal of Medicine*, since the late 1970s "the prevalence of HSV-2 infection has increased by 30 percent, and HSV-2 is now detectable in roughly one in five persons twelve years of age or older nationwide. Improvements in the prevention of HSV-2 are needed, particularly since genital ulcers may facilitate the transmission of the human immunodeficiency virus."[42]

Citing reasons for recent trends in the rise of STDs in the United States, the Alan Guttmacher Institute said in a recent report:

> Changes in sexual mores together with trends in marriage and divorce have helped fuel these increases. Earlier initiation of sexual intercourse and greater acceptance of sex outside marriage have combined with later age at marriage and more widespread divorce to increase the amount of time that individuals are sexually active and unmarried. During periods

when they are not married, many sexually active persons have several sex partners, which increases their chances of having intercourse with someone who is infected with an STD. For example, never-married sexually active women are *18 times more likely*, widows and separated women are *24 times more likely*, and divorced women are *38 times more likely* than married women to have had two or more partners in the last three months.[43]

And it isn't just the person(s) that a woman has sexual relations with that increases her risk of getting a sexually transmitted virus—it's all of the partners she has had *plus* all of the partners her partner has had during their lifetimes. Thus a woman can be indirectly exposed to multiple partners carrying HSV (as well as HPV) after marriage through her husband, and vice versa. Because viral STDs are incurable—continuously carried inside the body from the time of the primary (first) infection until death—*the risk of exposure is directly related to both spouses' total number of lifetime sexual partners.*

With at least four out of five of us harboring HSV type 1 and one in six of us carrying HSV type 2—the principal cause of genital herpes—getting a herpes diagnosis is not as unusual as it used to be.[44]

Symptoms. The first sign of a genital herpes outbreak is often a tingling, itching, or burning sensation at the affected site. Flulike symptoms—including backache, low-grade fever, chills, muscle aches, headache, pain in the groin, legs, or buttocks, and swollen lymph nodes (glands) in the groin area—are also likely during the outbreak. These symptoms of virally induced general malaise often begin within five days after exposure to HSV, become more pronounced within four days of the onset of the bumps or lesions, and taper off throughout the next seven days.[45] (Note: If you have any of the following danger signs during an initial HSV attack, it may signal an infection of the central nervous system. Seek medical attention immediately if you experience neck stiffness, fever, head pain, or eye irritation from normal sunlight.)

Within one to two days, a small patch of bumps appears at the infection site on the genitals, perineum, buttocks, anus, or urethra. Soon the bumps turn into tiny, fluid-filled blisters; these later burst open and weep, producing raw, ulcerated sores (lesions) that gradually develop scabs and dry up without leaving scars. Occasionally, new lesions crop up as the first group are healing. When lesions develop in a moist area such as the mouth or vagina, the lesions do not crust over but create new skin as the sores heal. The inflamed lesions may also cause painful urination and/or a vaginal discharge similar to a vaginal infection. Complete healing of the lesions usually occurs within one to three weeks. The average length of a primary HSV infection is about twelve days, with any recurrent episodes lasting about five days.[46]

Even when no blisters or lesions are present, herpes can be spread unknowingly by a man or woman who carries HSV through "viral shedding." If the virus is present, the infection is still contagious as viral particles are "shed" from the infected site. Asymptomatic shedding may also take place *before* any bumps or sores appear.

As the sores heal, the herpes simplex virus migrates through the nervous system until it reaches a cluster of nerve cells at the base of the spine called *ganglia*. During the infection's latent phase, HSV is harmless while it remains inactive. For most people with HSV, the virus does *not* cause a distressing outbreak of blisters. It simply travels to the ganglia and lies dormant there for an indefinite time.

With oral herpes, most people report that the first sign of an infection is a distinctive tingling, burning, itching sensation, or other feeling of slight discomfort on the lips or on the surrounding skin. Though very common, these warning signs, called *prodromal symptoms* in HSV infections anywhere on the body, are not always noticeable. Some women also experience flulike symptoms during an oral herpes infection.

The number of recurrent outbreaks is highly variable from woman to woman. Outbreaks may recur when the virus retraces its steps to the surface of the body, where new lesions develop. (The word *herpes* comes from the Greek term for "creeping," and that's exactly what this virus does. It literally comes out of hiding by creeping along sensory nerves.) According to one source, genital infections caused by HSV-2 have a recurrence rate of 60 to 88 percent; those caused by HSV-1 have a recurrence rate of 14 to 25 percent.[47] However, keep in mind that the rate significantly varies from one woman to the next, no matter what type of herpes virus is involved. Some people have nearly continuous outbreaks, whereas about 10 percent of those with HSV never experience an outbreak again.[48]

Recurrent infections, if they do occur, tend to be more prevalent in the first years after the primary infection. The number and severity of attacks tend to decrease over time. Many things can trigger a recurrence of the virus (see section below). It's essential to take good care of yourself if you have HSV to avoid triggering new infections.

Transmission and incubation. Genital herpes is primarily transmitted by vaginal, anal, and oral-genital contact. It may also be transmitted to the eyes (and elsewhere) by a contaminated finger. The primary infection may develop from one to twenty-six days after exposure to the virus. For the majority of women, there is a noticeable illness with definite symptoms. But please remember—it is estimated that at least three-quarters of the individuals who contract herpes are without symptoms or mistake their initial symptoms for the flu. Furthermore, if a woman has a herpes infection on the cervix or inside the vagina, she may be unaware of the infection or mistake her discomfort for vaginitis.

Diagnosis. If you detect new sores in your genital, vaginal, or anal area, seek medical attention immediately. Once the sores begin to heal, a false-negative report is possible, so it's important to see your doctor as soon as possible. Your physician will perform a pelvic exam and, if any sores are present, may be able to make a diagnosis by looking at the lesions. She will also gently scrape suspicious areas to obtain diagnostic samples that can be examined under a microscope. It usually takes at least twenty-four to forty-eight hours to receive the lab results.

Treatment. Unfortunately, there is no available drug treatment that can stop or eradicate the herpes simplex virus. However, the current drug of choice, acyclovir (Zovirax), can change the HSV's damage-causing potential when it leaves the nerve ganglia. Acyclovir can limit the duration of a symptomatic outbreak from nine to five days, reduce the healing period from three to two weeks, and cause viral shedding to last for only two days instead of ten.[49] During an attack, 200 milligrams of acyclovir is typically taken orally every four hours, five times a day. For women who become familiar with HSV's prodromal signs, acyclovir therapy taken within two days of an outbreak can be especially effective in decreasing the severity and pain of an active infection. This is referred to as "episodic" drug therapy. Acyclovir is also available as a topical cream that can be applied to affected areas. Although the cream may reduce discomfort, it will not speed healing.

Some women experience herpes outbreaks many times per year. In addition to aiding the immune system by taking natural supplements every day (Figure 93), they may find relief from trying "suppressive" acyclovir therapy. This regimen calls for 400 milligrams of the drug to be taken orally twice per day, every day. While this therapy has been shown to reduce outbreaks by at least 75 percent, it has not been demonstrated to eliminate viral shedding, and outbreaks are likely to resume once suppressive treatment ends.[50]

Complementary natural therapies. Since some women may be sensitive to one of the following treatments, please consult an appropriate textbook or specialist for more information. Try a variety of remedies to see which ones work best for you.

L-lysine. Dr. Richard Griffith, a professor of medicine at Indiana University, advocates a daily dosage of 500 milligrams of L-lysine per ten kilograms of body weight to treat HSV and 500 milligrams per day to prevent recurrences of cold sores. (Other sources suggest higher preventative dosages, ranging from 1,500 to 6,000 milligrams per day.) Foods rich in L-lysine include fish, shrimp, chicken, turkey, lamb, beef, beans, eggs, milk, yogurt, cheese, potatoes, mung beans (bean sprouts), legumes, brewer's yeast, fruits, and fresh vegetables. To help stop the herpes virus from becoming reactivated, Dr. Griffith also recommends decreasing one's intake of arginine-rich foods (especially cocoa, carob, chocolate, nuts and nut butters, chickpeas, sesame and sunflower seeds, wheat germ, grains, coconut, brown rice, and all caffeinated beverages).[51]

Topical treatments. Herpilyn cream, available at most health food stores or with a referral from the manufacturer (Enzymatic Therapy: 800-783-2286), can be applied to the affected area two to four times a day during an outbreak. Or you may want to try Oxy C-2 Gel, an effective antiviral, antifungal, and bacteriocidal topical agent. (It's available through American Biologics at 800-227-4473.)

Another possible alternative treatment, tea tree oil, an excellent natural antiseptic, can be dabbed directly on the affected area. You may dilute the oil with a little water if it's too strong, or combine the following oils and store them in a 25 (ml.) dropper bottle—8 milliliters tea tree oil, 5 milliliters lavender oil, and 12 ounces of sweet almond oil. Apply one to two drops of this mixture to the affected site; repeat every two to three hours as needed.

Carmex ointment, when applied to the affected area near the mouth at the first prodromal signs (tingling, burning, or itching) of an outbreak is also quite effective for many people. Another possible alternative skin treatment is salve made from equal parts marigold, golden seal, and myrrh.

Bathing. Using a bidet or taking sitz baths may offer temporary relief when lesions are present. Add three tablespoons of salt or one-half cup baking soda to two or three inches of warm tub water; soak for ten to fifteen minutes twice daily. To prepare an herbal bath, boil two ounces of Uva Ursi for five minutes in one gallon of water; then let it cool. Add this to cool bathwater (80°F or lower) and soak for twenty to thirty minutes twice daily, preferably in the morning and evening. You might buy a baby bathtub to use instead. Simply sit hip-deep in the water with your back and feet propped against some pillows. A basin filled with warm water that fits on your toilet stool (with the lid up) works great too, and it's much more convenient. You may add salt, baking soda, or essential oils (such as two drops each of lavender and thyme.)

Compresses. A compress is a cloth or cotton gauze pad soaked in hot or warm water to which a skin-soothing substance may be added. For quick relief when the blisters first appear, make homemade frozen compresses in advance. Soak sterile four-inch cotton gauze squares with clean water; place plastic wrap between each square; put the prepared squares in a plastic zippered bag, and store the entire package in your freezer. Keep these on hand to use if the need arises. Apply the compress to the affected area for five to ten minutes. Ice packs may also be used to relieve pain and itching.

Other compress ideas that may be beneficial—orange pekoe tea bags briefly soaked in warm water and applied to the affected area for up to ten minutes after squeezing out the excess water (the tannic acid in the tea reportedly has a soothing effect); baking soda compresses (stir one tablespoon of baking soda into four ounces of water and then soak a sterile gauze square in the liquid); herbal compresses (soak a piece of flannel cloth in a strong decoction of equal parts marigold and kava kava); or essential oil compresses (add a few drops of geranium, eucalyptus, and lemon oil to five milliliters of calendula oil; store in a dark-colored bottle and apply to the affected area on a sterile gauze square).

Pain relief. In most cases, a regimen of over-the-counter analgesics is recommended. Ask your physician for her advice on pain treatment at the time of your diagnosis.

General self-help measures. To speed healing, prevent the spread of HSV, and decrease the number of outbreaks:

- Keep the infected area clean and dry between baths and compress applications.
- Use a portable hair dryer (set on the coolest setting) to dry the area after bathing or soaking.
- Avoid tight-fitting clothing and synthetic underwear.
- Practice good hygiene. Wash your hands whenever you use the toilet or touch the affected area. You can avoid transmitting the virus to yourself or others by cleansing your hands often, as soap and water easily destroy the virus. Use gentle friction for at least ten seconds while you scrub.
- Abstain from intimate sexual contact during an outbreak of cold sores or genital herpes. Wait until all the sores have healed before resuming sexual activity, or at least avoid intimately touching any affected areas. Use condoms between outbreaks if your husband has been tested and does not have the same type of HSV.
- If urinating hurts, lean forward and direct the stream away from the sores, or use a "peri-bottle" rinse (fill a squirt bottle with warm water and spray over the genitals to dilute the urine) while urinating.

- Wear loose-fitting pajama bottoms during an outbreak. It's not unusual to touch itchy affected areas when half-asleep.

Follow-up. There are a number of effective ways to enhance your health and ease life with HSV after you receive the initial diagnosis.

Recognize and avoid triggers. Many women report having recurrences of HSV that are predictably "set off" by certain events, emotions, or environmental factors, such as:

- menstruation
- sunlight/sunburn
- illness, fever, and other infections
- hormonal irregularities
- emotional stress
- vigorous sexual activity
- nutritional imbalances and deficiencies
- surgery
- arginine-rich foods (especially chocolate)
- travel/jet lag
- school, work, and holiday deadlines
- depression
- moving
- family crises; relationship difficulties
- fatigue; irregular sleep patterns

Identify stress sources and implement effective coping strategies. A missed deadline, the holiday rush, overdue bill payments, sick children, and relationship difficulties are typical examples of triggers cited by women with HSV. Though it's impossible to avoid all of life's stresses and strains, the way a woman manages and responds to stress can ease or exacerbate its effects on her body, mind, and spirit. For more information, read *The Christian Woman's Guide to Sexuality* or another Christ-centered book that offers multiple ideas for coping with chronic stress.

Respond constructively to unhealthy, energy-zapping emotional states. Like stress, anxiety and depression are closely linked with immune system irregularities. Learning new ways to respond to life's difficulties and challenges is essential to promoting one's overall well-being. Consult your physician if your energy level is consistently low. As with any prescribed medication, if your physician recommends Prozac, Zoloft, St. John's-wort, or another appropriate treatment, be sure to discuss the treatment's benefits and possible alternative therapies.

Get regular Pap tests. Herpes may increase the risk of cervical cancer, so it's wise to have a Pap test every six to twelve months, depending on your health-care provider's recommendation.

If you're pregnant, let your doctor know that you have been infected with HSV. Your physician will want to monitor any outbreaks before the baby is born because the virus can harm an infant passing through the birth canal. A cesarean section may be required if you have an outbreak of HSV near the end of pregnancy.

Seek support. Women who receive a diagnosis for genital herpes commonly experience a variety of emotions as they come to terms with it. Be kind to yourself as you take time to adjust to what it will mean to alter your lifestyle in order to avoid future outbreaks.

Build up your immune system (see Figure 93).

Complementary Therapies
and Natural Treatments[52]
Figure 93

EAT FOODS HIGH IN ANTIOXIDANTS

Beta-carotene

Vegetables: beet greens, broccoli, carrots, pumpkins, spinach, sweet potatoes, cabbage, lettuce, yellow corn

Fruits: cantaloupe, apricots, and mangoes

Animal products: liver, eggs, milk, and yogurt

Vitamin A

Animal products: liver, eggs, milk, and yogurt

Vitamin C

Vegetables: brussels sprouts, cauliflower, peas, cabbage, and green peppers

Fruits: oranges, lemons, limes, pineapples, raspberries, strawberries, and grapefruit

Vitamin E

Vegetable oils, nuts, and whole grains (nuts and whole grains are also high in arginine)

TAKE ANTIOXIDANT SUPPLEMENTS

In *Advanced Nutritional Therapies,* preventative health expert Dr. Kenneth H. Cooper recommends these *minimum* daily dosages:[53]

Vitamin C: 500 milligrams, once or twice a day

Vitamin E: 400 IU, once a day

Folic acid: 400 *micro*grams, once a day

Selenium: 50 *micro*grams, three times a day

Beta-carotene: 25,000 IU through your diet (for example, one and a half medium-size carrots provide this amount)

Consult your favorite nutritional supplement text for further information.

TAKE EVENING PRIMROSE OIL

Essential fatty acids play an important role in regulating the immune system—and evening primrose oil carries the highest level of gamma-linoleic acid of any food. Use as directed on the bottle label.

USE GARLIC SUPPLEMENTS.

Garlic helps the body fight infections and disease. It has been used as a medicinal treatment since biblical times due to its potent properties as an immune system stimulant. With its special antiviral, antibiotic, and antifungal qualities, it is useful as a complementary therapy for any STD. Garlic may be eaten fresh, taken as a deodorized supplement, or used as an oil. During a herpes outbreak (including a cold sore attack), when you feel tingling at a herpes site, take twelve capsules of deodorized garlic (Kyolic is a commonly available brand), then three capsules every four hours during waking hours for four days.

TRY IMMUNE-STRENGTHENING HERBS

Echinacea

Golden seal (do not take during pregnancy!)

Blue flag

Note: See chapter 3 for contraindications.

PRACTICE IMMUNE-BOOSTING LIFESTYLE BEHAVIORS

Exercise regularly and sensibly.

Get enough rest and relaxation.

Eat regular, well-balanced, planned meals, taking time to enjoy mealtimes.

Eliminate as many sources of stress from your life as you can.

Practice sound sleep habits.

Drink six to eight cups (8 ounces each) of purified water daily.

Realize that overworking, expecting too much from others, and trying to be perfect can wreck your physical, emotional, social, and spiritual well-being. So give yourself (and others) a break, okay? Learn from the Lord's example and head for the hills. (See Figure 94.)

ADDRESS UNHEALTHY LIFESTYLE BEHAVIORS

Reduce or eliminate caffeinated and alcoholic beverages.

Stop smoking.

If you're in an out-of-bounds sexual relationship, it's time for a change. Pray for the Lord's strength and direction; make a fresh start with God's help; seek sound Christ-centered counseling; ask for prayer support from someone you trust; join an accountability group; read applicable texts for additional information; receive specific prayer to break spiritual bondage in your life.

If your husband was/is in an out-of bounds sexual relationship, it's time for a change. Give the broken fragments of your shattered dreams to Christ; call upon the Lord for renewal and guidance; pray for specific needs; assess relationship patterns that need changing; obtain Christ-centered counseling; be open to what God is teaching you through the life-changing experience of spiritual brokenness; join an accountability group; receive specific prayer to break spiritual bondage in your life.

Life in the Balance:
Is It Time to Head for the Hills?
Figure 94

The time we invest in meaningful moments with loved ones and with God in prayer reduces daily stress and yields lasting dividends, including spiritual renewal and significant long-term health benefits. Yet many of us spend little time simply enjoying the pleasure of being with our families or being alone with God. Except for specific, time-limited periods when overactivity is unavoidable, the way we live comes down to a series of personal choices we make on a daily basis. These decisions, in turn, have a direct impact on our physical, emotional, social, and spiritual well-being and on the well-being of those with whom we share close relationships. If you're interested in living a more balanced life, here are some things you may want to try.

MAKE AN ASSESSMENT

- Would you say that you are fairly calm, stable, and even-tempered most of the time, or do you often feel tense, moody, angry, anxious, and/or temperamental?
- Do you find it easy or difficult to relax, other than when sleeping? List five things you like to do that bring you relaxation and refreshment.
- Explain your current state of physical health. Are you facing any current health concerns, involved in any ongoing medical therapies, or taking regular medication? If so, please name them here.
- Describe your current workload, including housework and volunteer work.
- How active would you say you are in church-related activities?
- How often do you have regular quiet time with God? How often do you pray, other than at meals or during church services?
- If you are married, how satisfied are you with your marriage? If you are single, how satisfied are you with being single?
- Are you satisfied with the sexual relationship you have with your spouse? If so, why? If not, how would you change it?
- Do you have children? How are things going?
- Name at least three sources of stress in your life that you are facing right now.

DEVELOP A PLAN

Here are a few questions you may ask yourself about daily tasks and work responsibilities if your life seems to be swaying out of balance:

Can this task

(A) be eliminated?
(B) be done less often?
(C) be done at the same time as another task or activity?
(D) be delegated to someone else?
(E) be done later if I temporarily take a break?

Create a Household Task List

Who will:

Vacuum	____	Do dishes	____	Clean the bathroom	____
Make the bed	____	Do laundry	____	Cook	____
Change the linens	____	Do yard work	____	Take out garbage	____
Wash floor(s)	____	Get groceries	____	Pay bills	____
Other	____	Other	____	Other	____

HEAD FOR THE HILLS

Consider the number of times that Jesus is described as "heading into the hills." How many places can you find in the Gospels where Christ suddenly left the crowds and/or His disciples to be alone with God? Does your life take into account your need for quiet and rest? In the weeks ahead, how will you better accommodate your need for drawing near to Jesus away from the busyness of everyday demands and your work responsibilities?

REMEMBER GOD'S GOODNESS AND PROVIDENCE

- "What do people really get for all their hard work? I have thought about this in connection with the various kinds of work God has given people to do. God has made everything beautiful for its own time. He has planted eternity in the human heart, but even so, people cannot see the whole scope of God's work from beginning to end. So I concluded that there is nothing better for people than to be happy and to enjoy themselves as long as they can. And people should eat and drink and enjoy the fruits of their labor, for these are gifts from God" (Ecclesiastes 3:9-13 NLB).

- "Rejoice in the Lord always. I will say it again: Rejoice! Let your gentleness be evident to all. The Lord is near. Do not be anxious about anything, but in everything, by prayer and petition, with thanksgiving, present your requests to God. And the peace of God, which transcends all understanding, will guard your hearts and your minds in Christ Jesus. Finally, brothers, whatever is true, whatever is noble, whatever is right, whatever is pure, whatever is lovely, whatever is admirable—if anything is excellent or praiseworthy—think about such things" (Philippians 4:4-8).

- "Your love, O LORD, reaches to the heavens, your faithfulness to the skies. Your righteousness is like the mighty mountains, your justice like the great deep. O LORD, you preserve both man and beast. How priceless is your unfailing love! Both high and low among men find refuge in the shadow of your wings. They feast on the abundance of your house; you give them drink from your river of delights. For with you is the fountain of life; in your light we see light" (Psalm 36:5-9).

GET HELP

If you are struggling with fatigue, anger, depression, guilt, anxiety, or any other difficult-to-deal-with physical, emotional, or spiritual response to your current workload and family responsibilities, please pray for God's guidance. Consider asking your mentor, pastor, physician, or a Christ-centered counselor what steps you can begin to take that will help bring a healthy balance back into your life.

A WORD ABOUT STD-RELATED STIGMA

Any woman who acquires a sexually transmitted disease goes through a period of painful emotional and spiritual growth as she comes to terms with her infection. When she hears the news, her mind races through a list of possibilities, fears, and doubts. She may question the validity of the lab results and her doctor's diagnosis. Anger, grief, shame, disbelief, shock, sadness, and panic are commonly experienced to varying degrees.

For a chaste Christian woman who has abstained from sex outside marriage, getting an STD from her husband is likely to be a landmark event, representing a before-and-after crisis unlike any other. In many cases, getting an STD diagnosis will mean coming out of denial to face the gut-wrenching reality of a husband's infidelity, bringing about a necessary shift in life focus that provokes an in-depth reappraisal of one's marriage.

If this happens (or has happened) to you, I earnestly urge you to seek the help and healing Christ offers and desires for you. I realize that you may want to shake your fist at the Lord and yell at the top of your lungs, "What did I do to deserve this?" or collapse in a pool of tears while wondering how this could have happened to you. Please understand this though: *The virus that infected your body didn't choose you as its target.* STDs don't distinguish between "good" and "bad" sexual behavior—they simply act according to what their biological programming tells them to do.

This crisis may actually have a few important things to teach you, if you're willing to learn from it. Like a fork in the road, you will have several options awaiting your prayerful concern and attention. I can't tell you what the way ahead holds for you, but I can offer these words of encouragement. The Holy Spirit is intimately acquainted with the burdens of your marriage and is constantly available to lead, guide, and encourage you. Does the way ahead seem dark, confusing, unclear? Call upon God for help in your anguish. You will discover greater depths of His unfailing love in a place where the Lord wants you to depend upon Him, perhaps as never before. Please don't allow your anger to turn you away from the Lord's comfort and counsel. Allow the hurt you feel to carry you into His arms instead.

The stigma associated with getting an STD—whether it happens to be herpes, HPV, chlamydia, gonorrhea, syphilis, HIV, or any other disease—is something we can give to Christ, recognizing that He freely offers to help bear our heartache and grief. Thankfully, we can go to the Lord and seek His comfort, no matter how great the burden may be:

We do not have a high priest who is unable to sympathize with our weaknesses, but we have one who has been tempted in every way, just as we are—yet was without sin. Let us then approach the throne of grace with confidence, so that we may receive mercy and find grace to help us in our time of need.

—HEBREWS 4:15,16

How graciously our Shepherd tends the wounds of His flock! Remember, if you've made the heartbreaking mistake of having sex outside marriage, there's good news. God's Word promises that if we confess our sins, he is faithful and will forgive our sins and purify us from all unrighteousness (1 John 1:9). As we kneel before him, broken and sick at heart, He says, "Go now and leave your life of sin" (John 8:11). In exchange for the wrongs we have done in the past, He offers us new life and a brand-new chance to begin again as we walk with Him into the future.

Millions of Christian women today are learning what it means to live with an incurable STD; millions more have been successfully treated for sexually transmitted infections. Untold thousands daily face infertility as a result of PID. Will you pray with me for the sexual and reproductive health of our nation? Together, we can make a difference in our world as we compassionately extend the good news of Christ's unchanging love, grace, and freedom to one another.

Closing Thoughts

N ow for all the topics I haven't covered yet—everything from persis-
tent bladder infections, chronic yeast infections, endometrial hyperplasia,
HIV treatment, polycystic ovary disease, and "to douche or not to douche" (is
that the question?) . . .

Seriously, to make this book truly complete, it would have taken at least
1,000 pages—not 400—to include all of the topics I wanted to cover. I hope that
you will use this book wisely and often as an information resource and for
moral support when you feel that all you ever do is fight uphill battles, swim
against strong currents, and sound as if you're speaking in a foreign language
to those who can't/won't listen to you. I am more convinced than ever that
there are a lot of us out here—literally thousands of us, and probably even tens
of thousands—who desire to approach our health care from a life-affirming
perspective.

Is it any "less Christian" for women to be informed about their health care
than to passively submit to treatments they don't fully understand or agree
with? Is it "arrogant" to ask physicians questions related to reproduction? Is
it "too worldly" to compare physicians before purchasing their medical services? Of course not. In fact, *today's style of managed health care—as expensive and*

ethically complicated as it is—requires more prayer and thoughtfully considered involvement than ever before.

In closing, I want to encourage you to seek God's best for every aspect of your life. Your sexuality is a precious gift worth guarding, protecting, celebrating, and understanding. Yes, we live in a groaning world (Rom. 8:22), but this hard truth doesn't negate the marvelous fact that you and I are fearfully and wonderfully made, inside and out. It's easy to forget this, isn't it? We need to remind ourselves—often—of the intricate beauty of our bodies, giving thanks to our Creator for entrusting us with the gift of Christ's life within us. *What a privilege!*

$\mathscr{L}$ife-Affirming Ethical Codes in Traditional Medicine

DECLARATION OF GENEVA, WORLD MEDICAL
ASSOCIATION, 1948

At the time of being admitted as a member of the medical
profession:

> *I solemnly pledge myself to consecrate my life*
> *to the service of humanity;*
> *I will give to my teachers the respect and gratitude*
> *which is their due;*
> *I will practice my profession with conscience and dignity;*
> *The health of my patient will always be*
> *my first consideration;*
> *I will respect the secrets which are confided in me,*
> *even after the patient has died;*
> *I will maintain by all the means in my power,*
> *the honor and the noble traditions of the medical profession.*
> *My colleagues will be my brothers;*
> *I will not permit considerations of religion, nationality, race,*
> *party politics or social standing to intervene between*
> *my duty and my patient;*

*I will maintain the utmost respect
for human life from the moment of conception;
even under threat, I will not use my medical knowledge
contrary to the laws of humanity.
I make these promises solemnly, freely and upon my honor.*

"Adopted by the General Assembly of the World Medical Association at Geneva in 1948 and amended by the 22nd World Medical Assembly at Sydney in 1968, the Declaration of Geneva was one of the first and most important actions of the association. It is a declaration of physicians' dedication to the humanitarian goals of medicine, a declaration that was especially important in view of the medical crimes that had just been committed in Nazi Germany. The Declaration of Geneva was intended to update the Oath of Hippocrates, which was no longer suited to modern conditions."[1]

THE OATH OF HIPPOCRATES, SIXTH CENTURY B.C.
(EXCERPT)

I will keep [my patient] from harm and injustice. I will neither give a deadly drug to anybody if asked for it, nor will I make a suggestion to this effect. Similarly I will not give to a woman an abortive remedy. In purity and holiness I will guard my life and my art.

ECCLESIASTICUS 38:1-14
(*NEW ENGLISH BIBLE WITH THE APOCRYPHA*)

*Honor the doctor for his services; for the Lord created him.
His skill comes from the Most High,
and he is rewarded by kings.
The doctor's knowledge gives him high standing,
and wins him the admiration of the great.
The Lord has created medicines from the earth,
and a sensible man will not disparage them.
Was it not a tree that sweetened water,
and so disclosed its properties?
The Lord has imparted knowledge to men,
that by their use of his marvels he may win praise;
by using them the doctor relieves pain
and from them the pharmacist makes up a mixture.*

> There is no end to the works of the Lord,
> who spreads health over the whole world.
> My son, if you have an illness, do not neglect it,
> but pray to the Lord and he will heal you.
> Renounce your faults, amend your ways,
> and cleanse your heart from all sin.
> Bring a savory offering and bring flour for a token,
> and pour oil on the sacrifice; be as generous as you can.
> Then call in the doctor, for the Lord created him;
> do not let him leave you, for you need him.
> There may come a time when your recovery is in their hands;
> then they too will pray to the Lord
> to give them success in relieving pain and finding a cure
> to save the patient's life.

—BEN SIRA

THE OATH OF ASPAH, SIXTH CENTURY A.D.

Take heed that ye kill not any man with the sap of a root; and ye shall not dispense a potion to a woman with child by adultery to cause her to miscarry. . . . Put your trust in the Lord your God, the God of truth, the living God, for He doth kill and make alive, smite and heal. . . . Ye shall not cause the shedding of blood by any manner of medical treatment. Take heed that ye do not cause a malady to any man; and ye shall not cause any man injury by hastening to cut through flesh and blood with an iron instrument or by branding, but shall first observe twice and thrice and only then shall give your counsel.

—ASAPH JUDAEUS,

A HEBREW PHYSICIAN

ADVICE TO A PHYSICIAN, EIGHTH CENTURY A.D.

You are to prohibit the unsuited and the undeserving from studying medicine. A physician is to prudently treat his patients with food and medicine out of good and spiritual motives, not for the sake of gain. He should never prescribe a harmful drug or abortifacient. . . . He must not drink alcohol because it injures the brain. He must study medical books constantly and never grow tired of research. . . . A medical student should be constantly present in the hospital so as to study disease processes and complications under the learned professor and proficient physicians.

—HALY ABBAS,
PERSIAN ETHICIST AND PHYSICIAN

Sources: *The New English Bible* (Cambridge, England: The University Printing House, 1972); Daniel C. Overduin and John I. Fleming, *Life in a Test-Tube: Medical and Ethical Issues Facing Society Today* (Adelaide, Australia: Lutheran Publishing House, 1982).

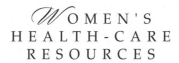

WOMEN'S
HEALTH-CARE
RESOURCES

PMS AND PAINFUL PERIODS

PMS Access, P.O. Box 9326, Madison, WI 53715. (800) 222-4PMS. Web site: www.womenshealth.com/. National group offering support for PMS sufferers.

Pope Paul VI Institute for the Study of Human Reproduction, 6901 Mercy Road, Suite 200, Omaha, NE 68106. (402) 390-6600. International research institute for issues related to human reproduction, including PMS, infertility, endometriosis, chronic miscarriage, and natural family planning.

Harvard Women's Health Watch, 164 Longwood Avenue, Boston, MA 02115-5818. (617) 432-1485. Offers a monthly newsletter with current information related to women's health issues. Note: Harvard Medical School publishes this newsletter, so expect the contents to reflect the school's secular standards. Worth reading if you want to stay updated and are willing to "pick out the bones."

For Further Reading

FDA, "Doing Something About Menstrual Discomforts." Common problems and treatments that are effective in relieving specific symptoms. Available free from the Consumer Information Center, P.O. Box 100, Pueblo, CO 81002. Request a copy of their current catalog.

Joseph Martorano and Maureen Morgan, *Unmasking PMS: The Complete Medical Treatment Plan* (New York: Berkley, 1994).

Penny W. Budhoff, *No More Menstrual Cramps and Other Good News* (New York: G. P. Putnam's Sons, 1980).

Katherina Dalton, *The Premenstrual Syndrome* (Springfield, IL: Charles C. Thomas, 1964) and Once a Month, 4th ed. (Claremont, CA: Hunter House, 1990).

Ann Navarro et al., *The PMS Solution: A Nutritional Approach to Premenstrual Syndrome* (New York: Harper and Row, 1985).

HYSTERECTOMY AND HOW TO AVOID UNNECESSARY SURGERY

Hysterectomy Educational Resources and Services Foundation (HERS), 422 Bryn Mawr Avenue, Bala Cynwyd, PA 19004. (215) 667-7757. Call between 9:00 A.M. and 5:00 P.M. EST.

For Further Reading

Stanley West with Paula Dranov, *The Hysterectomy Hoax* (New York: Doubleday, 1994).

Ivan K. Strauz, *You Don't Need a Hysterectomy: New and Effective Ways of Avoiding Major Surgery* (Reading, MA: Addison-Wesley, 1993).

Winnifred B. Cutler, *Hysterectomy: Before and After* (New York: Harper & Row, 1988).

Herbert A. Goldfarb with Judith Greif, *The No-Hysterectomy Option* (New York: Wiley, 1990).

Sidney Wolfe, *Women's Health Alert* (New York: Warner Books, 1991).

SECOND OPINIONS

Department of Health and Human Services, *Facing Surgery? Why Not Get a Second Opinion?* Includes a toll-free number for locating specialists. Available free from the Consumer Information Center (address above).

William H. Parker with Rachel L. Parker, *A Gynecologist's Second Opinion: The Questions and Answers You Need to Take Charge of Your Health* (New York: Plume, 1996).

ENDOMETRIOSIS

Endometriosis Association, 8585 N. 76th Place, Milwaukee, WI 53223. (800) 992-3636; call (414) 355-2200 for counseling or answers to specific questions. Web site: www.endometriosisassn.org/.

For Further Reading

Mary Lou Ballweg and the Endometriosis Association, *The Endometriosis Sourcebook* (Chicago, IL: Contemporary Books, 1995).

U.S.-Canadian Endometriosis Association, *Overcoming Endometriosis: New Help from the Endometriosis Association* (New York: Congdon & Weed, 1987).

HEALTH-CARE CONSUMER ISSUES

FDA Consumer. Covers recent developments in the regulation of foods, drugs, and cosmetics by the Food and Drug Administration. Also contains excellent articles on current health issues. Available through the Consumer Information Center (address above).

Health-care information on the Web. Dr. Koop's Community: *www.drkoop.com* is the best overall guide to understanding and managing your health-care options, obtaining information on specific drugs (the section on OCs is dynamite) and diseases, and chatting with others in health forums online. Dr. C. Everett Koop, the trusted medical authority who unequivocally affirms the value of human life from conception, writes a weekly "Dear-Abby-style" column for the Web site he developed.

HOW TO TALK TO AND SELECT HEALTH-CARE PROVIDERS AND PHARMACISTS

American Association of Retired Persons (in cooperation with the Federal Trade Commission), *Healthy Questions.* Available from the AARP, Consumer Affairs Section, 1909 K Street NW, Washington, DC 20049, or from the Consumer Information Center (free) as listed above.

CRISIS PREGNANCY, POSTABORTION SUPPORT, AND ADOPTION GROUPS

American Crisis Pregnancy Centers Helpline, (800) 67-BABY-6. Web site: www.thehelpline.org/.

American Victims of Abortion, Suite 402, 419 Seventh Street NW, Washington, DC 20004. (202) 626-8800.

Bethany Christian Services, 901 Eastern Avenue NE, Grand Rapids, MI 49503-1295. (800) BETHANY. Web site: www.bethany.org/.

Birthright, 11235 C Street NE, Chicago, IL 60643. (800) 550-4900. Web site: www.birthright.org/.

Crisis Pregnancy Centers Online, www.prolife.org/cpcs-online/.

Lifeline, (800) 368-3336.

National Life Center, Inc., 686 North Broad Street, Woodbury, NJ 08096. (800) 848-5683.

National Prolife Religious Council, c/o NAE, 1023 15th Street NW, Suite 50, Washington, DC 20005. (202) 789-1011.

The Nurturing Network, (800) 866-4666.

POSTABORTION SYNDROME (PAS) SYMPTOMS

Reexperiencing the Trauma of the Abortion

- Nightmares, recurrent dreams, flashback episodes.
- Anniversary reactions on the date the abortion took place.
- Emotional distress when exposed to events resembling some aspect of the abortion, such as during a pelvic exam, lovemaking, or childbirth.

Avoidance or Denial of the Abortion

- Blocking out thoughts or feelings concerning the abortion.
- Avoiding situations and activities that trigger thoughts about the abortion (exposure to pregnant friends or their babies, conversations about abortion or childbirth, medical exams, sex).
- Difficulty or inability to recall events related to the abortion.
- Emotional numbness, distancing from those around you, especially from your loved ones.

Increased Emotional Arousal

- Sleep disorders, irritability, angry outbursts, difficulty in concentrating, forgetfulness.
- Exaggerated startle response or hypervigilance.

Associated Symptoms

- Depression; frequent crying episodes; anxiety.
- Guilt and inability to forgive yourself.
- Self-destructive and/or addictive behaviors; substance abuse; suicide attempts or fantasies; sexual promiscuity; eating disorders.

Adapted from *The Mourning After* by Terry Selby (Grand Rapids, MI: Baker Book House, 1990), pp. 127-130.

Note: If you have had an abortion, no matter how long ago it has been, and you are experiencing PAS symptoms, contact one of the groups listed above now for help and support in taking the first steps toward recovery. When we bury our feelings instead of allowing ourselves to fully experience and face them, we bury them alive. Pain is always a part of the healing process. Don't be afraid to face it with a Friend who will accept you just as you are—the Lord Jesus Christ.

EDUCATIONAL SUPPLY CENTERS

American Life League, P.O. Box 1350, Stafford, VA 22554. (703) 659-4171 Web site: www.all.org/.

Couple to Couple League, P.O. Box 111184, Cincinnati, OH 45211-1184. (513) 471-2000. Web site: www.ccli.org/. Catalog orders: (800) 745-8252.

Focus on the Family, 8605 Explorer Drive, Colorado Springs, CO 80920. (800) A-FAMILY. Web site: www.fotf.org/.

For Further Reading

James Burtchaell, *Rachel Weeping* (San Francisco: Harper & Row, 1984).

Francis Schaeffer and C. Everett Koop, *Whatever Happened to the Human Race?* (Wheaton, IL: Crossway Books, 1979).

Curt Young, *The Least of These* (Chicago: Moody Press, 1983).

John Wilks, *A Consumer's Guide to the Pill and Other Drugs* (Stafford, VA: American Life League, 1997).

NATURAL FAMILY PLANNING

For individual NFP groups, practitioners, and instructors in your area, send a self-addressed, stamped envelope with your request to CCL or the Pope Paul VI Institute, or visit CCL's Web site.

Couple to Couple League (CCL); address and phone number is listed above. Headed by founders John and Sheila Kippley, CCL offers an excellent home study course in addition to an extensive network of individual NFP groups and instructors across the country. CCL currently provides services in 48 states and 13 foreign countries, with 20,000 active members in addition to more than 800 teaching couples and 200 volunteer PR representatives. Write or call for their catalogue and a reference to the group/instructor nearest you. In addition to the Home Study Course (which includes audio tapes, charts, books, and a basal body temperature thermometer), CCL serves as a book and audiovisual source for family education and Christian sexuality materials.

- *The Art of Natural Family Planning.* As written by John Kippley, this book presents arguments for NFP as a source of deep marital enrichment as well as a truly prolife approach to Spirit-led child spacing. Worth reading on these merits alone.
- "The Effectiveness of Natural Family Planning." Buy several copies of this smart little fifteen-page booklet and give it to your physician, your pastor, your mother, and your husband.
- "Birth Control and Christian Discipleship." Written by John Kippley and John Noonan. Long neglected because of their Catholic backgrounds. Other Christians are now catching on to these authors and for good reason. Read this brief-but-beautiful booklet to find out why.
- "Birth Control and the Marriage Covenant." More food for thought by NFP expert John Kippley.
- *Breastfeeding and Natural Child Spacing.* Sheila Kippley's classic work on the ecology of natural mothering and God's design for natural family planning.
- CCL's Pamphlet Series. A priceless collection of pamphlets on everything from the fruit of the Spirit and NFP to Margaret Sanger (how much more diversified can you get?). This collection offers a real bargain with prices ranging from just ten to fifty cents. Especially recommended: "A Physician's Reference to NFP," "The Case for NFP," "Practical Reasons for Chastity," "Reflections of a 17-Year-Old," and "From Contraception to Abortion."

Pope Paul VI Institute for the Study of Human Reproduction; address and phone number are listed above. Dr. Hilgers' unique Institute, besides being heavily involved in reproductive research from a thoroughly life-affirming perspective, provides teacher training in the Creighton NFP Model—a medically standardized version of the Ovulation Method of NFP. Available publications and audio cassettes include:

- *The Ovulation Method of Natural Family Planning.* An introduction to the Ovulation Method, this book is designed to supplement instruction in NFP and covers all the basics, from seminal fluid instruction to the impact of breastfeeding patterns on ovulation.

- *Picture Dictionary of the Ovulation Method.* Includes easy-to-understand color photographs of mucus symptoms, detailed charting information, and wonderful charts on women's fertility.

- NFP Audiotape Series. Dr. Hilgers' excellent tapes are available from the institute to enhance your understanding of moral, spiritual, and physiological aspects of NFP. Write for a catalog.

Billings Ovulation Method Association, 316 N. 7th Avenue, St. Cloud, MN 56303-3633. (888) NFP-NFP-1. Web site: www.billings-centre.ab.ca./. Provides education and instruction in the Ovulation Method throughout the world.

American Academy of Natural Family Planning, 615 S. Ballas Road, St. Louis, MO 63141-7018.(314) 569-6495.

Apple Tree Family Ministries, P.O. Box 2083, Artesia, CA 90702-2083. ATFM is an excellent source for natural family planning, birthing, and breastfeeding support from a Christian perspective. Founded by childbirth reform advocate Helen Wessel, ATFM is seeking to expand its educational and teacher training ministry into the twenty-first century, and understandably so, given the neopantheistic emphasis of most other natural birthing organizations. Write for a copy of their newsletter and catalog.

FOR FURTHER READING

Nona Aguilar, *The New No-Pill, No-Risk Birth Control* (New York: Rawson, 1986).

Toni Weschler, *Taking Charge of Your Fertility* (New York: HarperCollins, 1996).

SEXUALLY TRANSMITTED DISEASES

Office of Women's Health, Centers for Disease Control and Prevention, 1600 Clifton Road NE, MS: D-51, Atlanta, GA 30333. (404) 639-7230. Web site: www.cdc.gov/od/owh/whhome.htm/. One of eleven divisions of the CDC, the Office of Women's Health provides information on STDs, breast and cervical cancer, tobacco use, reproductive health, and violence.

National Institute of Allergy and Infectious Diseases, National Institutes of Health, Office of Communication, Building 31, Room 7A-50, 31 Center Drive, MSC2520,

Bethesda, MD 20892-2520. (301) 496-5717. Web site: www.niaid.nih.gov/. Offers free consumer pamphlets and a publications list on STDs upon request.

Medical Institute for Sexual Health, P.O. Box 4919, Austin, TX 78765. (800) 892-9484. Founded by Christian OB/GYN Dr. Joe S. McIlhaney, Jr., the institute is a nonprofit organization working to inform the public, educators, and medical professionals about the risks associated with STDs.

For Further Reading

Joe S. McIlhaney, *Sexuality and Sexually Transmitted Diseases* (Grand Rapids: Baker, 1990).

Philippa Harknett, *Herpes Simplex: The Self-Help Guide to Managing the Herpes Virus* (San Francisco: Thorson/HarperCollins, 1994).

HERBS AND VITAMINS

Ferry-Morse Seed Co., Box 200, Fulton, KY 42041. (800) 626-3392. Herbs, citrus fruit, flowers, and seeds. Grow your own!

Burgess Seed and Plant Co., 67 East Battle Creek Street, Galesburg, MI 49053. Herb seeds, garden supplies.

Indiana Botanic Gardens, Inc., Hammond, IN 46325. Herbs, herb preparations, gums, oils, and resins.

Northwestern Processing Co., 217 North Broadway, Milwaukee, WI 53202. Herbs, spices, teas, coffees, and nuts.

The Professional and Compounding Centers of America, Inc., P.O. Box 368, Sugar Land, TX 77487. Information and training for physicians and pharmacists regarding drug therapies related to reproductive health.

NUTRITION AND EXERCISE

Center for Science in the Public Interest, Suite 300, 1875 Connecticut Avenue NW, Washington, DC 20009-5728. Publishes the *Nutrition Action Health Letter.*

Food and Drug Administration (FDA): www.fda.gov/. The FDA on-line service.

President's Council on Physical Fitness and Sports, Walking for Exercise and Pleasure. Attractive twelve-page booklet on walking. Available from the Consumer Information Center (see address above).

For Further Reading

Jane Brody, *Jane Brody's Good Food Book* (New York: W. W. Norton, 1985).

Kenneth H. Cooper, *Advanced Nutritional Therapies* (Nashville: Thomas Nelson, 1996).

Julian Whitaker, *Dr. Whitaker's Guide to Natural Healing* (Rocklin, CA: Prima, 1996).

Jane Hirschman and Carol Hunter, *Overcoming Overeating* (New York: Fawcett Columbine, 1988).

Elizabeth Somer, *Food & Mood: The Complete Guide to Eating Well and Feeling Your Best* (New York: Henry Holt, 1995).

Debra Waterhouse, *Outsmarting the Female Fat Cell* (New York, Warner, 1994).

INFERTILITY

Infertility: Medical and Social Choices, available from the U.S. Superintendent of Documents. Along with the title, request stock number 052-003-01091-7 when calling the Government Printing Office at (202) 783-3238 for current pricing and ordering information.

A. Toth, *The Fertility Solution* (New York: Atlantic Monthly Press, 1991). Dr. Toth's startling suggestion for low-tech infertility treatment—antibiotic therapy—refutes other infertility specialists' recommendations for starting life in the lab. His revolutionary approach to reversing infertility is absolutely remarkable.

CANCER PREVENTION AND DETECTION

American Cancer Society. Check your phone book for a local chapter or contact ACS, 1599 Clifton Road, Atlanta, GA 30329. (800) ACS-2345. Hours: 8:30 A.M. to 5:00 P.M. EST. Web site: www.cancer.org/. This national organization provides a wide variety of educational materials, patient services, support groups, and rehabilitation resources.

National Cancer Institute, Office of Cancer Communications, National Institutes of Health, Building 31, Room 10A18, Bethesda, MD 20205. Web site: www.nci.nih.gov/. National organization that makes information, referral, and pamphlets available on cancer, including the latest treatment options. Ask for a list of available educational material from this branch of the U.S. Public Health Service or call 1-800-4-CANCER between 9:00 A.M. and 7:00 P.M. EST, Monday through Friday, except on Christmas.

American Institute for Cancer Research, Washington, DC 20069. National research and educational organization responsible for publishing a newsletter and pamphlets, including a summary of dietary guidelines for cancer prevention.

For Further Reading

"Everything Doesn't Cause Cancer," National Institutes of Health. Facts about the causes and prevention of cancer, with toll-free cancer information numbers. Available free from the Consumer Information Center (address above).

"Cancer Prevention: Good News, Better News, Best News," National Institutes of Health. How to protect yourself against cancer; includes nutritional information. Available free from the Consumer Information Center (address above).

Susan Love, *Dr. Susan Love's Breast Book* (Reading, MA: Addison-Wesley, 1990).

Kerry A. McGinn and Pamela J. Haylock, *Women's Cancers* (Alameda, CA: Hunter House, 1993).

Donald F. Tapley et al., *The Columbia University College of Physicians and Surgeons Complete Home Medical Guide* (New York: Crown, 1995).

Sidney J. Winawer and Moshe Shike, *Cancer Free: The Complete Cancer Prevention Program* (New York: Fireside, 1995).

$\mathscr{N}$ O T E S

Chapter 1

1. O. Chambers, *My Utmost for His Highest* (New York: Dodd, Mead & Co., 1935), 340. First Corinthians 6:19-20 is the biblical passage underlying Chambers's teaching.

2. G. Redmond, *The Good News About Women's Hormones* (New York: Warner, 1995), 26-27.

CHAPTER 3

1. J. R. Lee, *What Your Doctor May Not Tell You About Menopause: The Breakthrough Book on Natural Progesterone* (New York: Warner, 1996), 230.

2. *Diagnostic and Statistical Manual of Mental Disorders*, 4th ed. (Washington, D.C.: American Psychiatric Association, 1994), 716.

3. W. M. Harrison, J. Endicott, J. Nee et al., "Characteristics of Women Seeking Treatment for Premenstrual Syndrome," *Psychosomatics* 30:405-411, 1989; W. R. Keye, Jr., D. C. Hammond, and T. Strong, "Medical and Psychological Characteristics of Women Presenting with Premenstrual Problems," *Obstetrics & Gynecology* 68:634-637, 1986.

4. R. T. Frank, "The Hormonal Basis of Premenstrual Tension," *Archives of Neurology and Psychiatry* 26:1053-1057, 1931; K. Dalton, *The Premenstrual Syndrome* (Springfield, Ill.: Charles C. Thomas, 1964).

5. K. Dalton, *Premenstrual Syndrome and Progesterone Therapy*, 2nd ed. (London: William Heinemann Medical Books, 1984); K. Dalton, *Once a Month*, 4th ed. (Claremont, Calif.: Hunter House, 1990).

6. B. Andersch and L. Hahn, "Progesterone Treatment of Premenstrual Tension: A Double-blind Study," *Journal of Psychosomatic Research* 29:489-493, 1985; E. Freeman, K. Rickels, S. Sondheimer et al., "Ineffectiveness of Progesterone Suppository Treatment for Premenstrual Syndrome," *Journal of the American Medical Association* 264:349-353, 1990; S. Maddocks, P. Hahn, F. Moller et al., "A Double-blind Placebo-controlled Trial of Progesterone Vaginal Suppositories in the Treatment of Premenstrual Syndrome," *American Journal of Obstetrics and Gynecology* 154:573-581, 1986; M. Richter, R. Haltvick, and S. Shapiro, "Progesterone Treatment of Premenstrual Syndrome," *Current Therapeutic Research* 36:840-850, 1985; G. Sampson, "A Double-blind Controlled Trial of Progesterone and Placebo," *British Journal of Psychiatry* 135:209-215, 1979; Y. G. van der Meer, L. J. Benedek-Jaszmann, and A. C. Van Loenen, "Effect of High-Dose Progesterone on the Premenstrual Syndrome: A Double-blind Crossover Trial," *Journal of Psychosomatic Obstetrics and Gynaecology* 2-4:220-222, 1983.

7. L. Dennerstein, C. Spencer-Gardner, G. Gotts et al., "Progesterone and the Premenstrual Syndrome: A Double-blind Crossover Trial," *British Medical Journal* 290:1617-1621, 1985; S. Sneed and J. McIlhaney, *PMS: What It Is and What You Can Do About It* (Grand Rapids, Mich.: Baker, 1988), 119.

8. Lee, op. cit., 230.

9. Ibid., 231.

10. T. Hilgers, "PMS: Signs and Symptoms." Audiotape. (Omaha, Neb.: Pope Paul VI Institute).

11. Dalton, *The Premenstrual Syndrome*; Dalton, *Premenstrual Syndrome and Progesterone Therapy*; Hilgers, ibid.

12. Hilgers, ibid.

13. Ibid.

14. G. E. Abraham, "Nutritional Factors in the Etiology of Premenstrual Syndrome," *Journal of Reproductive Medicine* 28:446-464, 1983; *Total Health for Women,* ed. E. Michaud and E. Torg (Emmaus, Penn.: Rodale, 1995), 445; F. Facchinetti et al., "Oral Magnesium Relieves Premenstrual Mood Changes," *Obstetrics and Gynecology* 78:177-181, 1991; G. E. Abraham and J. T. Hargrove, "Effect of Vitamin B on Premenstrual Tension Syndrome: A Double-blind Crossover Study," *Infertility* 3:155, 1980; R. S. Landau et al., "The Effect of Alpha Tocopherol in Premenstrual Symptomatology: A Double-blind Trial," *Journal of the American College of Nutrition* 2:115-123, 1983.

15. Ibid.

16. R. L. Reid, "Endogenous Opiate Peptides and Premenstrual Syndrome," *Seminars in Reproductive Endocrinology* 5:191-197, 1987; C. J. Choung et al., "Neuropeptide Levels in Premenstrual Syndrome," *Fertility and Sterility* 44:760-760, 1985.

17. P. W. Budoff, "Zomepirac Sodium in the Treatment of Primary Dysmenorrhea Syndrome," *New England Journal of Medicine* 307:714-719, 1982; J. Poulakka et al., "Biochemical and Clinical Effects of Treating Premenstrual Syndrome with Prostaglandin Synthesis Precursors," *Journal of Reproductive Medicine* 30:149-153, 1985.

18. W. G. Crook, *Chronic Fatigue Syndrome and the Yeast Connection* (Jackson, Tenn.: Professional Books, 1992), 104-106.

19. Sneed and McIlhaney, op. cit., 33.

20. P. J. Schmidt, L. K. Nieman, M. A. Danaceau et al., "Differential Behavioral Effects of Gondal Steroids in Women with and in Those Without Premenstrual Syndrome," *New England Journal of Medicine* 338:209-216, 1998; J. F. Mortola, "Premenstrual Syndrome: Pathophysiologic Considerations," Editorial, *New England Journal of Medicine* 338:256-257, 1998.

21. W. S. Maxson, "The Use of Progesterone in the Treatment of PMS," *Clinical Obstetrics and Gynecology* 30:365-477, 1987; L. Dennerstein, C. Spencer-Gardner, and G. Potts, "Progesterone and the Premenstrual Syndrome: A Double-blind Crossover Trial," *British Medical Journal* 290:1617-1621, 1985.

22. S. J. Sondheimer et al., "Hormonal Changes in Premenstrual Syndrome," *Psychosomatics* 26:803-816, 1985.

23. J. Martorano and M. Morgan, *Unmasking PMS* (New York: Berkley, 1994), 120-123.

24. S. Thys-Jacobs, S. Ceccarelli, A. Bierman et al., "Calcium Supplementation in Premenstrual Syndrome: A Randomized Crossover Trial," *Journal of General Internal Medicine* 4:183-189, 1989; A. Stewart, "Clinical and Biochemical Effects of Nutritional Supplementation on the Premenstrual Syndrome," *Journal of Reproductive Medicine* 32:435-441, 1987.

25. P. M. S. O'Brien, D. Craven, C. Selby et al., "Treatment of Premenstrual Syndrome with Spironolactone," *British Journal of Obstetrics and Gynaecology* 86:142-147, 1979; I. D. Vellacott, N. E. Shroff, and M. Y. Pearce et al., "A Double-blind, Placebo-Controlled Evaluation of Spironolactone in the Premenstrual Syndrome," *Current Medical Research and Opinion* 10:450-456, 1987.

26. A. Rivera-Tovar, R. Rhodes, T. B. Pearlstein, and E. Frank, "Treatment Efficacy," in *Premenstrual Dysphorias,* ed. J. H. Gold and S. Severino (Washington, D.C.: American Psychiatric Press, 1994), 137-138; Martorano and Morgan, *Unmasking PMS,* 179-184.

27. J. Goodale, A. Domar, and H. Benson, "Alleviation of Premenstrual Symptoms with the Relaxation Response," *Obstetrics and Gynecology* 75:649-689, 1990.

28. M. Steiner, S. Steinberg, D. Stewart et al., "Fluoxetine in the Treatment of Premenstrual Dysphoria," *New England Journal of Medicine* 332:1529-1534, 1995; D. Rubinow, "The Treatment of Premenstrual Syndrome: Forward into the Past," *New England Journal of Medicine* 332:1574-1575, 1995;

J. F. Mortola, L. Girton, S. S. Yen, "Depressive Episodes in Premenstrual Syndrome," *American Journal of Obstetrics and Gynecology* 161:1682-1687, 1989; K. Rickels, E. Freeman, S. Sondheimer, "Fluoxetine in the Treatment of Premenstrual Syndrome," *Current Therapeutic Research* 48:161-166, 1990; A. B. Stone, T. Pearlstein, and W. Brown, "Fluoxetine in the Treatment of Late Luteal Phase Dysphoric Disorder," *Journal of Clinical Psychiatry* 152:290-293, 1991; Martorano and Morgan, op. cit., 217-219.

29. J. Willis, "Doing Something About PMS," *FDA Consumer*, June 1983.

CHAPTER 4

1. B. Andersch and I. Milson, "An Epidemiologic Study of Young Women with Dysmenorrhea," *American Journal of Obstetrics and Gynecology* 144:655-660, 1982.

2. M. Y. Daywood, "Dysmenorrhea," *Journal of Reproductive Medicine* 30:154-167, 1985.

3. A. Schwartz et al., "Primary Dysmenorrhea: Alleviation by an Inhibitor of Prostaglandin Synthesis," *Obstetrics and Gynecology* 44:709-712, 1974; F. H. Boehm and H. Sarralt, "Indomethacin for the Treatment of Dysmenorrhea: A Report on Two Independent Double-blind Trials," *Journal of Reproductive Medicine* 15:84-86, 1975; M. R. Henzl et al., "The Treatment of Dysmenorrhea with Naproxen Sodium: A Report on Two Independent Double-blind Trials," *American Journal of Obstetrics and Gynecology* 127:818-823, 1977; P. W. Budoff, "Use of Mefenamic Acid in the Treatment of Primary Dysmenorrhea," *Journal of the American Medical Association* 241:2713-2716, June 22, 1979; P. R. Owen, "Prostaglandin Synthetase Inhibitors in the Treatment of Primary Dysmenorrhea," *American Journal of Obstetrics and Gynecology* 148:96-103, 1984.

4. J. Willis, "Doing Something About Menstrual Discomforts," *FDA Consumer*, June 1983.

5. A. Berger and H. H. Schaumberg, "More on Neuropathy from Pyridoxine Abuse," *New England Journal of Medicine* 311:986-987, 1984.

6. K. Budd, "Use of D-Phenylalanine, an Enkephalinase Inhibitor, in the Treatment of Intractable Pain," *Advances in Pain Research and Therapy* 5:305-308, 1983.

CHAPTER 5

1. R. E. Frisch, "Body Fat, Puberty, and Fertility," *Biological Review* 59:161-188, 1984; R. E. Frisch and J. W. MacArthur, "Menstrual Cycles: Fatness as a Determinant of Minimum Weight for Height Necessary for Their Maintenance and Onset," *Science* 185:949-953, 1974; K. A. Halmi, "Anorexia Nervosa and Bulimia," *Annual Review of Medicine* 38:373-380, 1987; E. Kemman, S. A. Pasquale, and R. Skaf, "Amenorrhea Associated with Carotenemia," *Journal of the American Medical Association* 249:926, 929, 1983; K. M. Pirke et al., "Dieting Influences on the Menstrual Cycle: Vegetarian vs. Nonvegetarian Diet," *Fertility and Sterility* 46:1083-1088, 1986; Z. M. Van Der Spuy, "Nutrition and Reproduction," *Clinics in Obstetrics and Gynaecology* 12:579-604, 1985; K. A. Hutchinson-Williams and A. H. DeCherney, "Pathogenesis and Treatment of Polycystic Ovary Disease," *International Journal of Fertility* 32:421-430, 1987; G. Jarnerot, "Fertility, Sterility, and Pregnancy in Chronic Inflammatory Bowel Disease," *Scandinavian Journal of Gastroenterology* 117(1):1-4 (1982); S. B. Levine and R. C. Stern, "Sexual Function in Cystic Fibrosis: Relationship to Overall Health Status and Pulmonary Disease in 30 Married Patients," *Chest* 81:422-426, 1982; L. S. Neinstein, "Menstrual Dysfunction in Pathophysiologic States," *Western Journal of Medicine* 143:476-484, 1985; T. W. Seale, M. Flus, and O. M. Rennert, "Reproductive Defects in Patients of Both Sexes with Cystic Fibrosis: A Review," *Annals of Clinical and Laboratory Science* 15:152-158, 1985; S. M. Shalet, "Abnormalities of Growth and Gonadal Function in Children Treated for Malignant Disease," *Journal of the Royal Society of Medicine* 75:646-647, 1982; A. J. Hartz et al., "The Association of Smoking with Clinical Indicators of Altered Sex Steroids: A Study of 50,145 Women," *Public Health Reports* 102:254-259, 1987; H. Jick, J. Porter, and A. S. Morrison, "Relation Between Smoking and Age of Natural Menopause," *Lancet*, June 25, 1977, 1354-1355; J. Olson et al., "Tobacco Use, Alcohol Consumption, and Infertility," *International Journal of Epidemiology* 13:179-184, 1983; W. R. Phipps, D. W. Cramer, and I. Schiff, "The Association Between

Smoking and Female Infertility as Influenced by the Cause of Infertility," *Fertility and Sterility* 48:377-382, 1987; C. G. Smith and R. H. Asch, "Drug Abuse and Reproduction," *Fertility and Sterility* 48:355-373, 1987; R. J. Stillman, M. J. Rosenberg, and B. P. Sachs, "Smoking and Reproduction," *Fertility and Sterility* 46:545, 1986; E. Weisberg, "Smoking and Reproductive Health," *Clinical Reproduction and Fertility* 3:175-186, 1985; K. W. Hancock et al., "Significance of Low Body Weight in Ovulation Dysfunction After Stopping Oral Contraceptives," *British Medical Journal* 2:399-401, 1976; S. Harlap, "Are There Two Types of Post-Pill Anovulation?" *Fertility and Sterility* 31:486-491, 1979; T. Pardthaisong, R. H. Grey, and E. B. McDaniel, "The Return of Fertility Following Discontinuation of Oral Contraceptives in Thailand," *Fertility and Sterility* 35:532-534, 1981; T. Pardthaisong, R. H. Grey, and E. B. McDaniel, "Return of Fertility after Discontinuation of Depomeroxyprogesterone Acetate and Intrauterine Devices in Northern Thailand," *Lancet,* March 8, 1980, 509-511; C. Tietze, "Fertility After Discontinuance of Intrauterine and Oral Contraceptives," *International Journal of Fertility* 13:385-389, 1968; M. P. Vessey et al., "Fertility After Stopping Different Methods of Contraception," *British Medical Journal* 1:265-267, 1978; G. Waintraub, "Fertility After Removal of Intrauterine Ring," *Fertility and Sterility* 21:555-557, 1970; E. R. Baker, "Menstrual Dysfunction and Hormonal Status in Athletic Women: A Review," *Fertility and Sterility* 39:691-696, 1981; B. A. Bullen et al., "Induction of Menstrual Disorders by Strenuous Exercise in Untrained Women," *New England Journal of Medicine* 312:1345-1353, 1985; K. A. Carlberg, M. T. Buckman, and G. T. Peake, "Menstrual Dysfunction in Athletes," *Sports Medicine,* ed. O. Appenzeller and R. Atkinson (Munich, West Germany: Urband and Schwarzenberg, 1981); P. T. Ellison and C. Lager, "Moderate Recreational Running Is Associated with Lowered Salivary Progesterone Profiles in Women," *American Journal of Obstetrics and Gynecology* 154:1000-1003, 1986; A. R. Glass, P. A. Deuster, and S. B. Kyle, "Amenorrhea in Olympic Marathon Runners," *Fertility and Sterility* 48:740-745, 1987; A. B. Loucks, "Does Exercise Training Affect Reproductive Hormones in Women?" *Clinics in Sports Medicine* 5:535-557, 1986; J. C. Prior et al., "Reversible Luteal Phase Changes and Infertility Associated with Marathon Training," Letter. *Lancet,* July 31, 1982, 269-270; J. B. Mitchell et al., "The Relationship of Exercise to Anovulatory Cycles in Female Athletes: Hormonal and Physical Characteristics," *Obstetrics and Gynecology* 63:452-456, 1984; M. M. Shangold and H. S. Levene, "The Effect of Marathon Training upon Menstrual Function," *American Journal of Obstetrics and Gynecology* 143:862-868, 1982; M. M. Shangold et al., "The Relationship Between Long-Distance Running, Plasma Progesterone, and Luteal Phase Length," *Fertility and Sterility* 31:130-133, 1979; L. Zoldag, "Stress und Fortpflanzungsstorungen beim Rind. 1. Mitteilung: Einfluss von Stressoren auf den Geschlechtszyklus," *Deutsche tieratzliche Wochenschrift* 90:152-156, 1983; L. Zoldag, "Stress und Fortpflanzungsstorungen beim Rind. 2. Mitteilung: Einfluss von Stressoren auf die Trachtigkeit," *Deutsche tieratzliche Wochenschrift* 90:184-187, 1983; D. R. Mishell, Jr. and V. Davajan, *Infertility, Contraception and Reproductive Endocrinology,* 2nd ed. (Oradell, N.J.: Medical Economics, 1986); L. Speroff, R. H. Glass, and N. G. Kase, *Clinical Gynecological Endocrinology and Infertility,* 3rd ed. (Baltimore: Williams & Wilkins Co., 1983).

2. R. F. Valle, "Hysteroscopic Evaluation of Patients with Abnormal Uterine Bleeding," *Surgery, Gynecology & Obstetrics* 153:521-526, 1981.

CHAPTER 6

1. T. W. Hilgers, "The Scientific Foundations of Natural Family Planning." Audiotape No. NFP-3. See Resources for how to obtain this tape.

2. Ibid.

CHAPTER 7

1. T. W. Hilgers, G. E. Abraham, and D. Cavanaugh, "The Peak Symptom and Estimated Time of Ovulation," *Obstetrics and Gynecology* 52 (November 1978); Hilgers et al., "The Ovulation Method—Vulvar Observations as an Index of Fertility/Infertility," *Obstetrics and Gynecology* 53 (January 1979); Hilgers et al., "Natural Family Planning II. Basal Body Temperature and Estimated Time of Ovulation," *Obstetrics and Gynecology* 58 (March 1980); Hilgers et al., "Natural Family Planning III:

Intermenstrual Symptoms and Estimated Time of Ovulation," *Obstetrics and Gynecology* 58 (August 1981); Hilgers et al., "Natural Family Planning and the Identification of Postovulatory Infertility," *Obstetrics and Gynecology* 58 (September 1981).

2. Ingrid Trobisch and Elizabeth Roetzer, *An Experience of Love* (Old Tappan, N.J.: Fleming Revell, 1979), 12.

CHAPTER 8

1. L. T. Dennis, ed., *Letters of Francis A. Schaeffer* (Wheaton, Ill.: Crossway Books, 1986), 251-252.

2. Ibid., 229.

3. D. Bonhoeffer, *Ethics* (New York: Macmillan, 1955 [1975]), 175, 176.

4. Ibid., 176, 177.

5. Ibid., 179.

6. Raymond C. Van Leeuwen, "Breeding Stock or Lords of Creation?" *Christianity Today*, November 11, 1991, 36-37.

7. George K. Brushaber, "The Joy of Procreation," *Christianity Today*, November 11, 1991, 45.

CHAPTER 9

1. Department of Health and Human Services, *Facts About Oral Contraceptives* (Washington, D.C.: U.S. Government Printing Office, 1984), 3.

2. *FDA Consumer*, No. 76-3024, May 1976.

3. A. Guttmacher, "Prevention of Conception Through Contraception and Sterilization" in *Gynecology and Obstetrics*, vol. 1, C. H. Davis, ed. (Baltimore: Williams and Wilkins, 1966), 8.

4. R. Mishell, "Current Status of Oral Contraceptive Steroids," *Clinical Obstetrics and Gynecology* 19 (4):746 (1976).

5. Ortho Pharmaceutical Corporation, *A Guide to Methods of Contraception* (Raritan, N.J.: Ortho, 1979), 8.

6. S. R. Killich, "Ovarian Follicles During Oral Contraceptive Cycles: Their Potential for Ovulation," *Fertility and Sterility* 52:580, 1989.

7. *Random House College Dictionary*, rev. ed. (New York: Random House, 1982), 137.

8. *Physician's Desk Reference*, 50th ed. (Montvale, N.J.: Medical Economics, 1996).

9. *Cincinnati Post*, January 11, 1973.

10. *Federal Register* 41:236, December 7, 1976, 53634.

11. U.S. Department of Health, Education, and Welfare, "Family Planning Methods of Contraception," DHEW Publication No. HSA 78-5646 (Washington, D.C.: U.S. Government Printing Office, 1979).

12. American Medical Association, "What You Should Know About the Pill," patient pamphlet.

13. *Nursing '85 Drug Handbook* (Spring House Corporation, 1985), 470.

14. R. A. Hatcher, F. Guest, F. Stewart et al., *Contraceptive Technology, 1988-1989*, 14th rev. ed. (New York: Irvington, 1988), 252.

15. "Birth Control Breakthrough Almost Here: The Time-Release Capsule," *Self*, August 1989, 172.

16. *Physician's Desk Reference, 1996*, 1872.

17. Ortho, op. cit., 11.

18. Department of Health, Education, and Welfare, *Federal Register*, Part III, May 10, 1977, 23781.

19. Hatcher, op. cit., 268.

20. GynoPharma Inc., "Is an IUD the Right Birth Control for You?" (Somerville, N.J.: GynoPharma Inc., 1988).

21. R. G. Edwards, "The Physiologist and Contraception." Paper presented at the Family Research Conference at Exeter, Great Britain, 1971.

22. T. W. Hilgers, "The Intrauterine Device: Contraceptive or Abortifacient?" *Minnesota Medicine*, June 1974, 493-501.

23. Searle Laboratories, "For the Patient: Cu-7," (Chicago: Searle Laboratories, 1977), 3. For more evidence that the IUD may function as an abortion-inducing birth control technology, see the following references: *The Medical Letter*, vol. 22, no. 20, October 3, 1980; "Mechanism of Action of IUDs in Women," *American Journal of Obstetrics and Gynecology* 36 (3), September, 1970; *Population Report*, Series B, no. 4, July 1982; *Dorland's Illustrated Medical Dictionary*, 24th ed.; *World Almanac*, 1987; R. W. Kistner, *Gynecology: Principles and Practice*, 2nd ed., 673; W. T. Branch, *Office Practice of Medicine*, 1013; L. Parsons and S. Sommers, *Gynecology*, 2nd ed., 606; D. Hartford, T. Hilgers, and L. Frieder, *The New Abortionists: Chemical Abortion in Contemporary Culture* (Stafford, Va.: American Life League, 1994); D. Sterns, G. Sterns, and P. Yaksich, *The Birth Control Game: Gambling with Life* (Stafford, Va.: American Life League, 1990); *The PDR Family Guide to Women's Health and Prescription Drugs* (Montvale, N.J.: Medical Economics, 1994), 252-253, 261-263, 272-273.

24. B. M. Kahar, "Pharmaceutical Companies: The New Abortionists," *ALL About Issues*, February 1989, 30.

CHAPTER 10

1. Debra Evans, *Blessed Events: Christian Couples Share Their Experiences of God's Blessing Through Infertility, Natural Parenting, and Adoption* (Wheaton, Ill.: Crossway, 1990), 125-128. Portions of this chapter are adapted from *Blessed Events*, from *Without Moral Limits: Women, Reproduction, and the New Medical Technology* (Wheaton, Ill.: Crossway, 1989), and from articles I have written in *Christian Parenting Today* and *Clarity* magazines.

2. Evans, *Blessed Events*, 85-93.

3. Sue Halpern, "Infertility: Playing the Odds," *Ms.*, January/February 1989, 148.

4. Ibid.

5. Committee on Government Operations, *Medical and Social Choices for Infertile Couples and the Federal Role in Prevention and Treatment* (Washington, D.C.: U.S. Government Printing Office, 1989), 48-49.

6. U.S. Congress, Office of Technology Assessment, *Infertility: Medical and Social Choices* (Washington D.C.: U.S. Government Printing Office, May 1988, OTA-BA-358).

7. Dale Hanson Bourke, "Joni Turns 40," *Today's Christian Woman*, January/February 1990, 23-25, 69-69.

8. For a complete, fully documented history of IVF research, see D. Evans, *Without Moral Limits* (Wheaton, Ill.: Crossway, 1989); J. Rock and A. T. Hertig, "Some Aspects of Early Human Development," *American Journal of Obstetrics and Gynecology* 44:973-983, 1942; J. Rock and M. F. Menkin, "In Vitro Fertilization and Cleavage of Human Ovarian Eggs," *Science*, August 4, 1944, 105; M. F. Menkin and J. Rock, "In Vitro Fertilization and Cleavage of Human Ovarian Eggs," *American Journal of Obstetrics and Gynecology* 55:440-454, 1948; A. T. Hertig, "A Fifteen-Year Search for First-Stage Human Ova," *Journal of the American Medical Association*, January 20, 1989, 434-435; R. G. Edwards, "Maturation In Vitro of Mouse, Sheep, Cow, Pig, Rhesus Monkey and Human Ovarian Oocytes," *Nature*, October 23, 1965, 349-351; R. G. Edwards, "Maturation In Vitro of Human Ovarian Oocytes," *Lancet*, November 6, 1965, 926-929; R. G. Edwards, B. D. Bavister, and P. C. Steptoe, "Early

Stages of Fertilization In Vitro of Human Oocytes Matured In Vitro," *Nature*, February 15, 1969, 632-635; R. G. Edwards, "Mammalian Eggs in the Laboratory," *Scientific American* 215:81, 1966; R. G. Edwards, B. D. Bavister, and P. C. Steptoe, "Early Stages of Fertilization *In Vitro* of Human Oocytes Matured *In Vitro*," *Nature*, February 15, 1969, 632; L. Shettles, "Observations on Human Follicular and Tubal Ova," *American Journal of Obstetrics and Gynecology* 66 (2):235-247 (1953); L. Shettles, "A Morula Stage of Human Ova Developed In Vitro," *Fertility and Sterility* 6 (4):287-289 (1955); L. Shettles, "Corona Radiata and Zona Pellucida of Living Human Ova," *Fertility and Sterility* 9 (2):167-170 (1958); L. Mastroianni and C. Noriega, "Observations on Human Ova and the Fertilization Process," *American Journal of Obstetrics and Gynecology* 107 (5):682-690 (1970); J. F. Kennedy and R. P. Donahue, "Human Oocytes: Maturation in Chemically Defined Media," *Science* 164:1292-1293, 1969; P. Liedholm, P. Sundstrom, and H. Wramsky, "A Model for Experimental Studies on Human Egg Transfer," *Archives of Andrology* 5 (1):92 (1980); L. McLaughlin, *The Pill, John Rock and the Church* (Boston: Little, Brown and Company, 1982); R. G. Edwards and P. Steptoe, *A Matter of Life* (New York: William Morrow, 1980); R. G. Edwards and R. E. Fowler, "Human Embryos in the Laboratory," *Scientific American* 223:50, 1958; Richard G. Seed, Randolph W. Seed, and D. S. Baker, "Aspects of Bovine Embryo Transplant Directly Applicable to Humans: A Report of over 300 Procedures," *Fertility and Sterility* 28:313-314, 1977; Richard G. Seed and Randolph W. Seed, "Artificial Embryonation: Human Embryo Transplant," *Archives in Andrology* 5:90-91, 1980.

For studies involving embryo research, see J. E. Buster, Randolph W. Seed, and Richard G. Seed et al., "Nonsurgical Ovum Transfer as a Treatment in Infertile Women," *Journal of the American Medical Association*, March 2, 1984, 1171-1173; J. E. Buster et al., "An Instrument for the Recovery of Preimplantation Uterine Ova," *Obstetrics & Gynecology* 71:804-806, May 1988; J. E. Buster, Richard G. Seed, and Randolph W. Seed et al., "Nonsurgical Ovum Transfer of In Vivo Fertilized Donated Ova to Five Infertile Women: Report of Two Pregnancies," *Lancet*, July 23, 1983, 223-224; M. V. Sauer and J. E. Buster et al., "An Instrument for the Recovery of Preimplantation Uterine Ova," *Obstetrics & Gynecology* 71:804-806, 1988; M. V. Sauer, R. E. Anderson, and R. J. Paulsen, "A Trial of Superovulation in Ovum Donors Undergoing Uterine Lavage," *Fertility and Sterility* 51:131-134, 1989; J. D. Biggers, "In Vitro Fertilization and Embryo Transfer in Human Beings," *New England Journal of Medicine*, February 5, 1981, 336-341; A. Trounson and L. Mohr, "Human Pregnancy Following Cryopreservation, Thawing and Transfer of an Eight-Cell Embryo," *Nature*, October 20, 1983, 707-709; A. Trounson, "Pregnancy Established in an Infertile Patient After Transfer of a Donated Embryo Fertilized In Vitro," *British Medical Journal*, March 12, 1983, 835-838; A. Trounson et al., "Effect of Growth in Culture Medium on the Rate of Mouse Embryo Development and Viability In Vitro," *Journal of In Vitro Fertilization and Embryo Transfer* 4:265-268, 1987; A. Trounson, "Preservation of Human Eggs and Embryos," *Fertility and Sterility* 46:1-11, July 1986; A. Trounson, A. Peura, and C. Kirby, "Ultrarapid Freezing: A New Low-Cost and Effective Method of Embryo Cryopreservation," *Fertility and Sterility* 48:843-850, 1987; A. Trounson et al., "Ultrarapid Freezing of Early Cleavage Stage Human Embryos and Eight-Cell Mouse Embryos," *Fertility and Sterility* 49:822-826, May 1988; S. A. Hassani et al., "Cryopreservation of Human Oocytes," *Human Reproduction* 2:695-700, November 1987; A. Clark et al., "Social and Reproductive Characteristics of the First 100 Couples Treated by In-Vitro Fertilization Programme at National Women's Hospital, Auckland," *New Zealand Medical Journal*, June 24, 1987, 380-382; "Success Rates for IVF and Gift," *Contemporary OB/GYN*, May 1988, 89-106; J. E. Buster and M. V. Sauer, "Nonsurgical Donor Ovum Transfer: New Option for Infertile Couples," *Contemporary OB/GYN*, August 1986, 39-49; I. Craft et al., "Analysis of 1071 GIFT Procedures: The Case for a Flexible Approach to Treatment," *Lancet*, May 16, 1988, 1094-1097; I. Craft et al., "Successful Pregnancies from the Transfer of Pronucleate Embryos in an Outpatient In Vitro Fertilization Program," *Fertility and Sterility* 44:181-184, August 1985; A. H. DeCherney and G. Lavy, "Oocyte Recovery Methods in In-Vitro Fertilization," *Clinical Obstetrics and Gynecology* 29:171-179, March 1986; J. Deschacht et al., "In Vitro Fertilization with Husband and Donor Sperm in Patients with Previous Fertilization Failures Using Husband Sperm," *Human Reproduction* 3:105-108, January 1988; R. Frydman et al., "A New Approach to Follicular Stimulation for In Vitro Fertilization: Programmed Oocyte Retrieval," *Fertility and Sterility* 46:657-659, October 1986; R. Frydman et al., "An Obstetric Assessment of the First 100 Births from the In Vitro Fertilization Program at Clamart,

France," *American Journal of Obstetrics and Gynecology* 154:550-555, 1986; R. Frydman et al., "Programmed Oocyte Retrieval During Routine Laparoscopy and Embryo Cryopreservation for Later Transfer," *American Journal of Obstetrics and Gynecology* 155:112-117, July 1986; H. Jones, Jr., et al., "An Analysis of the Obstetric Outcome of 125 Consecutive Pregnancies Conceived In Vitro and Resulting in 100 Deliveries," *American Journal of Obstetrics and Gynecology* 154:848-854, 1986; H. Jones, Jr., H. Liu, and Z. Rosenwaks, "The Efficiency of Human Reproduction After In Vitro Fertilization and Embryo Transfer," *Fertility and Sterility* 49:649-653, 1988; H. Jones, Jr., et al., "The Program for In Vitro Fertilization at Norfolk," *Fertility and Sterility* 38:14-20, 1982; J. Leeton, A. Trounson, D. Jessup, and C. Wood, "The Technique for Embryo Transfer," *Fertility and Sterility* 38:156-161, 1982; "100 Test-Tube Babies Gather in Baltimore," *Lincoln Journal*, September 12, 1988, 6; "In Vitro Clinics Span Globe; Spawn New Treatments," *Lincoln Sunday Journal-Star*, July 24, 1988, 1A, 6A; R. P. Marrs, "Human In-Vitro Fertilization," *Clinical Obstetrics and Gynecology* 29:117, March 1986; R. P. Marrs, "Laboratory Conditions for Human In-Vitro Fertilization Procedures," *Clinical Obstetrics and Gynecology* 29:180-189, 1986; Medical Research International and the American Fertility Society Special Interest Group, "In Vitro Fertilization/Embryo Transfer in the United States: 1985 and 1986, Results from the National IVF/ET Registry," *Fertility and Sterility* 49:212-215, 1988; D. R. Meldrum et al., "Evolution of a Highly Successful In Vitro Fertilization-Embryo Transfer Program," *Fertility and Sterility* 48:86-93, 1987; S. Pace-Owens, "In Vitro Fertilization and Embryo Transfer," *JOGN Nursing*, Supplement, November/December 1985, 44S-48S; C. Ranoux et al., "A New In Vitro Fertilization Technique: Intravaginal Culture," *Fertility and Sterility* 49:654-657, 1988; C. Ranoux et al., "Intravaginal Culture and Embryo Transfer: A New Method for the Fertilization of Human Oocytes," *Review of French Gynecology and Obstetrics* 82:741-744, 1987; J. M. Rary et al., "Techniques of In Vitro Fertilization of Oocytes and Embryo Transfer in Humans," *Archives of Andrology* 5:89-90, 1980; V. Sharma et al., "An Analysis of Factors Influencing the Establishment of a Clinical Pregnancy in an Ultrasound-Based Ambulatory In Vitro Fertilization Clinic," *Fertility and Sterility* 49:468-478, 1988; P. H. Wessels et al., "Gamete Intrafallopian Transfer: A Treatment for Long-Standing Infertility," *Journal of In Vitro Fertilization and Embryo Transfer* 4:256-259, 1987; C. Wood et al., "Clinical Features of Eight Pregnancies Resulting from In Vitro Fertilization and Embryo Transfer," *Fertility and Sterility* 38:22, 1982; C. Wood et al., "Factors Influencing Pregnancy Rates Following In Vitro Fertilization and Embryo Transfer," *Fertility and Sterility* 43:245-250, 1985.

9. G. Kolata, "In Vitro Fertilization Goes Commercial," *Science* 221:1160-1161, 1983; F. Schumer Chapman, "Going for the Gold in the Baby Business," *Fortune*, September 17, 1984, 41; M. Novak, "Buying and Selling Babies: Limitations on the Marketplace," *Commonweal*, July 17, 1987, 406-407; G. Annas, "Making Babies Without Sex: The Law and the Profits," *American Journal of Public Health* 74:1415-1417, 1984; "Babies: No Sale," *Los Angeles Times*, February 4, 1988; C. A. Raymond, "IVF Registry Notes More Centers, More Births, Slightly Improved Odds," *Journal of the American Medical Association*, April 1, 1988, 1920-1921; Committee on Small Business, *Consumer Protection Issues Involving In Vitro Fertilization Clinics* (Washington, D.C.: U.S. Government Printing Office, 1988); A. Taylor Fleming, "New Frontiers in Conception," *New York Times Magazine*, July 20, 1980; G. Annas, "Redefining Parenthood and Protecting Embryos: Why We Need New Laws," *The Hastings Center Report*, October 1984, 50-52; G. Annas and S. Elias, "Social Policy Considerations in Noncoital Reproduction," *Journal of the American Medical Association*, January 3, 1986, 62-68; P. Bagne, "High-Tech Breeding," *Mother Jones* 8:23-29, 35, 1983; H. Jones, Jr., "The Impact of In Vitro Fertilization on the Practice of Gynecology and Obstetrics," *International Journal of Fertility* 31:99-111, 1986; J. E. Buster and M. V. Sauer, "Nonsurgical Donor Ovum Transfer: New Option for Infertile Couples," *Contemporary OB/GYN*, August 1986, 39-49; "Ovum Donor Transfer May See Wide Use in Treating Infertility," *Ob/Gyn News*, December 1, 1983, 1.

10. P. Ramsey, "Shall We 'Reproduce'? Part I. The Medical Ethics of In Vitro Fertilization," *Journal of the American Medical Association*, June 5, 1972, 1346-1350; P. Ramsey, "Shall We 'Reproduce'? Part II. Rejoinders and Future Forecast," *Journal of the American Medical Association*, June 12, 1972, 1484-1485; P. Ramsey, *Fabricated Man* (New Haven, Conn.: Yale University Press, 1970); R. G. Edwards, "Chromosomal Abnormalities in Human Embryos," *Nature*, May 26, 1983, 283; R. R. Angell et al., "Chromosome Abnormalities in Human Embryos After In Vitro Fertilization," *Nature*, May 26, 1983,

336-338; G. Vines, "New Insights into Early Embryos," *New Scientist*, July 9, 1987, 22-23; J. L. Watt et al., "Trisomy 1 in an Eight-Cell Human Pre-Embryo," *Journal of Medical Genetics* 24:60-64, 1987; P. M. Summers, J. M. Campbell, and M. W. Miller, "Normal In-Vivo Development of Marmoset Monkey Embryos After Trophectoderm Biopsy," *Human Reproduction* 3:389-393, 1988; P. Braude, V. Bolton, and S. Moore, "Human Gene Expression First Occurs Between the Four- and Eight-Cell Stages of Preimplantation Development," *Nature*, March 31, 1988, 459-461; R. G. Edwards and D. J. Sharpe, "Social Values and Research in Human Embryology," *Nature*, May 14, 1971, 87-88; R. G. Edwards, "Studies in Human Conception," *American Journal of Obstetrics and Gynecology*, November 1, 1973, 587, 599; R. G. Edwards and M. Puxon, "Parental Consent over Embryos," *Nature*, July 19, 1984, 179; K. Johnston, "Sex of New Embryos Known," *Nature*, June 18, 1987, 547; A. McLaren, "Can We Diagnose Genetic Disease in Pre-Embryos?" *New Scientist*, December 10, 1987, 44-45.

11. H. H. H. Kanhai et al., "Selective Termination in Quintuplet Pregnancy During First Trimester," *Lancet*, June 21, 1986, 1447; D. F. Farquharson et al., "Management of Quintuplet Pregnancy by Selective Embryocide," *American Journal of Obstetrics and Gynecology* 158:413-416, 1988; M. I. Evans et al., "Selective First Trimester Termination Octuplet and Quadruplet Pregnancies: Clinical and Ethical Issues," *Obstetrics & Gynecology* 71:289-296, 1988; R. L. Berkowitz et al., "Selective Reduction of Multifetal Pregnancies in the First Trimester," *New England Journal of Medicine*, April 21, 1988, 1043-1047; R. L. Berkowitz et al., "Selective Reduction of Multifetal Pregnancies (Reply)," *New England Journal of Medicine*, October 6, 1988, 950-951; J. M. Lorenz and J. S. Terry, "Selective Reduction of Multifetal Pregnancies," Letter, *New England Journal of Medicine*, October 6, 1988, 949-950; S. L. Romney, "Selective Reduction of Multifetal Pregnancies," Letter, *New England Journal of Medicine*, October 6, 1988, 949; J. Shalev et al., "Selective Reduction of Multifetal Pregnancies," Letter, *New England Journal of Medicine*, October 6, 1988, 949; E. F. Diamond, "Selective Reduction of Multifetal Pregnancies," Letter, *New England Journal of Medicine*, October 6, 1988, 950; D. H. James, "Selective Reduction of Multifetal Pregnancies," Letter, *New England Journal of Medicine*, October 6, 1988, 950; I. Craft et al., "Multiple Pregnancy, Selective Reduction, and Flexible Treatment," *Lancet*, November 5, 1988, 1087. "Selective Fetus Destruction Debated," *Lincoln Journal*, April 21, 1988, 5.

To find out how this heartbreaking subject is being detoxified for presentation in popular women's magazines, see "Tell Us What You Think: Is It Wrong to Terminate Some Fetuses During a Multiple Pregnancy?" *Glamour*, July 1988, 50; "This Is What You Thought: 57 Percent Say a Woman Should Have the Right to Terminate Some Fetuses," *Glamour*, September 1988, 197; "Choices," *Woman's World*, January 3, 1989, 44-45; R. Frydman et al., "Reduction of the Number of Embryos in a Multiple Pregnancy: From Quintuplet to Triplet," *Fertility and Sterility* 48:326-327, 1987.

12. J. Ashkenazi et al., "Abdominal Complications Following Ultrasonically Guided Percutaneous Transvesical Collection of Oocytes for In Vitro Fertilization," *Journal of In Vitro Fertilization and Embryo Transfer* 4:316-318, 1987; J. Ashkenazi et al., "Multiple Pregnancy After In-Vitro Fertilization and Embryo Transfer: Report of a Quadruplet Pregnancy and Delivery," *Human Reproduction* 2:511-515, August 1987; F. R. Batzer et al., "Multiple Pregnancies with Gamete Intrafallopian Transfer (GIFT): Complications of a New Technique," *Journal of In Vitro Fertilization and Embryo Transfer* 5:35-37, 1988; G. Byrne, "Artificial Insemination Report Prompts Call for Regulation," *Science*, August 19, 1988, 895; E. Chargaff, "Engineering a Molecular Nightmare," *Nature*, May 21, 1987, 199-200; H. Bequaert Holmes, "In Vitro Fertilization: Reflections on the State of the Art," *Birth* 15:134-1144, 1988; W. R. Phipps, C. B. Benson, and P. M. McShane, "Severe Thigh Myositis Following Intramuscular Progesterone Injections in an In Vitro Fertilization Patient," *Fertility and Sterility* 49:536-537, 1988; F. V. Price, "The Risk of High Multiparity with IVF/ET," *Birth* 15:157-163, 1988; J. J. Schlesselman, "How Does One Assess the Risk of Abnormalities from Human In Vitro Fertilization?" *American Journal of Obstetrics and Gynecology*, September 1, 1979, 135-148; D. H. Smith et al., "Tubal Pregnancy Occurring After Successful In Vitro Fertilization and Embryo Transfer," *Fertility and Sterility* 38:105-106, 1982; J. L. Yovich, S. R. Turner, and A. J. Murphy, "Embryo Transfer Technique as a Cause of Ectopic Pregnancies in In Vitro Fertilization," *Fertility and Sterility* 44:318-321, 1985.

13. R. G. Seed and R. Weiss, "Embryo Adoption: Technical, Ethical and Legal Aspects," *Archives in Andrology* 5, 1980; D. J. Cuisine, "Some Legal Implications of Embryo Transfer," *Lancet*, August 25,

1979, 407-408; J. E. Buster et al., "Survey of Attitudes Regarding the Use of Siblings for Gamete Donation," *Fertility and Sterility* 49:721-722, April 1988; H. I. Abdalla and T. Leonard, "Cryopreserved Zygote Intrafallopian Transfer for Anonymous Oocyte Donation," *Lancet,* April 9, 1988, 835; American Fertility Society Committee on Ethics, "Donor Eggs in In Vitro Fertilization," *Fertility and Sterility* 46, Supplement 1:42S-44S, 1986; American Fertility Society Committee on Ethics, "Donor Sperm in In Vitro Fertilization," *Fertility and Sterility* 46, Supplement 1:39S-41S, 1986; American Fertility Society Committee on Ethics, "Surrogate Gestational Mothers: Women Who Gestate a Genetically Unrelated Embryo," *Fertility and Sterility* 46, Supplement 1:58S-61S, 1986; L. B. Andrews, "Embryo Technology," *Parent's* Magazine 56:63-71, 1981; L. B. Andrews, "Legal and Ethical Aspects of New Reproductive Technologies," *Clinical Obstetrics and Gynecology* 29:190-204, March 1986. G. Annas and J. F. Henahan, "Fertilization, Embryo Transfer Procedures Raise Many Questions," *Journal of the American Medical Association*, August 17, 1984, 877-879, 882; J. E. Buster, "Survey of Attitudes Regarding the Use of Siblings for Gamete Donation," *Fertility and Sterility* 49:721-722, 1988; J. F. Correy, "Donor Oocyte Pregnancy with Transfer of Deep-Frozen Embryo," *Fertility and Sterility* 49:534-535, 1988; I. Craft and J. Yovich, "Implications of Embryo Transfer," *Lancet*, September 22, 1979, 642-643; I. Craft and P. F. Serhal, "Ovum Donation: A Simplified Approach," *Fertility and Sterility* 48:265-269, 1987; D. J. Cuisine, "Some Legal Implications of Embryo Transfer," *Lancet*, August 25, 1979, 407-408; "What Are the Moral Rights of Frozen Embryos?" *Health Progress*, October 1984, 54, 62; M. Johnston, "I Gave Birth to Another Woman's Baby," *Redbook*, May 1984, 44, 46; A. M. Junca et al., "Anonymous and Non-Anonymous Oocyte Donation Preliminary Results," *Human Reproduction* 3:121-123, 1988; J. F. Leeton et al., "Donor Oocyte Pregnancy with Transfer of Deep-Frozen Embryo," *Fertility and Sterility* 49:534-535, 1988; J. Leeton et al., "Successful Pregnancy in an Ovulating Recipient Following the Transfer of Two Frozen-Thawed Embryos Obtained from Anonymously Donated Oocytes," *Journal of In Vitro Fertilization and Embryo Transfer* 5:22-24, 1988; J. Leeton and J. Harman, "The Donation of Oocytes to Known Recipients," *Australia and New Zealand Journal of Obstetrics and Gynaecology* 27:248-250, 1987; "Woman Bears Own Grandchild," *Lincoln Journal*, October 1, 1987, 2; M. Madhevan, A. O. Trounson, and J. F. Leeton, "Successful Use of Human Semen Cryobanking for In Vitro Fertilization," *Fertility and Sterility* 40:340-343, 1983; M. C. Michelow, "Mother-Daughter In Vitro Fertilization Triplet Surrogate Pregnancy," *Journal of In Vitro Fertilization and Embryo Transfer* 5:31-34, 1988; J. Salat-Baroux et al., "Pregnancies After Replacement of Frozen-Thawed Embryos in a Donation Program," *Fertility and Sterility* 49:817-821, 1988; R. G. Seed and R. W. Seed, "Embryo Adoption: Technical, Ethical and Legal Aspects," *Archives in Andrology* 5, 1980.

14. John T. Noonan, "Christian Tradition and the Control of Reproduction," in *The Death Decision*, ed. Leonard J. Nelson (Ann Arbor, Mich.: Servant Books, 1984), 14.

15. L. B. Andrews, "Yours, Mine and Theirs," *Psychology Today*, December 1984.

16. U. S. Congress, Office of Technology Assessment, op. cit., 229.

17. S. Robinson and H. F. Pizer, *Having a Baby Without a Man* (New York: Simon & Schuster/Fireside Books, 1987); G. Hanscombe, "The Right to Lesbian Parenthood," *Journal of Medical Ethics* 9:133-135, 1983; B. Kritchevsky, "The Unmarried Woman's Right to Artificial Insemination: A Call for Expanded Definition of Family," *Harvard Women's Law Journal* 4:1-42, 1981; Lambda Legal Defense and Education Fund, Inc.; Lesbian Rights Project, San Francisco; Office of Gay and Lesbian Health Concerns, NYC Department of Health, and New York University Women's Center, *Lesbians Choosing Motherhood* (New York: Lambda Legal Defense and Education Fund, Inc., 1984); Lesbian Health Information Project, *Artificial Insemination: An Alternative Conception for the Lesbian and Gay Community* (San Francisco, Calif.: San Francisco Women's Centers, 1979); S. Stern, "Lesbian Insemination," *The CoEvolution Quarterly,* Summer 1980, 108-117.

18. S. Callahan, "Lovemaking and Babymaking," *Commonweal*, April 24, 1987, 237; S. Callahan, "Use of Third-Party Donors Threatens Basic Values," *Health Progress*, March 1987, 26-28; C. Krauthammer, "The Ethics of Human Manufacture," *The New Republic*, May 4, 1987, 17-21; B. Katz Rothman, "How Science Is Redefining Parenthood," *Ms.*, July/August 1982, 154, 156; A. Baran and R. Pannor, *Lethal Secrets: The Shocking Consequences and Unsolved Problem of Artificial Insemination* (New York: Warner, 1989); H. J. Muller, "Human Evolution by Voluntary Choice of Germ Plasm," *Science*, September 8,

1961, 643-649; H. D. Krause, "Artificial Conception, Legislative Approaches," *Family Law Quarterly* 19:185-206, 1988; R. P. S. Jansen, "Sperm and Ova as Property," *Journal of Medical Ethics* 11:123-126, 1985; R. Snowden and G. D. Mitchell, *Artificial Reproduction: A Social Investigation* (London: George Allen & Unwin, 1983); L. B. Andrews, *New Conceptions* (New York: Ballantine Books, 1985); R. Snowden and G. D. Mitchell, *The Artificial Family: A Consideration of Artificial Insemination by Donor* (London: George Allen & Unwin, 1981); R. C. Strickler, D. W. Keller, and J. C. Warren, "Artificial Insemination with Fresh Donor Semen," *New England Journal of Medicine,* October 23, 1975, 848-853; J. L. Yovich, "Surrogacy," *Lancet,* June 13, 1987, 1374; M. Curie-Cohen, L. Luttrell, and S. Shapiro, "Current Practice of Artificial Insemination by Donor in the United States," *New England Journal of Medicine,* March 15, 1979, 585-590.

19. R. Fitzhugh, "Where's Poppa?" *US Magazine,* October 22, 1984, 68-69. For a detailed discussion on the implications of deception about one's origins, read *Lethal Secrets,* op. cit.

20. Callahan, op. cit., *Commonweal,* 237.

21. U. S. Congress, Office of Technology Assessment, op. cit.

22. Hebrews 4:14-16.

CHAPTER 11

1. "The Soviet/U.S. Summit Data," *Newsweek,* December 14, 1987, 41; S. A. Alderman, E. Ackerman, and R. Rubin, "Abortions in America: So Many Women Have Them, So Few Talk About Them," *U.S. News & World Report,* January 19, 1998, page 1 of 2 (from www.usnews.com).

2. For example, the State of Georgia reported that among unmarried white women (ages thirty to forty-four) living in urban areas, the abortion ratio is 3,000 abortions for every 1,000 live births among women of the same age and marital/residential status. (*Georgia Epidemiology Report: The Epidemiology of Abortion in Georgia-Preliminary Report,* vol. 6, no. 11, November 1990.)

3. J. Rubin, "Where Are We Now? In the twenty-five years of *Roe v. Wade,* the abortion ruling has seen some changes, and so has the controversy surrounding it," *Los Angeles Times,* January 22, 1998, E1; L. M. Koonin et al., "Abortion Surveillance, United States, 1993 and 1994: Introduction, Methods, Results," vol. 46, *Morbidity and Mortality Weekly Report,* August 8, 1997, 37-42.

4. M. Wolfe, *Women's Health Alert* (New York: Addison Wesley, 1991), 73.

5. J. Placek, S. M. Taffel, and T. Liss, "Trends in the United States Cesarean Rate and Reasons for the 1980-1985 Rise," *American Journal of Public Health* 77:955-959, 1987.

6. R. Pokras, "Hysterectomy: Past, Present and Future," *Statistical Bulletin,* Metropolitan Life and Affiliated Companies, 70:12-21, October-December, 1989; 1995 Summary: National Hospital Discharge Survey.

7. P. Dranov, "An Unkind Cut," *American Health,* September 1990, 36.

8. Ibid., 39. KEY: Northeast 89,000 in 1988 for a total hysterectomy rate of 4.1 per 1,000 women fifteen years of age and older (ME, VT, NH, MA, CT, BI, NY, NJ, PA); Midwest 143,000 ('88) for a 5.8 rate (OH, IL, IN, MI, MN, IA, MO, ND, SD, KS, NE); South 251,000 ('88) for a 7.3 rate (DE, MD, DC, WV, VA, KY, NC, SC, GA, FL, TN, AL, MS, LA, OK, AR, TX); West 96,000 ('88) for a 4.9 rate (WA, OR, CA, NV, NM, AZ, ID, UT, CO, MT, WY, AK, HI).

9. Ibid., 39.

10. W. Cutler, *Hysterectomy: Before and After* (New York: Harper & Row, 1988), 2.

11. Dranov, op. cit., 40; S. M. Wolfe, op. cit., 52.

12. National Center for Health Statistics, "Hysterectomy in the United States: 1965-1984," *Vital and Health Statistics* (Washington, D.C.: U.S. Government Printing Office, 1987) Series 13, No. 92. DHHS Publication No. (PHS) 87-1753.

13. J. Placek and S. M. Taffel, "An Overview of Recent Patterns in Cesarean Delivery and Where We Are Today." Paper presented at the American Public Health Association annual meeting, Boston, November 13-17, 1988; P. J. Placek et al., op. cit.; R. H. Paul, "Toward Fewer Cesarean Sections: The Role of a Trial of Labor," *New England Journal of Medicine*, September 5, 1996, vol. 335, no. 10, 735-736.

14. J. Placek and S. M. Taffel, "Vaginal Birth After Cesarean (VBAC) in the 1980s," *American Journal of Public Health* 78:512, May 1988.

15. Wolfe, op. cit., 74.

16. *Washington Post*, January 23, 1983.

17. Torres and J. D. Forrest, "Why Do Women Have Abortions?" *Family Planning Perspectives* 20:169-188, July/August, 1988; S. A. Alderman, E. Ackerman, and R. Rubin, op. cit.

18. C. Wright, "Hysterectomy: Past, Present, and Future," *Obstetrics and Gynecology* 33:562-563, April 1969.

19. Adapted from R. G. Schneider, MD, *When to Say No to Surgery* (Englewood Cliffs, N.J.: Prentice-Hall, 1982), vii-viii.

CHAPTER 13

1. G. Annas, *The Rights of Hospital Patients* (New York: Avon, 1975); Joint Commission on Accreditation of Healthcare Organizations, *The 1991 Joint Commission Consolidated Standards Manual, Vol. 1* (Oakbrook Terrace, Ill.: JCAHO, 1991). This chapter is largely based upon information contained in these two works.

2. Ibid., 61. [*Schloendorff v. New York Hospital*, 211 N.Y. 127, 129, 105 N.E. 92, 93 (1914).]

3. JCAHO, op. cit.

4. Ibid., 80.

CHAPTER 14

1. S. M. Wolfe, *Women's Health Alert* (Reading, Mass.: Addison-Wesley, 1991), Appendix A.

2. Lincoln-Lancaster Commission on the Status of Women, *A Consumer Guide to Pregnancy and Childbirth Services in Lincoln-Lancaster County*, Lincoln, Neb., 1986.

3. V. Hufnagel, *No More Hysterectomies* (New York: Plume, 1989), 264-266.

4. National Institutes of Health.

5. Adapted from "How to Do Breast Self-Examination," American Cancer Society.

6. J. F. Newsome and R. McLelland, "A Word of Caution Concerning Mammography," *Journal of the American Medical Association* 255:528, 1986.

CHAPTER 15

1. M. E. Prilook, ed., "Endometriosis: New Views and Therapies," *Patient Care*, November 15, 1978, 24-96; G. D. Adamson, "Diagnosis and Clinical Presentation of Endometriosis," *American Journal of Obstetrics and Gynecology* 162: 568-569, 1990; W. P. Dmowski and E. Radwanska, "Current Concepts on Pathology, Histogenesis, and Etiology of Endometriosis," *ACTA Obstetrics and Gynecology Scandinavian Supplement* 123:29-33, 1984.

2. W. P. Dmowski and E. Radwanska, "Endometriosis and Infertility," *ACTA Obstetrics and Gynecology Scandinavian Supplement* 123:73-79, 1984.

3. American College of Obstetricians and Gynecologists, "Management of Endometriosis," *ACOG*

Technical Bulletin, No. 85, May 1985; R. L. Barberi, "Etiology and Epidemiology of Endometriosis," *American Obstetrics and Gynecology* 162:565-567, February 1990.

4. K. Lamb, R. G. Hoffman, and T. R. Nichols, "Family Trait Analysis: A Case Control Study of 43 Women with Endometriosis and Their Best Friends," *American Journal of Obstetrics and Gynecology* 154:596-601, 1986.

5. American College of Obstetricians and Gynecologists, op. cit.; C. A. Molgaard, A. L. Goldbeck, and L. Gresham, "Current Concepts in Endometriosis," *Western Journal of Medicine* 143:42-46, 1985.

6. D. L. Olive and K. L. Lee, "Analysis of Sequential Treatment Protocols for Endometriosis-Associated Infertility," *American Journal of Obstetrics and Gynecology* 154:613-619, 1986.

7. T. W. Hilgers, "Endometriosis: A Guide to the Disease and Its Treatment," Audiotape No. WH-4. Available from Dr. Thomas W. Hilgers at the Pope Paul VI Institute for the Study of Human Reproduction, 6901 Mercy Road, Omaha, NE 68106.

8. D. C. Martin and M. P. Diamond, "Operative Laparoscopy: Comparison of Lasers with Other Techniques," *Current Problems in Obstetrics, Gynecology and Fertility* 9:564, 1986; D. C. Martin and R. Vander Zwaag, "Excisional Techniques with the CO2 Laser Laparoscope," *Journal of Reproductive Medicine* 32:753, 1987; A. P. Chong and M. S. Baggish, "Management of Pelvic Endometriosis by Means of Intra-abdominal Carbon Dioxide Laser," *Fertility & Sterility* 41:70-74, January 1984.

9. M. E. Prilook, op. cit.; G. D. Adamson, op. cit.; W. P. Dmowski and E. Radwanska, op. cit.; American College of Obstetricians and Gynecologists, op. cit.; D. L. Olive and K. L. Lee, op. cit.; R. B. Greenblatt and V. Tzingounis, "Danazol Treatment of Endometriosis: Long-Term Follow-Up," *Fertility & Sterility* 32:518-520, November 1979; D. R. Meldrum, W. M. Partridge, and W. G. Karow, "The Hormonal Effects of Danazol and Medical Oophorectomy in Endometriosis," *Obstetrics and Gynecology* 62:480-485, October 1983; G. Rannevik and J. I. Thorell, "The Influence of Danazol on Pituitary Function and on the Ovarian Follicular Hormone Secretion in Premenopausal Women," *ACTA Obstetrics and Gynecology Scandinavian Supplement* 123:89-94, 1984; M. R. Henzl and L. Kwei, "Efficacy and Safety of Nafarelin in the Treatment of Endometriosis," *American Journal of Obstetrics and Gynecology* 162:570-574, February 1990; R. W. Shaw, "Nafarelin in the Treatment of Pelvic Pain Caused by Endometriosis," *American Journal of Obstetrics and Gynecology* 162:574-576, February 1990.

10. C. C. Bird, T. W. McElin, and P. Manalo-Estrella, "The Elusive Adenomyosis of the Uterus Revisited," *American Journal of Obstetrics and Gynecology* 112:583-593, 1972.

CHAPTER 16

1. F. DeStefano, J. R. Greenspan, and R. C. Dicker, "Complications of Interval Laparoscopic Tubal Sterilization," *Obstetrics and Gynecology* 61:153-158, 1983.

2. M. Ohligisser, Y. Sorokin, and M. Heifitz, "Gynecologic Laparoscopy. A Review Article," *Obstetrical and Gynecological Survey* 40:385-396, 1985; R. F. Mattingly and J. D. Thompson, *TeLinde's Operative Gynecology*, 6th ed. (Philadelphia: J. B. Lippincott & Co., 1985); A. A. Murphy, "Operative Laparoscopy," *Fertility and Sterility* 47:1-18, 1987.

3. V. Gomel et al., *Laparoscopy and Hysteroscopy in Gynecologic Practice* (Chicago: Year Book Medical Publishers, 1986).

4. P. J. Taylor and J. Hamou, "Hysteroscopy," *Journal of Reproductive Medicine* 28:359-388, 1983.

5. National Center for Health Statistics, E. J. Graves, "Utilization of Short-Stay Hospitals, United States, 1983 Annual Summary," *Vital and Health Statistics*, Series 13, No. 83, Department of Health and Human Services Publication Number (PHS) 85-1744, Public Health Service (Washington, D.C.: U.S. Government Printing Office, 1985).

6. D. A. Grimes, "Diagnostic Dilation and Curettage: A Reappraisal," *American Journal of Obstetrics and Gynecology* 142:1-6, 1982.

CHAPTER 17

1. R. Tuomala, "Hysterectomy," *Harvard Medical School Health Letter* 13:8, 1988; CDC Surveillance Summaries, August 8, 1997, 46:SS-4.

2. CDC Surveillance Summaries, August 8, 1997, 46:SS-4.

3. R. Dicker et al., "Complications of Abdominal and Vaginal Hysterectomy Among Women of Reproductive Age in the United States. The Collaborative Review of Sterilization," *American Journal of Obstetrics and Gynecology* 144:841-848, 1982; H. Amerika and T. Evans, "Ten-Year Review of Hysterectomies: Trends, Indications, and Risks," *American Journal of Obstetrics and Gynecology* 134:431-437, 1979; C. L. Easterday, D. A. Grimes, and J. A. Riggs, "Hysterectomy in the United States," *Obstetrics and Gynecology* 62:203-212, 1983.

4. For a detailed discussion on the benefits and risks of hysterectomy, read Dr. Winnifred B. Cutler's intensively researched book, *Hysterectomy: Before and After* (New York: Harper & Row, 1988).

5. S. S. Entman, "Uterine Leiomyomata and Adenomyosis," in *Novak's Textbook of Gynecology,* 11th ed. (Baltimore: Williams and Wilkins, 1988), 443.

6. H. W. Jones and G. S. Jones, "Sarcoma of the Uterus," in *Novak's Textbook of Gynecology,* 10th ed. (Baltimore: Williams and Wilkins, 1981), 452; V. C. Buttram and R. C. Reiter, "Uterine Leiomyomata: Etiology, Symptomatology and Management," *Fertility and Sterility* 433-445, 1981.

7. K. Buchi and P. J. Keller, "Estrogen Receptors in Normal and Myomatous Human Uteri," *Gynecology and Obstetric Investigations* 2:59-60, 1980; D. Shoup, F. J. Mont, and R. A. Lobo, "The Effects of Estrogen and Progestin on Endogenous Opioid Activity in Oophorectomized Women," *Journal of Clinical Endocrinology and Metabolism* 60:1:178-183, 1985; J. H. Strathy, C. B. Coulam, and T. C. Spelsburg, "Comparison of Estrogen Receptors in Human Premenopausal and Postmenopausal Uteri: Indication of Biologically Inactive Receptor in Postmenopausal Uteri," *American Journal of Obstetrics and Gynecology* 142:372-382, 1982; T. Tamaya, J. Fujimoto, and H. Okada, "Comparison of Cellular Levels of Steroid Receptors in Uterine Leiomyoma and Myometrium," *ACTA Obstetrics and Gynecology Scandinavia* 64:4:307, 1985; T. Tamaya et al., "Estradiol-17, Beta-progesterone and 5a-dihydrotestosterone Receptors of Uterine Myometrium and Myoma in the Human Subject," *Journal of Steroidal Biochemistry* 10:615-622, 1979; E. A. Wilson, F. Yang, and E. D. Rees, "Estradiol and Progesterone Binding in Uterine Leiomyomata and in Normal Uterine Tissues," *Obstetrics and Gynecology* 55:1:20-23, 1980.

8. A. Lemay, "Monthly Implant of Luteinizing Hormone-Releasing Hormone Agonist: A Practical Therapeutic Approach for Sex-Steroid Dependent Diseases," *Fertility and Sterility* 48:10-12, 1987; R. Maheux et al., "Luteinizing Hormone-Releasing Hormone Agonist and Uterine Leiomyoma: A Pilot Study," *American Journal of Obstetrics and Gynecology* 152:1034-1037, 1985; R. Maheux, A. Lemay, and P. Merat, "Use of Intranasal Luteinzing Hormone-Releasing Hormone Agonist in Uterine Leiomyomas," *Fertility and Sterility* 47:229-233, 1987; V. Perl et al., "Treatment of Leiomyomata Uteri with D-TRP6-Luteinizing Hormone-Releasing Hormone," *Fertility and Sterility* 48:383-389; C. P. West et al., "Shrinkage of Uterine Fibroids During Therapy with Goserelin (Zoladex), A Luteinzing Hormone-Releasing Hormone Agonist Administered as a Monthly Subcutaneous Depot," *Fertility and Sterility* 48:45-51, 1987.

9. A. Murphy, "Operative Laparoscopy," *Fertility and Sterility* 47:1-18, 1987.

10. D. Macleod and J. Hawkin's, *Bonney's Gynaecological Survey* (New York: Hoeber Medical Division, Harper & Row, 1964), 360-361.

11. Buttram and Reiter, op. cit.

12. R. F. Mattingly and J. D. Thompson, *TeLinde's Operative Gynecology*, 6th ed. (Philadelphia: J. B. Lippincott Co., 1985).

13. C. R. Garcia and R. W. Turek, "Submucosal Leiomyomas and Infertility," *Fertility and Sterility* 42:16-19, 1984.

14. C. R. Garcia, "Multiple Myomectomy: A Surgical Procedure," in *Obstetrics and Gynecology Illustrated* (Kalamazoo, Mich.: Learning Technology/Upjohn).

15. Wolfe, op. cit., 62.

16. Wolfe, ibid., 59; see also D. A. Drossman, "Patients with Psychogenic Pelvic Pain: Six Years' Observation in a Medical Setting," *American Journal of Psychology* 139: 1549-1557, 1982. (This study reports that a significant number of women who develop chronic pain do so *after* having a hysterectomy.)

17. R. C. Reiter and J. C. Gambone, "Demographic and Historic Variables in Women with Idiopathic Chronic Pelvic Pain," *Obstetrics and Gynecology* 75:428-432, 1990.

18. Quoted in Wolfe, op. cit., 60.

19. R. C. Reiter and J. C. Gambone, "Nongynecologic Somatic Pathology in Women with Chronic Pelvic Pain," *Journal of Reproductive Medicine,* 1990.

20. Quoted in Wolfe, op. cit., 60.

21. Wolfe, ibid., 47.

22. Dicker, op. cit.; Amerika and Evans, op. cit.; Easterday, Grimes, and Riggs, op. cit.; R. Pokras, "Hysterectomy: Past, Present and Future," *Statistical Bulletin,* Metropolitan Life and Affiliated Companies, 70:12-21, 1989; P. A. Wingo et al., "The Mortality Risk Associated with Hysterectomy," *American Journal of Obstetrics and Gynecology* 152:803-808, 1985; R. F. Mattingly, *Myomata Uteri in Operative Gynecology,* 5th ed. (Philadelphia: Lippincott, 1977); R. K. Laros and B. K. Work, "Female Sterilization III: Vaginal Hysterectomy," *American Journal of Obstetrics and Gynecology* 122:693-697, 1977; L. Zussman, S. Zussman, R. Sunley, and E. Bjornson, "Sexual Response After Hysterectomy-Oophorectomy: Recent Studies and Reconsideration of Psychogenesis," *American Journal of Obstetrics and Gynecology* 140:725-729, 1984; H. H. Reidel, E. Willenbock-Lehmann, K. Semm, "Ovarian Failure Phenomena After Hysterectomy," *Journal of Reproductive Medicine* 31:597-599, 1986; N. P. Roos, "Hysterectomies in One Canadian Province: A New Look at Risks and Benefits," *American Journal of Public Health* 74:39-46, 1984; H. G. Hanley, "The Late Urological Complications of Total Hysterectomy," *British Journal of Urology* 41:682-684, 1969; S. A. Farghaly, J. R. Hindmarsh, and P. H. L. Worth, "Post-Hysterectomy Urethral Dysfunction: Evaluation and Management," *British Journal of Urology* 58:299-302, 1986; J. Shaughnessy, "Enormous Hole Left in Woman's Bladder," *Medical Post,* July 8, 1986, 27; R. E. Miller, "Role of Hysterectomy in Predisposing the Patient to Sigmoidovesical Fistula Complicating Diverticulitis," *American Journal of Surgery* 147:660-661, 1984; W. H. Utian, "Effect of Hysterectomy, Oophorectomy, and Estrogen Therapy on Libido," *International Journal of Gynaecology and Obstetrics* 13:97-100, 1975; L. Dennerstein, C. Wood, and G. D. Burrows, "Sexual Response Following Hysterectomy and Oophorectomy," *Obstetrics and Gynecology* 49:92-96, 1977; S. Wolfe, *Women's Health Alert,* op. cit., 46-47.

23. F. Petraglia et al., "Endogenous Opioid Peptides in Uterine Fluid," *Fertility and Sterility* 46:2:247-251, 1986; C. A. Fox and B. Fox, "Comparative Study of Coital Physiology," *Journal of Reproduction and Fertility* 24:319-336, 1971; P. Kilkku et al., "Supravaginal Uterine Amputation vs. Hysterectomy: Effects on Libido & Orgasm," *ACTA Obstetrics and Gynecology Scandinavia* 62:147-151, 1983.

24. W. H. Masters, "The Sexual Response Cycle of the Human Female: Vaginal Lubrication," *Annals of the New York Academy of Science* 83:301-317, 1959; B. Charbonnel et al., "Human Cervical Mucus Contains Large Amounts of Prostaglandins," *Fertility and Sterility* 38:108-111, 1982.

25. T. Allen et al., "Vaginal Cervical Stimulation Selectively Increases Metabolic Activity in the Rat Brain," *Science* 211:1070-1072, 1981; T. Allen and N. T. Adler, "Localized Uptake of (14) Deogyglucose by the Preoptic Area of Female Rats in Response to Vaginocervical Stimulation," *Neuroscience Abstracts* 4, 1978.

26. Consider this statement from a recent medical textbook (*Novak's Textbook of Gynecology,* op. cit.): "Menstruation is a nuisance to most women, and if this can be abolished without impairing ovarian function, it would probably be a blessing to not only the woman but her husband."

27. Medical Education and Research Foundation, "Should You Be a Hysterectomy Holdout?" Printable Document-Electric Library, 1994; *Journal of the American Medical Association* 269:18, 1993.

28. National Women's Health Resource Center, "Emotional Aspects of Hysterectomy," 1994.

29. Adapted from "A Woman's Right to Know: Questions to Ask About Hysterectomy and the Alternatives," vol. 16, National Women's Health Report, March 1, 1994, 3.

CHAPTER 18

1. All cancer risks and statistics for this chapter are based on the following sources, with additional information noted as necessary in the text: *The PDR Family Guide to Women's Health and Prescription Drugs* (Montvale, N.J.: Medical Economics, 1994); S. J. Winawer and M. Shike, *Cancer Free: The Comprehensive Cancer Prevention Program* (New York: Fireside, 1995); K. A. McGinn and P. J. Haylock, *Women's Cancers* (Alameda, Calif.: Hunter House, 1993); K. J. Carlson, S. A. Eisenstat and T. Ziporyn, *The Harvard Guide to Women's Health* (Cambridge, Mass.: Harvard University, 1996); E. H. S. Page and A. J. Asire, *Cancer Rates and Risks*, NIH Publication 85-691, National Cancer Institute, 3rd ed., 1985; Silverberg and J. Lubera, "Cancer Statistics, 1987," *Ca: Cancer Journal for Clinicians* 37:2-19, 1987; R. K. Barber, "Ovarian Cancer," *Ca: Cancer Journal for Clinicians*, vol. 36, no. 3, May/June 1986, 150; *Mortality*, vol. 2 in *Vital Statistics of the United States, 1976*, National Center for Health Statistics; Council on Scientific Affairs, "Early Detection of Breast Cancer," *Journal of the American Medical Association* 252:3008-3011, 1984; H. Seidman et al., "Probabilities of Eventually Developing or Dying of Cancer: United States, 1985," *Ca: Cancer Journal for Clinicians* 35:36-56, 1985.

2. S. B. Sadeghi, E. W. Hsieh, and S. W. Gunn, "Prevalence of Cervical Intraepithelial Neoplasia in Sexually Active Teenagers and Young Adults," *American Journal of Obstetrics and Gynecology* 148:726-729, 1984; M. P. Vessey et al., "Neoplasia of the Cervix Uteri and Contraception: Possible Adverse Effect of the Pill," *Lancet* 2:930-934, 1983.

3. The Alan Guttmacher Institute, "Issues in Brief: Sexually Transmitted Diseases in the U.S.: Risks, Consequences and Costs," Printable Document-Electric Library, 3.

4. The Alan Guttmacher Institute, ibid., 5; C. P. Crum et al., "Human Papillomavirus Type 16 and Early Cervical Neoplasia," *New England Journal of Medicine* 310:880-883, 1984; "Condyloma Virus and Cervical Cancer: How Strong a Link?" *Contemporary OB/GYN*, February 1984, 210-224; D. Wagner et al., "Identification of Human Papilloma Virus in Cervical Swabs by Deoxyribonucleic Acid In Situ Hybridization," *Obstetrics and Gynecology* 64:767-772, 1984; F. Gagnon, "Contributions to the Study of the Etiology and Prevention of Cancer of the Uterus," *American Journal of Obstetrics and Gynecology* 60:516-522, 1960; "Risk of Cancer: STD Spread Mandates Treating Condyloma," *OB/GYN News* 20 (5), 1985; R. M. Richart, "Condyloma Viruses That Progress to Cancer Can Be Identified," *Contraceptive Technology Update* 4:143-144, 1983.

5. A. P. M. Heintz, N. F. Hacker, and L. D. Lagasse, "Epidemiology and Etiology of Ovarian Cancer: A Review," *Obstetrics and Gynecology* 66:127-135, 1985; M. S. Piver, "Alarming Trends in the Familial Ovarian Cancer Registry," *Contemporary OB/GYN*, February 1986, 120-129; D. A. Snowden, "Diet and Ovarian Cancer," *Journal of the American Medical Association* 254:356-357, 1985.

6. H. K. Ziel and W. D. Finkle, "Increased Risk of Endometrial Carcinoma Among Users of Conjugated Estrogens," *New England Journal of Medicine* 293:1167-1170, 1975; D. C. Smith et al., "Association of Exogenous Estrogen and Endometrial Carcinoma," *New England Journal of Medicine* 293:1164-1167, 1975; T. M. Mack et al., "Estrogens and Endometrial Cancer in a Retirement Community," *New England Journal of Medicine*, 294:1262-1267; S. Shapiro et al., "Risks of Localized and Widespread Endometrial Cancer in Relation to Recent and Discontinued Use of Conjugated Estrogens," *New England Journal of Medicine* 313:594-560, 1985; C. B. Coulam, "Why Ca Risk is Higher in Anovulatory Women," *Contemporary OB/GYN*, May 1984, 87.

7. B. Winkler et al., "Pitfalls in the Diagnosis of Endometrial Neoplasia," *Obstetrics and Gynecology* 64:185-194, 1984.

CHAPTER 19

1. 1 Corinthians 6:13b-18. Note: To make this passage more personal, I have substituted feminine for masculine pronouns and the word *prostitute* for wife and freely adapted these verses from the *New International Version*. Italics mine.

2. J. Nesmith, "Sexual Diseases Expected to Afflict 1 in 20 Worldwide," *The Atlanta Journal and Constitution*, December 21, 1990, A-6.

3. The Alan Guttmacher Institute, "Issues in Brief: Sexually Transmitted Diseases in the U.S.: Risks, Consequences and Costs," 1994, 1.

4. W. Cates, Jr., "Epidemiology and Control of Sexually Transmitted Diseases: Strategic Evolution," *Infectious Disease Clinics of North America* 1:1-23, 1987.

5. The Alan Guttmacher Institute, op. cit.; J. S. Bingham, *Sexually Transmitted Diseases* (Philadelphia: Williams & Wilkins, 1984).

6. Nesmith, op. cit., A-6.

7. D. A. Grimes, "Deaths Due to Sexually Transmitted Diseases: The Forgotten Component of Reproductive Mortality," *Journal of the American Medical Association* 255:1727-1729, 1986.

8. A. E. Washington, P. S. Amos, and M. A. Brooks, "The Economic Cost of Pelvic Inflammatory Disease," *Journal of the American Medical Association* 255:1735-1738, 1986.

9. Grimes, op. cit.

10. R. A. Hatcher, F. Guest, F. Stewart, G. K. Stewart et al., *Contraceptive Technology, 1988-1989,* 14th rev. ed. (New York: Irvington, 1988), 19.

11. Ibid.

12. R. C. Barnes and K. K. Holmes, "Epidemiology of Gonorrhea: Current Perspectives," *Epidemiology Review* 6:1-30, 1984.

13. Nesmith, op. cit.

14. K. Painter, "Syphilis Cases Hit 41-Year Peak," *USA Today*, February 2, 1990, D-1.

15. The Alan Guttmacher Institute, op. cit.

16. D. T. Fleming et al., "Herpes Simplex Type 2 in the United States, 1976-1994," *New England Journal of Medicine* 337:1105-11 1997.

17. J. S. McIlhaney, *Sexuality and Sexually Transmitted Diseases* (Grand Rapids: Baker, 1990), 14.

18. Ibid., 114.

19. *The PDR Family Guide to Women's Health* (Montvale, N.J.: Medical Economics, 1994), 106.

20. The Alan Guttmacher Institute, op. cit.

21. Centers for Disease Control and Prevention, "Chlamydia trachomatis Genital Infection," *Morbidity and Mortality Weekly Report*, 46:9, March 7, 1997; Institute of Medicine, *The Hidden Epidemic: Confronting Sexually Transmitted Diseases* (Washington, D.C.: National Academy Press, 1996).

22. Centers for Disease Control and Prevention, Office of Women's Health, "Sexually Transmitted Diseases," Printable Document-Electric Library, 1998.

23. T. Murphy, ed., "FDA Approves New Chlamydia Identification Tests," *Contraceptive Technology Update* 5:97-99, 1984.

24. Hatcher, op. cit., 35; M. Abramowicz, ed., "Treatment of Sexually Transmitted Diseases," *The Medical Letter on Drugs and Therapeutics* 26:653, 1984, 7; *PDR Family Guide to Women's Health and Prescription Drugs*, op. cit., 117.

25. The Alan Guttmacher Institute, op. cit.; *The PDR Family Guide to Women's Health and Prescription*

Drugs, op. cit., 118; K. J. Carlson, S. A. Eisenstat, and T. Ziporyn, *The Harvard Guide to Women's Health*, 264.

26. The Centers for Disease Control and Prevention, "Sexually Transmitted Disease Surveillance 1995," Table 11.

27. Hatcher, op. cit., 30

28. Ibid.; *The PDR Family Guide to Women's Health and Prescription Drugs*, op. cit., 119.

29. Centers for Disease Control: "Penicillinase-producing *Neisseria gonorrhea:* United States, 1986," *Morbidity and Mortality Weekly Report* 36:107-108, 1987.

30. Carlson, Eisenstat, and Ziporyn, op. cit., 266.

31. Ibid.; *The PDR Family Guide to Women's Health and Prescription Drugs*, op. cit.

32. The Alan Guttmacher Institute, op. cit., 5.; Grimes, op. cit.

33. Abramowicz, op. cit., 8; *The PDR Family Guide to Women's Health and Prescription Drugs*, 54.

34. The Alan Guttmacher Institute, op. cit., 5.

35. Ibid.

36. *The PDR Family Guide to Women's Health and Prescription Drugs*, op. cit., 106.

37. CDC, Office of Women's Health, op. cit.

38. A. P. Ball, *Notes on Infectious Diseases* (London: Churchill Livingstone, 1982).

39. C. G. Prober, "Herpetic Vaginitis in 1993," *Clinical Obstetrics and Gynecology* 36:1, 1993, 178.

40. *The PDR Family Guide to Women's Health and Prescription Drugs*, op. cit., 110.

41. Harvard Women's Health Watch, "Genital Herpes," September 1997, 6.

42. D. T. Fleming et al., "Herpes Simplex Virus Type 2 in the United States, 1976 to 1994," *The New England Journal of Medicine*, 337:1105-1111, 1997.

43. The Alan Guttmacher Institute, op. cit., 1. (Italics mine.)

44. D. T. Fleming, op. cit.

45. C. G. Prober, op. cit., 180.

46. *The PDR Family Guide to Women's Health and Prescription Drugs*, op. cit., 111.

47. C. G. Prober, op. cit., 178.

48. *The PDR Family Guide to Women's Health and Prescription Drugs*, op. cit., 110.

49. Ibid., 111.

50. Ibid.

51. Medical Education and Research Foundation, "Lysine and Cold Sores," Printable Document-Electric Library, 1995, 1.

52. K. H. Cooper, *Advanced Nutritional Therapies* (Nashville: Thomas Nelson), 1996; J. F. Balch and P. A. Balch, *Prescription for Nutritional Healing*, 2nd ed. (Garden City Park, N.J.: Avery, 1997).

53. Cooper, op. cit., 14, 45, 50, 56.

APPENDIX A

1. D. C. Overduin and J. I. Fleming, *Life in a Test Tube: Medical and Ethical Issues Facing Society Today* (Adelaide, Australia: Lutheran Publishing House, 1982), 224.

$\mathscr{G}$ LOSSARY

abortifacient: Any drug or substance capable of inducing abortion.

abortion: The spontaneous or deliberate ending of a pregnancy before the developing baby can survive outside the mother's womb.

abortion rate: The number of abortions during a specific time in relation to the total number of women between the ages of fifteen and forty-four in a given population. (Usually expressed as the number of abortions per 1,000 women ages fifteen to forty-four.)

abortion ratio: The number of abortions during a specific period of time in relation to the total number of live births in a given population. (Usually expressed as the number of abortions per 1,000 live births.)

acrosome: The lead end of the head of a sperm that releases enzymes to dissolve the surface of the ovum.

adenomyosis: Noncancerous, invasive growth of the uterine lining into the muscle of the uterus.

adhesion: New connective tissue produced by inflammation, surgery, or injury. This tissue holds together two structures that are normally separate.

American College of Obstetricians and Gynecologists [ACOG]: National organization of certified specialists in obstetrics and gynecology.

amenorrhea: The absence of menstruation.

amniocentesis: Diagnostic sampling of amniotic fluid during pregnancy, especially for the purpose of genetic analysis. The fluid is obtained by puncturing the mother's abdomen and womb with a special needle.

amnion: The fluid-filled sac or membrane enclosing the developing baby within the womb, also referred to as the "bag of waters."

amniotic fluid: A colorless liquid surrounding the baby within the womb.

amniotomy: The artificial rupture of the amniotic sac by a physician.

anesthesia: The partial or complete loss of sensation with or without loss of consciousness as a result of injury, disease, or the administration of a drug or gas.

anovulation: The absence of ovulation.

antenatal: Occurring before birth.

antepartum: Around the time of birth; a term used to describe the labor and delivery functions and staff of a hospital.

anti-HCG vaccine: Long-acting vaccine designed to block the action of HCG on the uterine lining during pregnancy, thereby inducing abortion.

antiprostaglandin: Any substance capable of acting to reduce or inhibit the effects of prostaglandins within the body.

artificial insemination [AI]: Semen deposited in the vagina by a mechanical instrument rather than a man's penis.

artificial insemination by donor [AID]: Artificial insemination using sperm obtained from a donor.

artificial insemination by husband [AIH]: Artificial insemination using sperm obtained from one's husband.

aspermia: The absence of sperm and semen.

azoospermia: The absence of sperm in semen.

bacterial vaginosis: Vaginal inflammation caused by bacteria.

basal body temperature: The temperature of the body taken orally, rectally, or vaginally after at least three hours of sleep, taken before rising.

basal body temperature method of family planning [BBT]: A method of family planning that relies on identifying the fertile period of a woman's menstrual cycle for the purpose of attempting or avoiding pregnancy.

basal thermometer: Specially calibrated instrument designed to measure resting body temperature in relation to ovulation.

benign: Noncancerous.

biopsy: The surgical removal of a sample of tissue for diagnostic purposes.

birth: The process by which a new human being enters the world and begins life outside the mother's body.

birth center: A facility designed to prevent interference in the natural process of childbirth; may be freestanding or connected to a hospital. Many obstetrical departments are now naming redesigned in-hospital units "birthing centers" for consumer appeal. If continuous electronic fetal monitoring, induction of labor, artificial rupture of the membranes, epidural anesthesia, and routine episiotomies are frequently being conducted in a facility using this name, it is not a birth center. It is a hospital.

birth control: The prevention of birth.

birth rate: The number of births during a specific period of time in relation to the total population of a certain area.

blastocyst: The fertilized ovum during its second week of development; name means "many-celled hollow ball."

bonding: The deepening of intimacy over time between two people through emotional, physical, and spiritual interactions. Touch, eye contact, speech, and loving gestures create, sustain, and magnify human bonds within the family.

breast self-examination (BSE): A method in which a woman may routinely check her breasts and surrounding areas for signs of change that could indicate cancer.

calendar method: A highly ineffective method of family planning that involves abstaining from intercourse during the fertile time of the month as determined by the calendar. Also called *rhythm*.

cancer: A malignant and invasive growth or tumor.

candidiasis: Vaginal infection and irritation caused by *candida*, or yeast.

cannula: A hollow tube or sheath.

carcinoma: Cancer of the tissue overlying internal and external body surfaces.

cardiovascular fitness: Well-being of the heart and circulatory system promoted through diet, weight management, and aerobic exercise; these measures enhance the oxygen level in the blood.

catheter: A thin, plastic tube designed to perform invasive medical procedures upon the body.

cautery: The burning away of damaged cell tissue via electrical current.

celibacy: A way of life that involves commitment to sexual abstinence.

certified nurse-midwife [C.N.M.]: A registered nurse who is a graduate of an approved training program and who has passed a certification examination.

cervical canal: The opening within the uterine cervix that protrudes into the vagina.

cervical cap: A small latex cap designed to be worn directly over the cervix during intercourse to prevent sperm from entering the uterus.

cervical dysplasia: Abnormal changes in the cells covering the cervix.

cervical crypts: Indentations within the lining of the cervical canal that act as storage compartments for sperm.

cervicitis: Inflammation of the cervix caused by irritation, infection, or injury.

cervicography: Technique using photographs of the cervix to obtain a diagnosis.

cervix: The fixed, lower necklike segment of the uterus that forms the passageway into the vagina.

cesarean section, C-section: The surgical removal of a baby through an incision in the mother's abdominal tissue and uterine wall.

chancriod, chancre: Infectious sore or ulcer caused by syphilis.

chastity: The practice of sexual purity inside or outside of marriage, characterized by self-control, high moral standards, esteem for self, and respect for others.

chlamydia: A generic term for infection caused by the organism *Chlamydia trachomatis*, a sexually transmitted disease characterized by a thick yellow discharge from the cervix that may result in pelvic abscesses, pelvic inflammatory disease, and involuntary sterility. Also called *mucopurulent cervicitis*.

chorion: The outermost membrane covering the developing baby during the first trimester. The chorion encloses the amnion, lies closest to the wall of the uterus, and eventually becomes the placenta.

chromosome: Threadlike bodies within the nucleus of every cell that make up strands of DNA. These structures contain the genetic material that is passed from parents to their children. Each normal human cell contains forty-six chromosomes arranged in twenty-three pairs from the time of conception.

cilia: Hairlike filaments lining the inner wall of the fallopian tubes. These filaments beat rhythmically to create a current that takes the egg toward the uterus.

clitoris: The female organ devoted entirely to increasing sexual tension and providing pleasurable sensations when stimulated; plays a key role in a woman's sexual response; the structure in the female that corresponds to the glans penis in the male.

clomiphene citrate [Clomid, Serophene]: A drug used to induce ovulation in anovulatory women. Its precise mechanism of action is unknown.

coitus: See *sexual intercourse.*

coitus interruptus: See *withdrawal method.*

colposcopy: Gynecological diagnostic technique employing a binocular-like instrument called a colposcope that allows a physician to obtain a magnified view of the cervix.

conception: The fertilization of the egg by a sperm that initiates the growth of a human being and triggers the onset of pregnancy. ACOG changed the definition of conception in 1965 to mean implantation of a fertilized egg. This allows birth control methods that prevent implantation of fertilized ova to be called contraceptives rather than contragestives or abortifacients.

conceptus: Fertilized ovum or "pre-embryo"; term often is used by researchers to dehumanize the earliest stages of human development following conception.

cone biopsy: A minor surgical procedure in which a cone-shaped section of the cervix around the cervical canal is removed.

condom: A soft, flexible sheath worn over an erect penis during sexual intercourse to prevent sperm from entering the vagina.

contraception: The act of preventing conception.

contraceptive: Any type of technology (drug, device, or surgery) that prevents conception.

contrafetal: Any type of technology (drug, device, or surgery) that is designed to act against the fetus and induce abortion.

contragestive: Any type of technology (drug, device, or surgery) that interrupts pregnancy and induces an abortion.

contranidational: Any type of technology (drug, device, or surgery) that disrupts the implantation of an embryo and induces abortion.

copulation: Sexual intercourse.

corpus luteum: Name means "yellow body"; the temporary gland created within a ruptured ovarian follicle; secretes hormones to protect and maintain pregnancy until the placenta matures and takes over this role.

cryobank: Place where frozen sperm is stored; a commercial business selling frozen sperm.

cryopreservation: The storage of living cells by the use of special chemicals and ultrarapid freezing.

cryosurgery: Use of a cold source to freeze and destroy damaged cell tissue.

curettage: Scraping of the uterine lining with a spoon-shaped, sharp instrument called a curette.

cyst: A closed sac or pouch with a definite wall that contains fluid, semifluid, or solid material.

cystitis: Inflammation of the bladder and urinary tract. See *urinary tract infection.*

cystocele: The bulging of the bladder and front wall of the vagina into the vagina as a result of giving birth, advanced age, or surgery.

DES [diethylstilbestrol]: A synthetic estrogen used during the 1950s and 1960s to prevent miscarriage. In 1971 it was found to cause a rare form of vaginal cancer, and vaginal changes were found in a significant number of the daughters born to women who had taken DES during pregnancy.

diaphragm: A dome-shaped latex device worn over the cervix with spermicide during intercourse to prevent sperm from entering the uterus.

dilation: The process of opening. In labor, uterine contractions press the baby against the cervix to open the womb. In gynecological procedures, metal rods of increasing size are inserted into the cervix to stretch it open. In either case, cervical dilation is accompanied by a menstrual-like cramping sensation.

dilation and curettage [D&C]: Name literally means "opening, cutting, and scraping." A surgical procedure in which the cervix is forcibly opened and the inside of the uterus is scraped with a sharp, spoonlike instrument called a curette. Used to remove polyps or an overgrowth of uterine tissue, as a way of diagnosing cancer, and after childbirth to remove tissue retained in the womb. Also a method of abortion involving the dismemberment of the developing child by suction and extraction from the uterus.

dilation and evacuation [D&E]: A surgical procedure used to abort a child during the second trimester of pregnancy requiring crushing of the skull and surgical dismemberment of the baby's body before removal from the womb.

diuretic: Any drug that increases the rate of passage of urine from the body. Used to prevent the excess accumulation of fluid and commonly used as a treatment for high blood pressure.

douche: Cleansing of the vagina with fluid.

dysmenorrhea: Painful menstruation resulting from the shape of the uterus and/or the process of menstruation. Prostaglandins have been linked to menstrual pain, and antiprostaglandin medication such as ibuprofen often substantially relieves the pelvic discomfort associated with menstrual cramps.

dyspareunia: Painful or difficult intercourse.

dysplasia: Abnormal development of cells that may grow as a precursor to cancer.

ectopic pregnancy: A pregnancy occurring outside the uterus, usually in a fallopian tube.

ejaculation: The sudden release of semen from the male urethra.

embryo: In humans, an unborn child before the eighth week of pregnancy; a period that involves rapid growth, initial development of the major organ systems, and early formation of the main external features.

embryo transfer [ET]: The placement of an embryo into a woman's uterus. The embryo being transferred may have been fertilized *in vitro* (within the laboratory) or *in vivo* (within the reproductive tract of an egg donor).

endocervical curettage: Scraping of the lining of the cervical canal.

endocervix: The membrane that lines the inner canal of the cervix.

endocrine system: The system of glands within the body, including the thymus, pituitary, parathyroid, thyroid, adrenals, ovaries (in females), and testicles (in males).

endocrinologist: A physician specializing in diseases of the endocrine system.

endocrinology/infertility: The branch of obstetrics and gynecology dealing with the hormones, diseases, and conditions that affect fertility.

endometrial biopsy: Removal of a small piece of tissue from the uterine lining for microscopic evaluation and diagnosis.

endometrial hyperplasia: Overgrowth of the uterine lining.

endometriosis: A growth of endometrial tissue outside the uterus, thought to occur in about 15 percent of women. Women who do not get pregnant until later in life are more likely to acquire this disease, with the average age of diagnosis being thirty-seven. Pregnancy seems to prevent or delay the onset of this problem. The most common symptoms of endometriosis are severe menstrual cramps, painful intercourse, painful bowel movements, and soreness above the pubic bones. Endometriosis is a factor in many cases of female infertility.

endometrium: The inner lining of the uterus.

endorphin: Any one of the substances of the nervous system made by the pituitary gland producing morphine-like effects as a way of reducing pain within the body.

epidemic: A disease spread rapidly throughout the population.

episiotomy: A surgical procedure performed during childbirth in which the opening of the vagina is enlarged with a cut.

Epostane: See *RU486*.

estrogen: A hormone secreted by the ovaries that regulates the development of secondary sexual characteristics in women and produces cyclic changes in tissue lining the vagina and the uterus. Natural estrogens include estradiol, estrone, and their metabolic product, estriol. When used therapeutically, estrogens are usually given in a conjugated form, such as ethinyl estradiol, conjugated estrogens (USP), or the synthetic estrogen DES (diethylstilbestrol).

estrogen replacement therapy: Medical treatment using estrogen to restore hormonal balance. Because the therapy increases the risk of uterine cancer, it is usually prescribed only for women who have had a hysterectomy.

ethics: A system of moral principles or standards governing conduct.

eugenic abortion: The deliberate killing of a preborn child for eugenic reasons.

eugenics: The science that deals with the physical, moral, and intellectual improvement of the human race through genetic control.

fallopian tube: The duct that conveys the egg from the ovary to the womb. Also called oviduct.

family physician: A physician who has completed a three-year residency in family practice medicine.

ferning test: A test for the presence of estrogen in cervical mucus, which is an indication of fertility.

fertilization: See *conception*.

fertile: Having the ability to conceive and bear offspring; fruitful; not sterile.

fertile mucus: A substance secreted by the cervix that is capable of facilitating the transport of sperm through a woman's reproductive tract.

fertile period: The time during the menstrual cycle in which conception may take place, beginning three to six days before ovulation and ending two to three days afterward.

fetus: The term applied to a developing baby after the eighth week of pregnancy until birth.

fibrocystic breast disease: Noncancerous lumps in the breast that usually develop in response to hormonal changes during the menstrual cycle.

fibroid: A noncancerous lump or growth composed of fibrous tissue.

fimbria: The fringelike borders of the open ends of the fallopian tubes.

follicle: A pouchlike recessed structure in the ovary containing an immature ovum called an oocyte and the cells surrounding the oocyte.

follicle-stimulating hormone [FSH]: A hormone secreted by the pituitary gland that is responsible for stimulating the growth of ovarian follicles in women and the development of sperm (spermatogenesis) in men.

FSH: See *follicle stimulating hormone*.

fundus: The rounded portion of the uterus from which contractions originate during labor.

gamete: A mature male or female reproductive cell; the spermatozoan or ovum.

gamete intrafallopian transfer [GIFT]: The placement of sperm and oocytes into an unblocked fallopian tube through a laparoscope for *in vivo* fertilization.

gender: The specific sex of a person; male or female.

gene: The basic unit of heredity in a chromosome that carries characteristics from parent to child.

genetic: A condition or quality determined or influenced by a person's genes.

general anesthesia: Medically induced loss of feeling and sensation, including the loss of memory and consciousness.

genic: Of or resembling a gene or genes.

genitals: External sex organs.

germ cells: Ova or sperm.

gestation: The period between conception and birth.

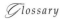

gland: An organ of highly specialized cells capable of releasing material not related to its normal metabolism.

gonad: A primary sex organ; an ovary or a testis.

gonadotropin: A hormone capable of stimulating the gonads, or primary sex organs.

gonorrhea: A specific, contagious inflammatory infection of the genital mucus membrane, mouth, or anus of either sex. It is transmitted by intimate sexual contact.

graafian follicle: A mature ovarian sac that ruptures during ovulation to release a mature egg.

gynecologist: A physician who specializes in the problems of the female sexual organs.

gynecology: The branch of medicine dealing with diseases and problems of the female reproductive tract.

gyne-, gyno-: Prefix meaning woman, female.

gynetech: A new form of medicine specializing in the technological control of human reproduction.

HCG: See *human chorionic gonadotropin.*

healing: The process or act in which health is restored to the body, emotions, mind, or spirit.

health: A state of physical, emotional, mental, and spiritual well-being.

health-care provider: A person who provides health services to health-care consumers.

hemorrhoids: Dilated veins in the rectal tissue that may produce itching and pain.

herpes genitalis: An infection caused by the herpes simplex II virus that is usually transmitted by sexual contact and causes painful blisters on the skin and mucous membranes of the male and female genitals.

herpes simplex II: See *herpes genitalis.*

heterologous insemination: See *artificial insemination by donor.*

homologous insemination: See *artificial insemination by husband.*

high-risk pregnancy: Term describing the probability that complications may occur during pregnancy and childbirth.

home birth: Birth taking place at home. As used by those who advocate home birth for healthy childbearing women, the term indicates a planned home birth attended by skilled maternity-care providers. As used by those seeking to eliminate home birth, the term is used to indicate all births taking place outside the hospital, including miscarriages, early arrivals during transport, unattended and unplanned home births, and involuntary home births among women too poor to afford hospitalization.

hormone: Chemical substances, produced by ductless glands in one part of the body, that affect an organ or group of cells in another area of the body.

hormone replacement therapy (HRT): Medical treatment using both estrogen and a progestin, a form of progesterone, to restore hormonal balance in women who have not had a hysterectomy.

hospital birth: Birth taking place in a hospital.

human chorionic gonadotropin [HCG]: A hormone produced by the chorionic villi that is responsible for triggering the release of progesterone and estrogen; measured during a pregnancy test through urine. HCG is extracted from the urine of pregnant women and administered by injection to stimulate ovarian and testicular function.

Human immunodeficiency virus (HIV): The virus that causes AIDS.

hymen: The fold of mucous membrane, fibrous tissue, and skin that partially covers the vaginal entrance. When broken, small elevations remain. These are referred to as hymenal tags.

hypertension: High blood pressure.

hyster-, hystero-: Prefix: womb; hysteria.

hysterectomy: The surgical removal of the uterus.

hystero-oophorectomy: The surgical removal of the uterus and one or both ovaries.

hysterosalpingogram: X-ray study of the uterus and fallopian tubes after injecting radiopaque material into these organs; used for diagnosis of infertility or sterility.

hysterosalpingo-oophorectomy: The surgical removal of the uterus, fallopian tubes, and ovaries.

hysteroscopy: Inspection of the inside of the uterus by means of a lighted instrument called a hysteroscope.

hysterotomy: 1. Incision of the uterus. 2. Cesarean section. 3. A method of induced abortion conducted through incisions in the mother's abdominal wall and uterus.

iatrogenic: Produced or caused by a physician.

idiopathic infertility: Infertility of unknown cause.

infection: Multiplication of parasitic organisms inside the body.

implantation: Embedding of the developing baby in the lining of the uterus.

incest: Sexual relations between family members.

induced abortion: An intentional termination of a pregnancy before an unborn child has developed to the point where he or she can survive outside the uterus.

induction of labor: The artificial production of labor.

infertile: The inability to conceive or produce offspring.

infertility: The state of being infertile or unable to carry a pregnancy. Medically defined as the inability of a couple to conceive after twelve months of intercourse without contraception.

intrauterine device [IUD]: A form of contraception in which a bent strip of plastic or copper is inserted into the uterus to prevent pregnancy; does not act to prevent ovulation or conception.

IVF/ET: See *in vitro fertilization* and *embryo transfer*.

invasive techniques: Any medical procedure that penetrates the boundaries of the body.

in vitro fertilization [IVF]: Conception occurring in laboratory apparatus; name literally means "in-glass" fertilization.

in vivo fertilization: Fertilization within the human body.

Kegel exercises: Conscious contractions of pelvic floor muscles done for the purpose of improving muscle tone and sexual response; named after Dr. Arnold Kegel, a physician whose research proved the value of these exercises in improving the strength of the pelvic floor.

labia: The fleshy, liplike folds of skin at the opening of the vagina—the labia majora, forming the border of the vulva, and the labia minora, which extend from the clitoris backward on both sides of the vagina.

labor: The series of stages during the process of childbirth through which the baby is born and the uterus returns to a normal state; contractions of the uterus that result in the birth of a baby.

lactation: The process by which milk is produced and secreted by the breasts for nourishing an infant.

laparoscopy: Exploration of the pelvic cavity by means of a lighted instrument called a laparoscope.

laparotomy: The surgical opening of the abdomen; an abdominal operation.

laser: Acronym for *light amplification by stimulated emission of radiation*.

laser surgery: Any operative procedure that employs a laser rather than a scalpel to excise body tissue.

lay midwife: A birth attendant who has acquired her skills through apprenticeship and experience rather than formalized schooling.

liable: To be legally responsible.

litigate: To seek remedy through a court of law, including the act of carrying out a lawsuit, by means of presenting evidence of damage or harm.

low-risk pregnancy: Term used to describe the probability that pregnancy and childbirth will be normal and uneventful.

luteal: Referring to the corpus luteum, its functions, or its effects.

luteinizing hormone [LH]: A hormone produced by the pituitary gland in both males and females. It stimulates the production of testosterone in men and the secretion of estrogen in women.

luteal phase: The second half of the menstrual cycle, following ovulation, when the corpus luteum secretes progesterone.

malignant: Cancerous.

malpractice, medical: The failure of a health-care professional to render proper services; reprehensible ignorance, negligence, or criminal intent toward a client; bad, wrong, or injudicious treatment resulting in injury, unnecessary suffering, or death; the misconduct or misuse of medicine.

mammary gland: The milk-secreting gland in the breast.

mammogram: X-ray of the soft tissue of the breast used to identify various cysts or tumors.

menarche: The onset of menstruation; the beginning of the first menstrual cycle.

menopause: The end of menstruation when the menses stop as a normal result of the decline of monthly hormonal cycles.

menses: The normal flow of blood and discarded uterine cells that takes place during menstruation.

menstrual cycle: The cycle of hormonal changes that begins at puberty and repeats itself on a monthly basis unless interrupted by pregnancy, lactation, medication, or metabolic disorders.

menstruation: The natural process by which the lining of the nonpregnant uterus is cast off, resulting in a discharge of blood and mucosal tissue from the vagina.

menstrual extraction: Removal of the lining of the uterus by suction before menstruation occurs; also a method of induced abortion.

metastasis: The spread of cancer from one area of the body to another.

microsurgery: Surgery performed while a physician observes through a microscope.

midwife: A birth attendant who respects nature while supporting and supervising the natural processes of labor during childbirth; a woman who practices the art of midwifery.

midwifery: The traditional practice of providing help and assistance to women during childbirth, characterized by watching and waiting upon nature's design for labor.

mini-pill: Oral contraceptive containing progestin only.

miscarriage: The spontaneous loss of a baby before the twenty-eighth week of pregnancy.

mittelschmerz: The painful sensation that occurs on one side of the lower abdomen during ovulation.

monogamous: Marrying once for life; having one sexual partner.

morbidity: A state of illness or disease.

morning-after pill: A very large dose of estrogen taken orally within twenty-four to seventy-two hours after intercourse to terminate a pregnancy.

mortality: Death.

mortality rate: The number of deaths during a specific time within a given population. When dealing with fetuses and babies, the rate is based on number of deaths per 1,000 live births; when considering mothers, the rate quoted represents the number of deaths per 100,000 pregnancies.

mucus: The slippery, sticky secretion released by mucous membranes and glands.

myometrium: The muscular wall of the uterus.

natal: Referring to birth.

natural family planning [NFP]: Any method of family planning that does not use drugs or devices to prevent conception.

nipple: A small cylindrical bump positioned just below the center of each breast and containing fourteen to twenty openings to the milk ducts.

noninvasive: Referring to any test, treatment, or procedure that does not penetrate the boundaries of the body.

Norplant: See *progestin skin implants.*

nurse-midwife: See *certified nurse-midwife.*

obstetrics: The branch of medicine dealing with the management of pregnancy and childbirth.

oligogenics: The limitation of offspring through utilizing some form of birth control.

oligospermia: Deficient levels of sperm in seminal fluid; may be temporary or permanent.

oocyte: The early or primitive human egg before it has completed development.

oogenesis: The growth and development of female eggs.

oophorectomy: The surgical removal of an ovary.

oral contraceptive: A steroid drug taken to induce infertility.

os: Opening of the cervical canal.

osteoporosis: Increased porosity of bone tissue; the loss of normal bone density marked by a thinning of bone tissue and the growth of small openings in the bone.

OTC: Over-the counter; refers to medication sold without a prescription.

ova: Human eggs; female reproductive or germ cells; a cell capable of developing into a new organism of the same species. (Singular: *ovum.*)

ovary: One of the pair of primary sexual organs in females located on each side of the lower abdomen beside the uterus. The ovaries produce the reproductive cell, or ovum, and two known hormones, estrogen and progesterone.

ovariectomy: The removal of an ovary or a portion of the ovary.

oviduct: See *fallopian tube.*

Ovulation Method of family planning: A method of family planning that relies on the observation of the type and amount of cervical mucus secreted during the menstrual cycle as a means of predicting fertility.

ovum donor: See *egg donor.*

ovum transfer [OT]: See *embryo transfer.*

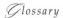

Pap test: A method of collecting tissue cells in the vagina and at the opening of the cervix and examining them for abnormality.

peak mucus: A cloudy to clear mucus coating the vaginal area during times of high estrogen levels at the most fertile point in the menstrual cycle.

pelvic floor: The muscles and tissues that form the base of the pelvis.

pelvic inflammatory disease [PID]: Inflammation of the female reproductive organs in the pelvis, often resulting in scarring, blocked fallopian tubes, and infertility.

pelvic floor: The muscles and tissues that form the base of the pelvis.

pelvis: The bowl-shaped lower portion of the trunk of the body.

penis: The male organ of urination and sexual intercourse made up of three circular masses of spongy tissue covered with skin.

perimenopause: Period during which menstruation slowly tapers off before stopping (menopause).

perinatal: The period from the twenty-eighth week of pregnancy to one week after the baby's birth.

perinatologist: A physician who specializes in maternal-fetal medicine.

perineum: The part of the body lying between the inner thighs, with the buttocks to the rear and the genitals to the front.

PID: See *pelvic inflammatory disease.*

pituitary gland: A small gland lying at the base of the brain that supplies many hormones to regulate a variety of processes within the body, including growth, reproduction, and lactation.

placenta: A temporary organ created to exchange waste products and carry nutrients between mother and baby during pregnancy; produces hormones to protect and maintain gestation.

polyp: A small, tumorlike growth that protrudes from a mucous membrane surface.

postcoital test: Samples of deposited semen and vaginal-cervical discharge removed from different areas along the length of the cervical canal for diagnostic analysis; the microscopic analysis of vaginal and cervical secretions within several hours of sexual intercourse.

postpartum: After childbirth.

pregnancy: The growth and development of a new human being inside a woman's uterus.

premenstrual dysphoric disorder [PDD]: Depressive disorder distinguished by severe, recurrent sadness that disrupts daily activities and occurs during the late luteal phase of the menstrual cycle.

premenstrual syndrome [PMS]: The presence of a set of interrelated symptoms that recur regularly during the same phase of each menstrual cycle.

premenstrual tension: The presence of emotional symptoms that recur regularly at the same phase of the menstrual cycle.

prenatal: The period before birth.

progesterone: Hormone produced by the corpus luteum and, during pregnancy, the placenta; prepares the uterine lining for implantation and the breasts for lactation; relaxes smooth muscles to prevent uterine contractions and subsequent pregnancy loss.

progestin: Any one of a group of hormones, natural or synthetic, that have progesterone-like effects on the reproductive system.

progestin skin implants: Nonbiodegradable plastic cylinders containing progestin, designed to be inserted into a woman's upper arm by a physician under local anesthesia for the purpose of preventing birth for up to three years.

progestogen: See *progestin.*

prolactin: The hormone responsible for milk secretion that is released in response to the suckling of an infant at the breast.

proliferative phase: The portion of the menstrual cycle between menstruation and ovulation.

prostaglandins: A group of strong hormonelike fatty acids that act on certain body organs. Used as a method of inducing labor or abortion.

pubic bone: One of two bones that form the front part of the pelvis.

pubic lice: Parasitic infestation of the outer genital area.

rape: Third-degree sexual assault, involving penetration of the body with the penis without consent.

rectocele: The bulging of the rectum and the back wall of the vagina into the vagina as the result of giving birth, advanced age, or surgery.

reproductive endocrinologist: An obstetrician-gynecologist who specializes in diagnosing and treating infertility.

rhythm: See *calendar method.*

RU486: A drug capable of inducing abortion by inhibiting the secretion of progesterone.

saline abortion: Abortion induced by injecting a salt solution directly into the amniotic sac, thereby poisoning the fetus.

sanitary pad: An absorbent pad designed to be worn during menstruation to collect the menstrual flow.

sarcoma: Cancer of the connective tissue.

semen: The thick, white-colored fluid released by the male sex organs for the purpose of transporting sperm.

seminal fluid: See *semen.*

septate uterus: Uterus with a dividing membrane.

serotonin: A natural body chemical concentrated within the nervous system that plays a role in transmitting nerve impulses, constricting blood vessels, and stimulating smooth muscles.

sex: A division of humans into male or female based on many characteristics, including body parts and genetic differences.

sex-linked: A genetic characteristic controlled by genes in sex chromosomes.

sexual assault: Sexual contact without consent.

sexual intercourse: The sexual union of two people of the opposite sex during which the penis is placed inside the vagina.

sexuality: The sum total of the physical, emotional, intellectual, and spiritual traits that are shown through a person's identity and behavior, whether related to the reproductive organs or to procreation.

sexually transmitted disease [STD]: A contagious disease spread through intimate sexual contact.

sexually transmitted infertility: The inability to conceive or produce children as a result of damage to the reproductive organs due to a sexually transmitted disease.

side effect: A reaction resulting from medical treatment or therapy.

slough: To cast off or shed dead cells from living tissue.

sonogram: Another term for an ultrasound diagnostic test.

sperm: The male cell of reproduction, also called a *spermatozoa* or *gamete.*

sperm bank: See *cryobank.*

sperm count: An estimate of the number of sperm in a given sample of seminal fluid.

sperm donor: A man who produces sperm through masturbation for use in artificial insemination, usually for a fee.

spermatogenesis: The process of sperm production.

spermatozoan: The mature male sex or germ cell formed within the seminiferous tubules of the testes. (Singular: *spermatozoa.*)

spermicide: Any chemical substance that kills sperm cells.

sperm antibody test: Antibodies to sperm may be present in a woman's vaginal secretions; this test examines the sperm-mucus interaction.

sperm count: An estimate of the number of sperm within a given sample.

sperm motility: The rate at which sperm move from one point to another.

staphylococcus aureus: A type of bacteria that produces a poison responsible for causing toxic shock syndrome.

sterile: The inability to produce children.

sterilization: An act or process that renders a person incapable of reproduction.

stress: Any factor that requires a response or change on the part of an organism or an individual.

stressor: Anything capable of causing wear and tear on the body's mental, physical, emotional, or spiritual resources.

symptom: Something felt or noticed by an individual that can be used to detect what is going on within the body.

sympto-thermal method: A method of family planning requiring fertility awareness based on the ovulation and basal body temperature methods of family planning.

syphilis: A sexually transmitted disease caused by an organism called a spirochete.

tampon: A compact pack of absorbent material designed to soak up the menstrual flow within the vagina.

teaching hospital: A hospital associated with a medical institution in which students train and work with patients.

technician: A person skilled in a particular technique.

technique: The body of specialized procedures and methods used in any particular field.

technological, technology, high-tech: The branch of knowledge that deals with industrial arts, applied science, and engineering; a technological process, invention, method, or the like; in obstetrics and gynecology, medical care characterized by the use of invasive techniques and man-made interventions.

testes: The two male reproductive glands located in the scrotum that produce sperm and the male sex hormone, testosterone. (Singular—*testicle* or *testis.*)

testosterone: A naturally secreted hormone in both males and females that is capable of producing masculine sexual characteristics.

therapy: The treatment of an abnormal condition.

thromboembolism: A condition in which a blood vessel is blocked by a clot.

toxic shock syndrome: A potentially fatal sudden disease associated with the use of super-absorbent tampons during menstruation; caused by the bacteria *staphylococcus aureus.*

trimester: Period of three months; one of the three phases of pregnancy.

trophoblast: A strand of single cells ringing the blastocyst that will later become the placenta.

tubal cautery: Sterilization of a woman by burning both fallopian tubes.

tubal ligation: Sterilization of a woman via surgical removal of a small segment of each fallopian tube.

tubal pregnancy: A pregnancy in which the early embryo implants within the fallopian tube and cannot develop normally.

ultrasonography: Inaudible high-frequency sound waves used to outline the shape of body organs or a developing baby.

ultrasound: See *ultrasonography.*

urethra: The canal that carries urine from the bladder.

urinary stress incontinence: The involuntary passage of urine when coughing, sneezing, or laughing; results from poor sphincter control of the urethra.

urinary tract: All of the structures involved in the release and elimination of urine from the body.

urinary tract infection [UTI]: An infection of the urinary tract marked by frequency of urination, a painful burning sensation while voiding, and possibly pus in the urine.

urogenital: Of or relating to the urinary and reproductive systems.

urology: The branch of medicine concerned with the care of the urinary tract in men and women and of the male genital tract.

use-effectiveness: The actual level of effectiveness of a birth control method.

uterine lavage: Flushing of the uterus performed by use of a catheter inserted into the cervix.

uterine prolapse: Falling or dropping of the uterus.

uterus: The thick-walled, hollow, muscular female organ of reproduction.

vacuum aspiration: A method of inducing abortion using a suction machine to remove the developing baby, placenta, and amniotic sac from the uterus.

vacuum extractor: An instrument used as an alternative to forceps that adheres to the baby's scalp and forcibly pulls the baby out of the birth canal.

vagina: The muscular tubelike membrane that forms the passageway between the uterus and genital entrance. It receives the penis during lovemaking and becomes the canal through which the baby passes during childbirth.

vaginal discharge: Any discharge from the vagina.

vaginal suppository: A solid cone of medicated material designed to dissolve slowly when inserted into the vagina.

vaginitis: Inflammation of the vagina usually caused by infection, poor hygiene, or chemical irritation.

vas deferens: One of a pair of tubes within the male reproductive tract through which sperm pass.

vasectomy: A surgical procedure that produces male sterility by cutting a section out of each vas deferens.

viable: Capable of living, growing, and developing; a baby capable of living outside the uterus; a pregnancy capable of sustaining itself.

virgin: A person who has never had sexual intercourse.

virginity: The state of being a virgin.

vulva: The external female genitals, including the labia majora, labia minora, and the clitoris.

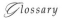

wet smear: Small amount of tissue placed on a slide for microscopic evaluation and diagnosis.

withdrawal method: A technique of contraception in which the penis is withdrawn from the vagina before ejaculation. Highly unreliable since the pre-ejaculatory fluid released through the male urethra contains sperm. Also called *coitus interruptus*.

womb: See *uterus*.

wrongful life action: A lawsuit brought against a physician or health facility because an unwanted child was born.

X-chromosome: The sex-determining chromosome carried by all ova and approximately one-half of sperm.

X-ray: Short wavelength radiation that can penetrate solid forms and leave a photographic image on plates or film.

Y-chromosome: The sex-determining chromosome carried by about one-half of all sperm, never by an egg, that produces a male child.

yeast infection: A fungal infection resulting in itching and inflammation of the vagina, characterized by a thick white discharge and caused by the overgrowth of *Candida albicans*.

zygote: The developing egg between the time of fertilization and implantation in the wall of the uterus.

$\mathcal{I}$ N D E X